DESIGNING RESISTANCE TRAINING PROGRAMS

SECOND EDITION

Steven J. Fleck, PhD
Fleck's Rx, Colorado Springs, Colorado

William J. Kraemer, PhD
The Pennsylvania State University

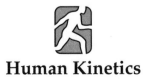

Human Kinetics

Library of Congress Cataloging-in-Publication Data

Fleck, Steven J., 1951-
    Designing resistance training programs / Steven J. Fleck, William
J. Kraemer. -- 2nd ed.
        p.   cm.
    Includes bibliographical references and index.
    ISBN 0-87322-508-2
    1. Exercise. 2. Isometric exercise. I. Kraemer, William J.,
1953-   .   II. Title.
GV505.F58   1997
613.7'1--dc21   96-46413
                                                        CIP

ISBN: 0-87322-508-2

Copyright © 1987, 1997 by Steven J. Fleck and William J. Kraemer

Acquisitions Editor: Rick Frey, PhD, Scott Wikgren; **Developmental Editor:** Kristine Enderle; **Assistant Editors:** Sandra Merz Bott, Coree Schutter; **Editorial Assistant:** Laura Majersky; **Copyeditor:** Karen Bojda; **Proofreader:** Erin Cler; **Indexer:** Barbara E. Cohen; **Graphic Designer:** Robert Reuther; **Graphic Artist:** Denise Lowry; **Photo Editor:** Emily Mann; **Cover Designer:** Jack Davis; **Illustrator:** Jennifer Delmotte; **Printer:** Edwards Brothers

Printed in the United States of America   10 9 8 7 6 5

Human Kinetics
Web site: http://www.humankinetics.com/

United States: Human Kinetics, P.O. Box 5076, Champaign, IL 61825-5076
1-800-747-4457
e-mail: humank@hkusa.com

Canada: Human Kinetics, 475 Devonshire Road, Unit 100, Windsor, ON N8Y 2L5
1-800-465-7301 (in Canada only)
e-mail: humank@hkcanada.com

Europe: Human Kinetics, P.O. Box IW14, Leeds LS16 6TR, United Kingdom
+44 (0)113-278 1708
e-mail: humank@hkeurope.com

Australia: Human Kinetics, 57A Price Avenue, Lower Mitcham, South Australia 5062
(08) 82771555
e-mail: humank@hkaustralia.com

New Zealand: Human Kinetics, P.O. Box 105-231, Auckland Central
09-523-3462
e-mail: humank@hknewz.com

Dedication

To my wife Maelu, for her understanding of the time needed to complete a book.

To my mother Elda and father Marvin, for their support and understanding through the ups and downs of my life and career.

—Steven J. Fleck

First and foremost to my wife Joan, for her love and tenacious support as a partner in life. To my children Daniel, Anna, and Maria who have given us love and added different perspectives to our lives.

To my parents Ray and Jewell Kraemer, who taught me what hard work and dedication can accomplish in life. As I watched my father, a consummate jazz musician, work to make ends meet, I learned the concept of sacrifice and the joy of doing a job you love. From my mother I learned what nurture and love can do when a child's dreams are taken seriously by a parent.

To my sister Judy, who has always been a source of unending love and support throughout my life and was always there when others were not. To my mother-in-law Marian and late father-in-law "Barney" Bernabei, for their love and support over the years. To my sister-in-law Maelu Fleck and brother-in-law Louis Bernabei, who have always been there and supported us—I thank you.

To my uncle Dominic T. Wong, who showed me the basics of weight training as a young boy. To my grade school football coach, the late Howard Metz, an ex-Marine who took a group of boys and taught them what being a man was all about and who showed us when and where "toughness" counted on the field of competition.

To my high school buddy and college roommate Rick Griffin, who shared with me thousands of training sessions over the years as we played high school and college football together and grew to be men. To my high school football coach Jack Jansen, a consummate coach, role model, and friend, who gave me a vision beyond high school. To my many friends in high school and college who shared the joy of resistance training with me.

To Roger Harring, my college football coach at the winningest Division III program in the United States, at the University of Wisconsin-LaCrosse, who valued weight training for his players over two and a half decades ago when it was not yet popular.

To my friend Carl Maresh, without whose encouragement, perpetual optimistic view of life, and support as a friend I would not be who I am today—thanks, Carl, for that one foot of laboratory desk space. To my friend Dan Steffen, for the many years we spent together coaching football and teaching at Carroll College, where as strength coach I learned the practical basics for my insights into the conditioning of athletes.

To Bruce Noble, who took a chance on a young graduate student and did not laugh when I told him I wanted to study the physiology and biochemistry of resistance training. To Mike Clark, Tom Richardson, Mike Nitka, and Mike Kemp, for making the weight room a laboratory—I thank you for your support. To Jim Vogel, who gave me my first opportunity to study and lead scientific research efforts on resistance training—I will always remember your class as a human being, your support, and your quiet eloquence.

To John Patton, Everett Harman, Joe Dziados, and my laboratory staff at USARIEM, who worked so hard on projects with me in the early days, and to Howard Knuttgen, who allowed me to develop as a scientist—I thank you all.

iii

To my friends Keijo Häkkinen, Robert Staron, Gary Dudley, and Robert Newton, for their intense collaborative efforts with my laboratory on the study of resistance training—I thank you.

To my coauthor Steve Fleck, who has been there over the years from the days of college football to our working together as scientists—it is still special!

At the great risk of slighting any of my scientific colleagues, friends, and collaborators, I thank you all and have valued your support and friendship over the years.

To my present and former graduate students, I thank each of you, as you have been an integral part of the discovery process and the quest in my laboratory for greater understanding of the study of resistance training.

To all my many friends and colleagues here at Penn State University, who are too many to list, I am honored to be a part of one of the most fertile scientific environments for scholarly work in the areas of molecular biology, physiology, exercise physiology, and exercise and sport sciences—I thank you all and owe my refined efforts on this book to you.

Finally, to my humble belief in God, for always showing me the way and for showing me that a vocation can be something of great joy—not because of the science but because of all the people who touch one's life and the simple message of "be nice to everyone."

This book is in part the result of these combined influences in my life and it is a great joy to see this work—with my friend and colleague Steve Fleck—come into print in its second edition.

—William J. Kraemer

Contents

Part III   Resistance Training and Special Populations   181

Preface

When we wrote the first edition of *Designing Resistance Training Programs*, which was published in 1987, we had two primary purposes in mind. We wanted to provide readers with a view of resistance training based on scientific literature and to promote the use of a more structured, scientific approach in the prescription of exercise. These remain the primary goals for this second edition.

Since the publication of the first edition, the amount of information about resistance training has exploded: More research on resistance training has been published in the past decade than in the *five* decades prior to 1987. We have tried to utilize selected studies that best represent the current knowledge of a particular topic inasmuch as it would be an insurmountable task to present every piece of literature published on resistance training. This second edition, then, developed from the recent expansion of scientific literature and the more sophisticated understanding it provides both scientists and practitioners. The dramatic amount of new information published in the peer-reviewed scientific literature, however, unfortunately has a counterpart of an increased amount of misinformation in the field. Too often misinformation contributes to confusion and less than optimal exercise prescriptions of resistance training. The important challenge thus remains what it was 10 years ago: to provide a factual basis from which to make program-design decisions.

The need for a structured approach to exercise prescription has been paramount in determining the content of this textbook. The process of exercise prescription involves using good judgment based both on experience and a solid, factual understanding of resistance training. Experience combined with solid, scientific information for decision making leads to the best individualized programs and optimal results from training. This book should help provide you with the necessary understanding and theoretical framework to use a structured approach in the exercise prescription of resistance training.

The second edition of *Designing Resistance Training Programs* is organized into three parts.

Part I develops the foundation by helping you gain a basic understanding of the major principles and underlying biological basis for resistance training. You'll find the basic terms, definitions, and principles used in resistance training presented in chapter 1, information that is vital as a foundation for subsequent chapters. Chapter 2 reviews the different types of resistance training. With the proliferation of modalities now available for resistance exercise, understanding some of the types used most frequently is important to designing and developing exercise prescriptions to meet different goals. Chapter 3 presents an up-to-date view of the fundamentals of muscle physiology. The neuromuscular unit is the primary target for almost all resistance training programs; knowing the factual basis of muscle function, muscle fiber types, and neurology gives you an understanding of how the body functions. In chapter 4 we overview aspects of fitness related to endurance exercise, anaerobic sprint and interval training, and flexibility. Most resistance training programs are not performed alone, so it is essential to know how to successfully integrate other fitness programs into a resistance training program to ensure success of the total conditioning program.

In part II the focus is on the information necessary for designing optimal resistance training. Chapter 5 sets the stage by developing the structured approach used in individualized program design. It explains how a *needs analysis* is made, overviews the acute program variables, discusses what changes can be made in the program with long-term chronic training, and overviews the administrative and safety concerns in implementing a resistance training program. Chapter 6 describes and evaluates the multitude of resistance training systems that have evolved over the past century, setting the context of how variables in the acute programs have been manipulated. In chapter 7 we discuss the adaptations that might be expected from various resistance training programs, seeking to provide you with realistic expectations of what resistance training can accomplish. In chapter 8 you'll learn about the consequences of detraining. Understanding what can happen when resistance training is stopped—and the course of time of any losses in physiological adaptations and performance—can help you design in-season programs that best maintain the gains accomplished in earlier training phases.

In part III we look more closely at resistance training for special populations, including differences that exist and and needs they create. In chapter 9 we examine the development of resistance training programs for women, considering differences in strength and physiology between men and women and their impact on training adaptations. We also discuss some misconceptions related to prescribing resistance training for women. In chapter 10 we turn to resistance training for children. Although resistance training programs for children can observably improve fitness, prevent injury, and enhance sport performance, nevertheless specific differences are appropriate in the exercise prescriptions for children compared with those for adults. Resistance training for older men and women has been shown to increase functional abilities and improve health status, so we have added chapter 11 in this second edition. In this chapter we discuss the normal decline in physiological function and how resistance training can offset these age-related declines and fight the aging process. In chapter 12 we show how three resistance training sports have

developed and influenced resistance training today: the sports of weight lifting, power lifting, and body building. We examine the differences in program design for these three sports and give example programs.

Program design in resistance training requires one to develop very specific training goals and then to match these goals with the necessary program design to achieve desired results, that is, taking a structured approach. It involves a constant and challenging decision-making process that must be based on a scientific understanding of resistance training and proper evaluation of the progress being made with a particular program. Ultimately, designing a successful program requires a mind open to monitoring a program and modifying it as necessary if progress toward training goals is not occurring.

It is our hope that resistance training will be more than an emotional response to one style of training or piece of equipment, and that having a training philosophy will be augmented with having an approach to resistance training based on facts and responses to the individual trainee. We are excited about this second edition and hope it will help you design optimal resistance training programs. Good luck and good training!

Steven J. Fleck, PhD
William J. Kraemer, PhD

Acknowledgments

We would first like to thank all the athletes, coaches, and strength coaches we have worked with and with whom we have had the opportunity to discuss training over the years. These opportunities have provided insights and have stimulated challenging discussions that in some cases provided fundamental ideas for eventual research in resistance training.

As with any book, as authors we are faced with the dramatic challenge of deciding who to acknowledge for their influence and contributions to this work. Obviously, it would take an inordinate amount of space for both of us to do justice to the many people who have directly or indirectly contributed over the years to our careers, professional development, and scientific understanding of resistance training. We owe a huge debt of gratitude to the many esteemed colleagues with whom we have worked, collaborated, and published. This second edition would not have been possible but for the scientific efforts over the past 10 years of our colleagues, who have helped the strength and conditioning profession to focus on the design of resistance training programs based on the results of laboratory research. We also thank the many bright and talented graduate students we have had the honor to be associated with and who have shaped our everyday lives with their contributions.

At the high risk of slighting someone, we would also like to thank a number of individuals who directly impacted the development and writing of the second edition of this book: in particular, Dr. Gary Dudley, Dr. Carl Maresh, Dr. Robert Staron, Dr. Keijo Häkkinen, Dr. Robert Newton, and Mr. Mike Clark. We thank you.

As with any book, a great many people were involved in the creation of *Designing Resistance Training Programs*. Over the past 10 years the production of such a scholarly work has dramatically changed in terms of its challenges and demands. We thank many people at Human Kinetics, starting with Dr. Rainer Martens, who many years ago saw value in our desire to write a text on resistance training that was based on the scientific literature instead of writing just another book that focused only on resistance exercise techniques. We thank our developmental editor, Kristine Enderle, who grew with us over the course of the project and worked so hard in the day-to-day struggles of putting this book together and coordinating its production with all of the different departments at Human Kinetics. We also thank assistant editors Sandra Merz Bott and Coree Schutter for their attention to details and kind assistance in helping to bring this work to completion. We want to thank all of the people at Human Kinetics who made spectacular professional contributions to the creation of all aspects of this book.

Finally, we thank you, the reader, for your interest in this book, which proves that designing resistance training programs takes a thirst for an understanding beyond exercise techniques and fad programs. We wish you good luck and good training.

Steven J. Fleck and William J. Kraemer

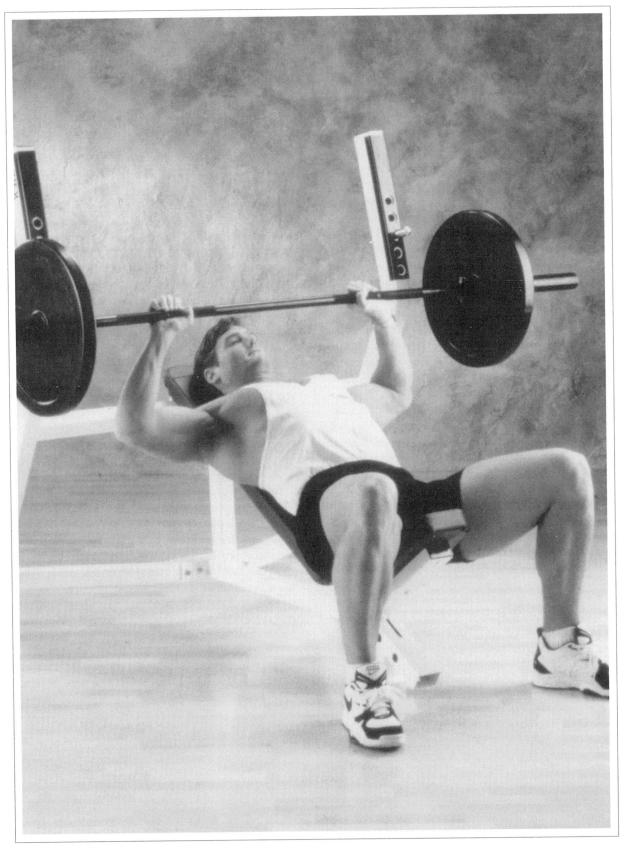

PART I

FOUNDATIONS OF RESISTANCE TRAINING

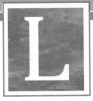

ike all fields of study, the study of resistance training is based on underlying principles and concepts. The information presented in the first four chapters is needed to understand and successfully design any resistance training program. Chapter 1 presents principles needed to safely and effectively perform and design resistance training programs. The characteristics of the various types of resistance training are detailed in chapter 2. The characteristics of a particular type of resistance training may make it desirable or undesirable for use by a certain population. Chapter 3 describes how muscles function and are controlled. This information is needed to gain insight for optimally designing resistance training programs. Resistance training should be a part of a total fitness program, and how resistance training fits into a total training program is discussed in chapter 4.

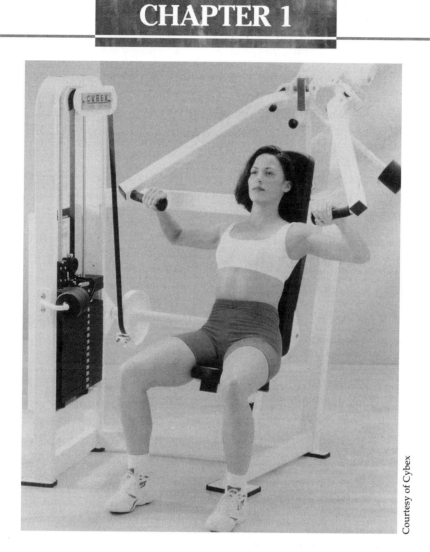

CHAPTER 1

Courtesy of Cybex

Basic Principles of Resistance Training and Exercise Prescription

Resistance training, also known as strength or weight training, has become one of the most popular forms of exercise both for enhancing an individual's physical fitness and for conditioning athletes. The terms strength, weight, and resistance training have all been used to describe a type of exercise that requires the body's musculature to move (or attempt to move) against an opposing force, usually presented by some type of equipment. The terms resistance and strength training encompass a wide range of training modalities, including plyometrics and hill running. Weight training typically is used to refer only to normal resistance training using free weights or weight machines. The increasing number of health club, high school, and college resistance training facilities attests to the popularity of this form of physical conditioning. Individuals who participate in a resistance training program expect the program to produce certain benefits, such as increased strength, increased muscle size, improved sport performance, increased fat-free mass, and decreased body fat. A well-designed and consistently performed resistance training program can produce all these benefits.

Both the recreational weight trainer and the athlete expect gains in strength or muscle size (muscular hypertrophy) from a resistance training program. Many different types of resistance modalities (e.g., isokinetic, variable resistance, isometric) can produce gains in strength. In addition, many different training systems (e.g., combinations of sets, repetitions, and resistances) can produce significant increases in strength or muscular hypertrophy, as long as the system presents and can continue to present an effective training stimulus to the muscle. The effectiveness of a specific type of resistance modality or training system depends on its proper use in the total exercise prescription or training program.

Most athletes and many recreational lifters expect the gains in strength and power produced by a resistance training program to lead to improvements in sport performance. Resistance training can improve motor performance (e.g., ability to sprint, to throw an object, or to jump); these improvements in basic motor skills can lead to better performance in various games and sports. The amount of carryover from a resistance training program to a specific sport performance depends on the *transfer specificity* or *transfer carry-over* between the training program and the sport skills. For example, a multijoint exercise, such as hang-cleans from the knees, would have greater transfer carry-over to vertical jump ability or to a linebacker's ability to tackle a running back head on than would isolated, single-joint exercises such as knee extensions and knee curls. Both multijoint and single-joint exercises increase the strength of the thighs and hamstring muscle groups. However, a greater similarity of biomechanical movements and muscle recruitment patterns between a multijoint exercise and a sporting activity results in greater transfer specificity. Thus, in general, multijoint exercises have a greater transfer specificity than single-joint exercises.

Body compositional change is also a goal of many recreational lifters and athletes engaged in resistance training programs. Normally the changes desired are a decrease in the amount of body fat and an increase in muscle mass. However, some individuals desire a gain or a loss in total body weight. All these changes can be achieved by a properly planned and performed resistance training program. The success of a program depends on the effectiveness of the exercise prescription, which ultimately produces the training stimulus.

Resistance training can produce the changes in body composition, strength, muscular hypertrophy, and motor performance desired by many individuals. To produce optimal changes in these areas it is necessary to adhere to some basic principles. These principles apply regardless of the resistance modality or the type of system used.

BASIC DEFINITIONS

Before discussing the basic principles of resistance training, it is necessary to define some basic terms commonly used in describing resistance training programs or principles.

Repetition. A repetition is one complete movement of an exercise. It normally consists of two phases: the concentric muscle action, or lifting of the resistance, and the eccentric muscle action, or lowering of the resistance.

Set. This is a group of repetitions performed continuously without stopping. While a set can be made up of any number of repetitions, sets typically range from 1 to 15 repetitions.

Repetition Maximum (RM). This is the maximum number of repetitions per set that can be performed at a given resistance with proper lifting technique. Thus, a set at a certain RM implies the set is performed to momentary voluntary fatigue. 1 RM is the heaviest resistance that can be used for one complete repetition of an exercise. 10 RM is a lighter resistance that allows completion of 10, but not 11, repetitions with proper exercise technique.

Power. Power is the rate of performing work. Power during a repetition is defined as the weight lifted times the vertical distance the weight is lifted divided by the time to complete the repetition. If 100 lb (45 kg or 445 N) are lifted vertically 3 ft (0.9 m) in 1 s, the power is 100 lb $\times$ 3 ft $\div$ 1 s = 300 ft $\cdot$ lb $\cdot$ s^{-1} (or about 400 W). Power during a repetition can be increased by lifting the same weight the same vertical distance in a shorter period of time. Power can also be increased by lifting a heavier resistance the same vertical distance in the same period of time as a lighter resistance.

Strength. Strength is the maximal amount of force a muscle or muscle group can generate in a specified movement pattern at a specified velocity of movement (Knuttgen and Kraemer 1987). In an exercise such as a bench press, 1 RM is a measure of strength at a relatively slow speed of movement.

Concentric Muscle Action. When a weight is being lifted, the muscles involved normally are shortening. This is termed a concentric muscle action (figure 1.1a). During a concentric muscle action, shortening of the muscle occurs, and therefore the word *contraction* for this type of muscle action is also appropriate.

Eccentric Muscle Action. When a weight is being lowered in a controlled manner, the muscles involved are lengthening in a controlled manner

(figure 1.1b). Muscles can only shorten or lengthen in a controlled manner; they cannot push against the bones to which they are attached. In most exercises, gravity will pull the weight back to the starting position. To control the weight as it returns to the starting position, the muscles must lengthen in a controlled manner, or the weight will fall abruptly.

Isometric Muscle Action. When a muscle is activated and develops force but no movement at a joint occurs, an isometric muscle action takes place (figure 1.1c). This can occur when a weight is held stationary or when a weight is too heavy to lift any higher.

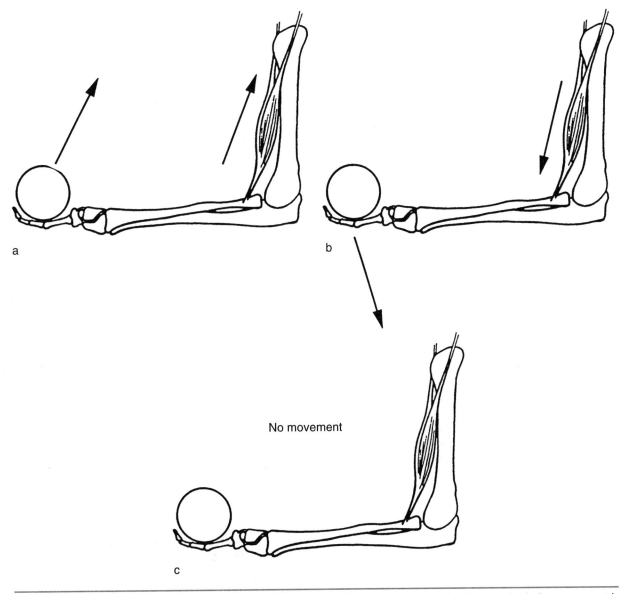

a

b

No movement

c

Fig. 1.1   Major types of muscle actions: a. During a concentric muscle action a muscle shortens; b. during an eccentric muscle action the muscle lengthens in a controlled manner; c. during an isometric muscle action no movement of the joint occurs and no shortening or lengthening of the muscle takes place.

VOLUNTARY MAXIMAL MUSCULAR ACTIONS

Voluntary maximal muscular actions appear to be the most effective way to increase muscular strength (Fleck and Schutt 1985). This does not mean that the maximal resistance possible for one complete repetition (1 RM) must be lifted by the individual. Performing voluntary maximal muscular actions means that the muscle must move with as much resistance as its present fatigue level will allow. The force that a partially fatigued muscle can generate during a voluntary maximal muscular contraction is not as great as that of a nonfatigued muscle. The last repetition in a set to momentary concentric failure is thus a voluntary maximal muscular action. The force produced is not the maximum, because the muscle is partially fatigued. Many resistance training systems use momentary concentric failure or RM resistances as a gauge to ensure the performance of voluntary maximal muscular actions. This ensures that the desired increases in strength, power, or local muscular endurance will occur. Performing voluntary maximal muscular actions in resistance training is often referred to as *overloading* the muscle. The muscle must act against a resistance that it normally does not encounter if physiological changes resulting in the desired training effects are to take place.

Some resistance training machines have been specifically designed to force the muscle to perform voluntary maximal actions either through a greater range of motion (see chapter 2, "Variable Resistance Training") or for more repetitions in a set to momentary voluntary fatigue (see chapter 2, "Isokinetics"). Developments in equipment such as variable resistance and isokinetic equipment attest to a belief in the necessity for voluntary maximal contractions. All competitive Olympic weight lifters, power lifters, and body builders use voluntary maximal muscular actions at some point in their training programs. Competitive lifters realize the need for voluntary maximal contractions to bring about optimal gains in strength or muscular hypertrophy.

INTENSITY

Closely related to voluntary maximal muscular actions is the intensity and power output of training. Power can be increased by using a heavier resistance and performing repetitions at the same speed of movement in some exercises or by lifting or moving a given resistance faster in other exer-

cises. The closer the velocity is to maximal at which a given resistance is moved, the greater the power. This is true for both single-joint and multijoint exercises (Komi 1979). Increasing the power of an exercise by increasing the velocity of movement is important when a major goal is to increase the power output of the muscle and not just its ability to lift maximal resistances (1-RM weights).

Intensity of an exercise can be estimated as a percentage of the 1 RM or any RM for the exercise. The minimal intensity that can be used to perform a set to momentary voluntary fatigue to result in increased strength is 60% to 65% of the 1 RM (McDonagh and Davies 1984). This means that performing a large number of repetitions with a very light resistance will result in no strength gain. It also means that the maximal number of repetitions per set of an exercise that will result in increased strength will vary from exercise to exercise and from muscle group to muscle group. For example, the maximal number of repetitions possible at 60% of 1 RM for the leg press is 34 and for a knee curl is 11 (Hoeger et al. 1987).

Unlike endurance exercise, intensity of resistance training cannot be estimated by heart rate during the exercise. Heart rate during resistance exercise does not consistently vary with the exercise intensity (figure 1.2). Heart rate attained during sets to momentary voluntary fatigue at 50% and 80% of 1 RM are higher than heart rates attained during sets at 1 RM or sets performed to momentary volun-

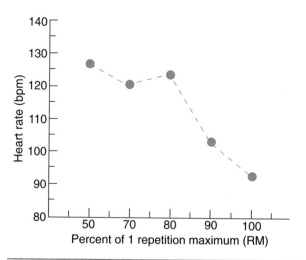

Fig. 1.2 Maximal heart rate of a moderately trained group of males during knee-extension sets to momentary voluntary fatigue at various percentages of the 1 RM. The heart rate does not reflect the intensity (% of 1 RM) of the exercise.

Adapted, by permission, from S.J. Fleck and L.S. Dean, 1987, "Previous resistance-training experience and the pressor response during resistance exercise," *Journal of Applied Physiology* 63(1): 118.

tary fatigue at higher percentages of 1 RM (Fleck and Dean 1987).

TRAINING VOLUME

Training volume is a measure of the total amount of work (Joules) performed in a training session, in a week of training, in a month of training, or in some other time period. Frequency (number of training sessions per week, month, or year) and duration (length of each training session) have a direct bearing on the training volume. The simplest method to estimate volume is to sum the number of repetitions performed in a specific time period, such as a week or month of training. Volume can also be estimated by the total amount of weight lifted. For example, if 100 lb (45 kg) are used to perform 10 repetitions, the volume of training is 1000 lb (450 kg) = 10 repetitions $\times$ 100 lb (45 kg).

Training volume is more precisely determined by calculating the work performed. Total work in a repetition is the weight times the vertical distance the weight is lifted. Thus, if 100 lb (45 kg or 445 N) is lifted vertically 3 ft (0.9 m) in a repetition, volume or total work is 100 lb $\times$ 3 ft = 300 ft · lb (445 N $\times$ 0.9 m = 400 J). Training volume for a set of 10 repetitions in this example is 300 ft · lb (400 J) per repetition $\times$ 10 repetitions = 3000 ft · lb (4000 J). The calculation of training volume is useful in determining the total training stress.

A relationship exists between training volume and muscular hypertrophy; body builders who use large training volumes develop large muscles. Larger training volumes appear to be important when the goal of a resistance training program is a decreased percentage of body fat, increased lean body mass, or muscular hypertrophy (Hather et al. 1992; Stone, O'Bryant, and Garhammer 1981; Stone et al. 1982). Larger training volumes may also result in a slower loss of strength gains after cessation of training (i.e., detraining) (Hather et al. 1992). Training volume is discussed in greater detail in chapter 2.

PERIODIZATION

Variation in the training volume and intensity (periodization) is extremely important for optimal gains in strength (Matveyev 1981; O'Bryant, Byrd, and Stone 1988; Stone, O'Bryant, and Garhammer 1981; Willoughby 1993). Periodization is discussed in more detail in chapter 5.

Slight variations in the position of the foot, hand, or other body parts that do not affect the safety of the lifter can be valuable in producing continued gains in strength (Garhammer 1981b). The use of several exercises to vary the conditioning stimulus of a particular muscle group is also a valuable means to ensure continual increases in strength (see chapter 3, "Muscle Fiber–Type Recruitment"). Periodization is needed to achieve optimal gains in strength and power.

PROGRESSIVE OVERLOAD

Progressive resistance exercise or progressive overload refers to the practice of continually increasing the stress placed on the muscle as it becomes capable of producing greater force or has more endurance. At the start of a training program the 5 RM for arm curls might be 50 lb (23 kg), a sufficient stimulus to produce an increase in strength. Later in the training program five repetitions at 50 lb (23 kg) would not be a sufficient stimulus to produce further gains in strength, because the individual can easily perform five repetitions with 50 lb (23 kg); consequently this stimulus is no longer a 5 RM. If the training stimulus is not increased at this point, no further gains in strength will occur.

There are several methods to progressively overload the muscle. The resistance (amount of weight used) to perform a certain number of repetitions can be increased. The use of RM automatically provides progressive overload, because as the muscle's strength increases, the amount of resistance necessary to perform a true RM also increases. For example, a 5 RM may increase from 50 lb (23 kg) to 60 lb (27 kg) after several weeks of training.

Another method to progressively overload the muscle is to increase the training volume (i.e., the number of sets and repetitions of a particular exercise). Because of the possibility of overtraining, care must be exercised when progressively overloading the muscle. This is especially true when the progressive overload is in the form of an increased training volume (Stone et al. 1982). Therefore, as a general rule large increases in the resistance or volume of training should be avoided, especially for individuals with little resistance training experience. A reasonable guideline is to increase the resistance for a particular number of repetitions or training volume by no more than 2.5% to 5% at one time.

REST PERIODS

Recovery between sets of an exercise, between exercises, and between training sessions is an important factor for the success of the program. The rest periods allowed between sets and between exercises during a training session are in large part determined by the goals of the training program. The rest periods between sets and exercises, the resistance used, and the number of repetitions performed per set all affect the design and the goals of the program (see chapter 5). In general, if the goal is to increase the ability to exhibit maximal strength, relatively long rest periods (several minutes), heavy resistances, and three to six repetitions per set should be used. When the goal is to increase the ability to perform high-intensity exercise for a period of several seconds, rest periods between sets should be less than 1 min. Repetitions and resistance can range from 5 to 15 RM, depending on the exact type of high-intensity ability one wishes to enhance. If enhancement of long-term endurance (aerobic power) is the goal, then circuit-type resistance training with short rest periods (less than 30 s), relatively light resistances, and 10 to 15 repetitions per set is prescribed.

Traditionally, one day of recovery is allowed between training sessions for a particular muscle group. This is still a good general rule, though some evidence indicates that other patterns of training sessions and recovery periods are equally beneficial (see chapter 5, "Rest Periods Between Workouts"). Residual muscular soreness, when it interferes with performance of the following training session, is a good indication that the rest between workouts was insufficient.

SPEED SPECIFICITY

Most coaches and athletes maintain that some resistance training should be performed at the velocity required during the actual sporting event. For many sporting events this means a high velocity of movement. This belief is based on the concept that resistance training produces its greatest strength gains at the velocity at which the training is performed. There is scientific evidence that supports this view (see chapter 2, "Isokinetics"). However, an intermediate training velocity is best if the aim of the program is to increase strength at all velocities of movement (Kanehisa and Miyashita 1983a). Thus, for an individual interested in general strength, an intermediate training velocity is recommended. However, training at a fast velocity results in gains in strength and power at a fast velocity to a slightly greater extent than does training at a slow velocity, and vice versa (Kanehisa and Miyashita 1983a, 1983b). Thus, velocity-specific

training to maximize strength and power gains at a specific velocity is appropriate for athletes at some points in their training.

MUSCLE ACTION

If an individual trains isometrically and progress is evaluated with a static muscle action, a large increase in strength may be apparent. However, if this same individual's progress is determined using concentric or eccentric muscle actions, little or no increase in strength may be demonstrated. This is called testing specificity (see chapter 2, "Comparison of Training Types"). This testing specificity indicates that gains in strength are specific to the type of muscle action used in training (e.g., isometric, variable resistance, isokinetic). This specificity of strength gains is caused by learning to recruit the muscles to perform that particular type of muscle action (see chapter 3). Therefore, a training program for a specific sport should include the types of muscle actions encountered in that sport. For example, isometric muscle actions are frequently performed while wrestling, so it is beneficial to incorporate some isometric training into the resistance training program for wrestling.

MUSCLE-GROUP SPECIFICITY

Muscle-group specificity simply means that each muscle group requiring strength gains must be trained. If an increase in strength is desired in the flexors (biceps group) and extensors (triceps) of the elbow, exercises for both groups need to be included in the program. Exercises in a training program must be specifically chosen for each muscle group in which an increase in strength, local muscular endurance, or hypertrophy is desired.

ENERGY-SOURCE SPECIFICITY

There are two anaerobic sources and one aerobic source of energy for muscle actions (see chapter 3). The anaerobic sources of energy supply the majority of energy for high-powered, short-duration events, such as sprinting 100 m, whereas the aerobic energy source supplies the majority of energy for longer-duration, lower-power events, such as running 5000 m. If an increase in the ability of a muscle to perform anaerobic exercise is desired, the bouts of exercise should be of short duration and high intensity. To increase aerobic capability, training will be of a longer duration and lower intensity. Resistance training is most commonly used to bring about adaptations of the anaerobic energy sources. The number of sets and repetitions and the length of rest periods between sets and exercises need to be appropriate for the energy source in which training adaptations are desired. This is discussed in more detail in chapter 5.

SAFETY ASPECTS

Successful resistance training programs have one prominent feature in common—safety. Resistance training has some inherent dangers, as do all physical activities. The chance of injury can be greatly reduced or completely removed by using correct lifting techniques, spotting, and proper breathing, by maintaining equipment in good working condition, and by wearing appropriate clothing.

The chance of being injured while performing resistance training is very slight. In college football players (Zemper 1990) the weight-room injury rate was very low (0.35 per 100 players per season). Weight-room injuries accounted for only 0.74% of the total reported time-loss injuries during the football season. This injury rate may be reduced to even lower levels through more rigorous attention to proper procedures in the weight room (Zemper 1990).

Spotting

Proper spotting is necessary to ensure the safety of the participants in a resistance training program. Spotters serve two major functions: to assist the trainee with the exercise and to summon help if an accident does occur.

Briefly, several factors should be considered when spotting.

- The spotter must be strong enough to assist the trainee if needed.
- During the performance of certain exercises (e.g., back squats) more than one spotter may be necessary to ensure the safety of the lifter.
- Spotters should know proper spotting technique and the proper technique for the lift for which they are spotting.
- Spotters should know how many repetitions the trainee is going to attempt.
- Spotters must be attentive at all times to the

lifter and to his or her performance of the exercise.
- Spotters should summon help if an accident or injury occurs.

Following these simple guidelines will aid in the avoidance of weight-room injuries (see chapter 5 for more information). A detailed description of spotting techniques for all exercises is beyond the scope of this text, but spotting techniques for a wide variety of individual resistance training exercises have been presented elsewhere (Kraemer and Fleck 1993).

Breathing

Excessively holding one's breath with a closed glottis (Valsalva maneuver) during performance of resistance training is not recommended. Blood pressure rises substantially during resistance training exercises (Fleck and Dean 1987a, 1987b; MacDougall et al. 1985). Figure 1.3 depicts the intraarterial blood pressure response during maximal isometric muscle actions during one-legged knee extensions. The blood pressure response during an isometric muscle action in which breathing

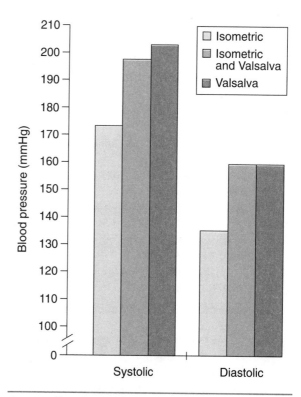

Fig. 1.3 Systolic and diastolic blood pressures during an isometric action only, simultaneous isometric action and Valsalva maneuver, and Valsalva maneuver only.
(Unpublished data of authors, $n = 6$)

was allowed is lower than the response observed during either an isometric action performed simultaneously with a Valsalva maneuver or a Valsalva maneuver in the absence of an isometric muscle action. This demonstrates that the elevation of blood pressure during resistance training is lower if breathing occurs during the muscle action than if a Valsalva maneuver is performed during the muscle action. Elevated blood pressure makes the heart's work harder (pumping blood through the body is more difficult) and requires substantially more energy.

Exhaling during the lifting of the resistance and inhaling during the lowering of the resistance in each repetition are normally recommended. During an exercise at 1 RM or during the last few repetitions of a set performed to momentary voluntary fatigue, some breath holding will occur. However, excessive breath holding should be discouraged.

Proper Technique

Proper technique for resistance training exercises is partially determined by the specific muscle groups that one desires to train. Altering the proper form of an exercise allows other muscle groups to help perform the exercise movement. This decreases the training stimulus on the muscles normally associated with a particular exercise. Proper technique is altered in several advanced resistance training systems (e.g., burn system, forced repetition system), but these systems are not recommended for beginning resistance trainers (see chapter 6).

Proper technique is also necessary to prevent injury, especially in exercises such as squats, deadlifts, and power cleans. Improper technique in these types of exercises places undue stress on the lower back region and should be avoided. Improper form often occurs when the lifter performs an exercise with resistances that exceed his or her present strength capabilities.

Full Range of Motion

Exercises normally are performed with the full range of motion allowed by the body's position and the joints involved. Although no definitive studies are available, it is assumed that to develop strength throughout a joint's full range of motion, training must be performed through the joint's full range of motion. Studies involving joint-angle specificity with isometric training indicate that if training is performed only at a specific joint angle,

strength gains will be realized in a narrow range around that specific joint angle and not throughout the joint's full range of motion (see chapter 2, "Isometrics"). Thus, performing exercises through a full range of motion ensures strength gains throughout the full range and is important to proper exercise technique.

Equipment Maintenance

Maintaining equipment in proper operating condition is of utmost importance for a safe resistance training program. Pulleys and cables or belts should be checked for wear frequently and replaced as needed. Equipment should be lubricated as indicated by the manufacturer. Cracked or broken free-weight plates or plates in a machine's weight stack should be replaced. Upholstery should be disinfected daily. The sleeves on Olympic bars should revolve freely so that skin is not torn off a lifter's hands. An injury resulting from improper equipment maintenance should never happen in a well-run resistance training program.

Resistance Training Shoes

A safe shoe for resistance training does not have to be specifically designed for Olympic-style or power lifting but should have a good arch support, a non-slip sole, proper fit, and little or no shock-absorbing capability of the sole. The first three of these factors are for safety reasons. The last factor is important for a simple reason: Force produced by the leg muscles to lift the weight should not be wasted in compressing the shoe's sole.

Resistance Training Gloves

Gloves for resistance training are designed without fingers, so the glove covers only the palm area. This design protects the palms from catching or scraping on barbells and machine handles but still allows a good grip of the bar or handle. Gloves help prevent blisters and the ripping of calluses on the hand. However, they are not mandatory equipment for safe resistance training.

Training Belt

Training belts have a wide back portion, which supposedly helps support the lumbar area or lower back. Training belts do help support the lower back, but not because of the wide back area. Instead, the belt gives the abdominal muscles something to push against. This helps to raise intraabdominal pressure, which supports the lumbar vertebrae from the front (Harman et al. 1989; Lander, Hundley, and Simonton 1992; Lander, Simonton, and Giacobbe 1990). A training belt can be used for exercises that involve the lumbar region heavily, such as squats and deadlifts. However, a belt is not necessary for safe performance of these exercises. A belt should not be used to alleviate technique problems caused by weak abdominal or lower-back musculature. If exercises that greatly involve the lower back are to be performed, exercises to strengthen the lower back and abdominal regions need to be included in the training program.

Wearing a tightly cinched belt during an activity increases blood pressure compared with blood pressure during the same activity performed without a training belt (Hunter et al. 1989). This increased blood pressure can result in increased cardiovascular stress. Thus, a training belt should not be worn during activities such as riding a stationary bike or for exercises in which the lumbar area is not heavily involved. Furthermore, belts should normally not be worn when performing exercises that do not require back support or that use moderate to light resistances (> 6 RM).

SELECTED READINGS

Kraemer, W.J., and Fleck, S.J. 1993. *Strength training for young athletes.* Champaign, IL: Human Kinetics.

McDonagh, M.J.N., and Davies, C.T.M. 1984. Adaptive responses of mammalian skeletal muscle to exercise with high loads. *European Journal of Applied Physiology* 52:139-55.

Willoughby, D.S. 1993. The effects of mesocycle-length weight training programs involving periodization and partially equated volumes on upper and lower body strength. *Journal of Strength and Conditioning Research* 7:2-8.

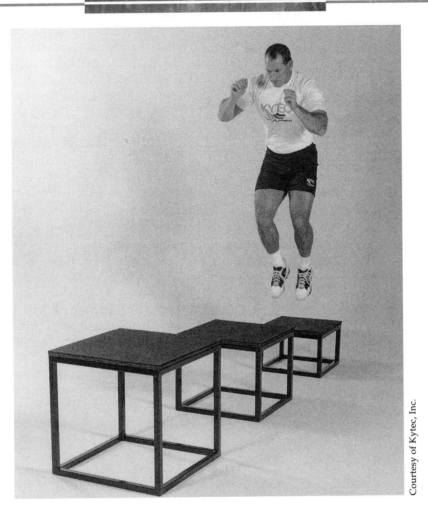

CHAPTER 2

Courtesy of Kytec, Inc.

Types of Strength Training

Most athletes perform strength training as a portion of their overall training program. Their main interest is not how much weight they can lift, but whether increased strength brought about by training results in better performances in their sport. There are several factors to consider when selecting a type of strength training. Does this type of training increase motor performance? Vertical jump tests, a 40-yd dash, and throwing a ball for distance are common motor performance tests.

Is strength increased throughout the range of motion and at all velocities of movement? Most sports require strength through a joint's entire range of motion, or at least a major portion of it. If strength is not increased throughout the entire range of motion, performance may not be enhanced as much as possible by a particular type of training. The majority of athletic events require strength at a variety of movement speeds, particularly at fast velocities. If strength is not increased over a wide range of movement speeds, once again improvements in performance may not be optimal.

Does this type of training cause changes in percentage of body fat or lean body mass and, if so, to what extent? How much of an increase in strength can be expected over a specified training period with this type of training? How does this type of training compare with other types of training in the preceding factors?

There has been a considerable amount of research concerning resistance training. The emergence of conclusions from this research, however, is hampered by several factors. The vast majority of studies have been of short-term duration (8 to 12 wk) and used untrained or moderately trained individuals as subjects, which makes direct application of the studies' results to long-term training (years) and athletes controversial.

As an example, elite Olympic-style weight lifters during 1 yr of training show an increase in 1 RM snatch of 1.5% and in 1 RM clean and jerk of 2% and show an increase in lean body mass of 1% or less and a decrease in percentage body fat of up to 1.7% (Häkkinen et al. 1987; Häkkinen et al. 1988b). Over 2 yr of training, elite Olympic weight lifters show an increase in total (1 RM snatch plus 1 RM clean and jerk) of 2.7% and an increase in lean body mass of 1.0% and a decrease in percentage body fat of 1.7% (Häkkinen et al. 1988b). These changes are much smaller than those shown by untrained or moderately trained individuals in strength

(tables 2.3 and 2.4) and body composition (table 7.6) over much shorter training periods of 8 to 20 wk. This indicates that bringing about changes in strength and body composition in elite athletes may be more difficult than in untrained or moderately trained individuals. The fact that it is more difficult to bring about an increase of strength in highly trained individuals is clearly shown in figure 2.1.

Other factors that can affect gains in strength are the number of muscular actions (sets and repetitions) performed and the resistance or intensity utilized in training. These factors vary considerably from study to study and make interpretation of the results difficult. Enough research has been conducted, however, to reach some tentative conclusions concerning the types of strength training. This chapter addresses the major research concerning types of strength training and the conclusions that it demonstrates.

ISOMETRICS

Isometrics, or static resistance training, refers to a muscular action during which no change in the length of the muscle takes place. This type of resistance training is normally performed against an immovable object such as a wall, a barbell, or a weight machine loaded beyond an individual's maximal concentric strength. Isometrics can also be performed by having a weak muscle group contract against a strong muscle group, for example, by contracting the left elbow flexors maximally to try to bend the left elbow while simultaneously resisting the movement by pushing down on the left hand with the right hand with just enough force to stop any movement at the left elbow. If the left elbow flexors are weaker than the right elbow extensors, the left elbow flexors would perform an isometric action at 100% of a maximal voluntary action. The cost of isometrics can range from minimal when using a wall as the immovable object to quite expensive when using a loaded weight machine as the immovable object.

Isometrics came to the attention of the American public in the early 1950s, when Steinhaus (1954) introduced the work of two Germans, Hettinger and Muller (1953). Hettinger and Muller concluded that gains in strength of 5% per week were produced by one daily two-thirds maximal isometric action 6 s in duration. Gains in strength of this magnitude with such little training time and effort seemed unbelievable. Review of subsequent studies demonstrates that isometric training leads to static strength gains but that the gains are substantially less than 5% per week (Fleck and Schutt 1985).

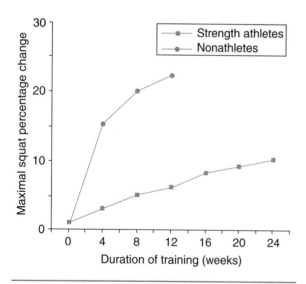

Fig. 2.1 The percentage of change in maximal squat ability from the pretraining value depends on the pretraining status of the trainees and duration of training.

Adapted, by permission, from K. Häkkinen, 1985, "Factors influencing trainability of muscular strength during short-term and prolonged training," *National Strength and Conditioning Association Journal* 7:33.

Increases in strength from isometric training are related to the number of muscle actions performed, the duration of the muscle actions, whether the muscle action is maximal or submaximal, and the frequency of training. Most studies involving isometric training manipulate several of these simultaneously. It is therefore difficult to evaluate the importance of any one factor. Enough research has been conducted, however, to allow some recommendations concerning isometric training.

Maximal Voluntary Muscle Actions

Increases in strength can be achieved with submaximal isometric muscle actions (Alway, Sale, and MacDougall 1990; Davies, Parker, Rutherford, and Jones 1988; Davies and Young 1983; Hettinger and Muller 1953). However, it is generally believed and supported, although not fully substantiated, by the majority of research that maximal voluntary muscle actions (MVMAs) are superior to submaximal voluntary isometric muscle actions in bringing about increases in strength (Rasch and Morehouse 1957; Ward and Fisk 1964). The majority of sport scientists and practitioners now use 100% of MVMA for training purposes.

Number of Muscle Actions and Training Duration

Hettinger and Muller (1953) proposed that only one 6-s muscle action per day was necessary to produce maximal gains in strength. As shown in table 2.1, many combinations in the number and duration of MVMAs can result in strength gain. The majority of research has utilized MVMAs of 3 to 10 s in duration and a relatively small number of muscle actions per day. The duration of the muscle action and the number of training muscle actions per day individually show weaker correlations to increases in strength than do duration and number combined (McDonagh and Davies 1984). This means that the length of time a muscle is activated is directly related to increased strength. It also indicates that optimal gains in strength are the result of either a small number of long-duration muscle actions or a high number of short-duration muscle actions. As an example, seven daily one-minute muscle actions at 30% of MVMA or 42 three-second MVMAs per training day over a 6-wk training period both result in about a 30% increase in isometric MVMA (Davies and Young 1983).

Studies in table 2.1 also indicate that one muscle action per day is ineffective in causing increases in strength. Collectively this information indicates that the most efficient use of training time is to perform MVMAs when using isometric training, that the duration of the MVMAs should be a minimum of 3 to 5 s, and that a minimum of 15 to 20 MVMAs should be performed per training session.

Frequency of Training

Three training sessions per week result in a significant increase of a muscle's MVMA (Alway, MacDougall, and Sale 1989; Alway, Sale, and MacDougall 1990; Carolyn and Cafarelli 1992; Davies, Parker, Rutherford, and Jones 1988; Garfinkel and Cafarelli 1992). Increases in isometric MVMA over 6 to 16 wk of training range from 14% to 44% in these studies. However, whether three training sessions per week bring about maximal increases in strength is not fully substantiated. Hettinger (1961) calculated that alternate-day isometric training is 80% as effective as daily training sessions and that once-a-week training is 40% as effective. Hettinger also concluded that training once every 2 wk does not cause increases in strength, though it does serve to maintain strength. The exact percentages are controversial, but the superiority of daily training with isometrics is well established (Atha 1981). To increase maximal strength, the optimal isometric program should consist of MVMAs performed on a daily basis.

Muscular Hypertrophy

Increases in limb circumferences from training are usually associated with muscular hypertrophy. Significant increases in strength accompanied by increased limb circumferences have been reported from isometric training (Kanehisa and Miyashita 1983a; Kitai and Sale 1989; Meyers 1967; Rarick and Larson 1958). One study concludes that changes in limb circumference do not necessarily accompany increased strength (Ward and Fisk 1964).

More recently computerized tomography has been used to measure muscle cross-sectional area changes due to isometric training. Cross-sectional area of the elbow flexors is increased 5.4% and isometric strength increased 14.5% after 6 wk of isometric training. Nevertheless, no correlation between the increased strength and cross-sectional area was shown (Davies, Parker, Rutherford, and Jones 1988). A second study using computerized tomography reported a 28% increase in isometric strength and a 14.6% increase in the cross-sectional area of the knee extensors after 8 wk of isometric training and reported a relationship between the increased strength and cross-sectional area (Garfinkel and Cafarelli 1992).

TABLE 2.1
Effect of 100% Maximal Voluntary Contractions on Isometric Strength

Reference	Duration of contraction(s)	Contractions per day	Duration × contractions per day	Number of training days	MVIA increase (%)	MVIA increase % per day	Muscles
Ikai and Fukunaga 1970	10	3	30	100	92	0.9	Elbow flexors
Komi and Karlsson 1978	3-5	5	15-25	48	20	0.4	Quadriceps
Bonde-Petersen 1960	5	10	50	36	15	0.4	Elbow flexors
Alway, MacDougall, and Sale 1989	10	5-15	50-150	48	44	0.9	Triceps surae
Bonde-Petersen 1960	5	1	5	36	0	0	Elbow flexors
McDonagh, Hayward, and Davies 1983	3	30	90	28	20	0.7	Elbow flexors
Grimby et al. 1973	3	30	90	30	32	1.1	Triceps
Davies and Young 1983	3	42	126	35	30	0.9	Triceps surae
Carolyn and Cafarelli 1992	3-4	30	90-120	24	32	1.3	Quadriceps
Garfinkel and Cafarelli 1992	3-5	30	90-150	24	28	1.2	Quadriceps

MVIA = maximal voluntary isometric action

Note. Adapted, by permission, from M.J.N. McDonagh and C.T.M. Davies, 1984, "Adaptive responses of mammalian skeletal muscle to exercise with high loads," European Journal of Applied Physiology 52:140. Additional data from Garfinkel and Cafarelli 1992, Carolyn and Cafarelli 1992, Alway et al. 1989.

Whether hypertrophy occurs and the extent to which it occurs may vary from muscle to muscle, as shown by the following studies. Type I and Type II muscle fiber diameters in the vastus lateralis (one of the knee extensors) did not change after 9 wk of isometric training at 100% of MVMA (Lewis et al. 1984). Type I and Type II fiber areas increased in the soleus approximately 30% after 16 wk of isometric training with either 30% or 100% of MVMA (Alway, MacDougall, and Sale 1989; Alway, Sale, and MacDougall 1990), whereas only the Type II fibers of the lateral gastrocnemius increased in area 30% to 40% after the same length and intensity of training (Alway, MacDougall, and Sale 1989; Alway, Sale, and MacDougall 1990).

Collectively this information indicates that muscular hypertrophy of both the Type I and Type II muscle fibers can occur from isometric training with submaximal and maximal muscle actions. Increases in strength not related to muscular hypertrophy may also occur from isometric training. Thus, increases in strength may also occur from neural adaptations (see chapter 7). Isometric training can bring about increases in hypertrophy and neural adaptations, both of which can increase strength.

Joint-Angle Specificity

When isometric training is performed, the gains in strength occur predominantly at the joint angle at which the isometric training is performed; this is *joint-angle specificity*. The majority of research indicates that static strength increases from isometric training are joint-angle specific (Bender and Kaplan 1963; Gardner 1963; Kitai and Sale 1989; Lindh 1979; Meyers 1967; Thepaut-Mathieu, Van Hoecke, and Martin 1988; Williams and Stutzman 1959), although lack of joint-angle-specific gains in strength have also been shown (Knapik, Mawdsley, and Ramos 1983; Rasch and Pierson 1964; Rasch, Preston, and Logan 1961). Many factors may affect the degree to which joint-angle specificity occurs, including the muscle group(s) trained, the joint angle at which the training is performed, and the intensity and duration of the isometric actions.

Isometric training of the elbow extensors at an elbow joint angle of 90° results in increased isometric MVMA at an elbow angle of 90° (Knapik, Mawdsley, and Ramos 1983). There is, however, a smaller but significant increase at elbow angles of 70° and 110°. Thus, there is a carry-over of strength increases up to at least 20° on either side of the training angle. Isometric training of the plantar flexors

with the ankle joint at 90° results in increased strength at the training angle and significant carry-over of strength increases at only ± 5° of the training angle (Kitai and Sale 1989). Training of the elbow flexors at an elbow angle of 80° results in a carry-over of strength increases over a large range of elbow angles (Thepaut-Mathieu, Van Hoecke, and Martin 1988), whereas training of the elbow flexors at an elbow angle of 25° or 120° results in a much smaller carry-over to other joint angles (figure 2.2).

Joint-angle specificity (figure 2.2) is most marked when the training is performed with the muscle in a shortened position (25° angle) and occurs to a smaller extent when the training occurs with the muscle in a lengthened position (120° angle) (Gardner 1963; Thepaut-Mathieu, Van Hoecke, and Martin 1988). When training occurs at the midpoint (80° angle), joint-angle specificity may occur within a greater range of motion (Kitai and Sale 1989; Knapik, Mawdsley, and Ramos 1983; Thepaut-Mathieu, Van Hoecke, and Martin 1988) or may not occur (Rash and Pierson 1964; Rasch, Preston, and Logan 1961). In addition, twenty 6-s muscle actions result in greater carry-over to other joint angles than six 6-s muscle actions (Meyers 1967). This indicates that the longer the total duration of isometric training (number of muscle actions × duration of each muscle action), the greater the carry-over to other joint angles.

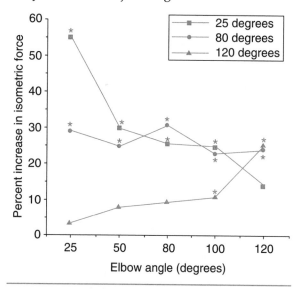

Fig. 2.2   Percent gain in isometric strength of elbow flexors due to isometric training at different elbow angles.

* = significant increase (*p* ≤ .05).

Adapted, by permission, from C. Thepaut-Mathieu, J. Van Hoecke, and B. Maton, 1988, "Myoelectrical and mechanical changes linked to length specificity during isometric training," *Journal of Applied Physiology* 64:1502.

Isometric training of the elbow flexors at four different joint angles increases static strength at all four joint angles and significantly increases dynamic power of the elbow flexors (Kanehisa and Miyashita 1983a). Thus, it is possible to increase dynamic power with isometric training if the isometric actions are performed at several points in the joint's range of motion.

This information from studies of joint-angle specificity indicates some practical guidelines for increasing strength and power throughout the entire range of motion. First, the training should be performed at joint-angle increments of approximately 10° to 20°. Second, the total duration (duration of each muscle action × number of muscle actions) of the isometric training per session should be long (3- to 5-s actions, 15 to 20 actions per day). Third, if isometric actions cannot be performed throughout the entire range of motion, it is best to perform them with the muscle in a lengthened position rather than a shortened position.

It is possible to take advantage of isometric training's angle specificity. Every dynamic exercise has a *sticking region*, the place within the exercise's range of motion where the mechanical advantage is at its lowest point. The sticking region is therefore the portion of the exercise where it is most difficult to continue to move the resistance. Performance of isometric training within this region of the range of motion will increase strength at these particular joint angle(s) and may therefore aid in the performance of the dynamic exercise.

Motor Performance

Isometric training at one joint angle does not increase motor performance ability (Clarke 1973; Fleck and Schutt 1985). This may be the result of several factors. Isometric training at one joint angle does not increase a limb's maximal velocity of movement with little or no resistance (DeKoning et al. 1982) and may reduce a limb's maximal speed of movement (Swegan 1957). Many motor performance tests (e.g., vertical jump, softball throw for distance) involve moving at maximal speeds with little or no resistance to movement. If a limb's maximal speed of movement is not increased or is decreased, improvement in motor performance will not occur.

Because dynamic power can be increased with isometric training if the isometric actions are performed at several points within the range of motion (Kanehisa and Miyashita 1983a), a possibility of improving motor performance exists. If isomet-

ric actions are used, training should be performed at 10° to 20° intervals throughout a movement's range of motion. This will increase the possibility of increasing motor performance.

Other Considerations

As with all resistance training, a Valsalva maneuver will occur but should not be encouraged. A Valsalva maneuver will result in an exaggerated blood pressure response. A maximal isometric deadlift for 30 s results in systolic and diastolic blood pressures of 230 and 155 mmHg, respectively (Vitcenda et al. 1990). Isometric knee extensions at 100% of MVMA with no breath holding result in systolic and diastolic blood pressures of 174 and 135 mmHg, respectively (see figure 1.3). The same isometric action with breath holding results in systolic and diastolic blood pressures of 198 and 158 mmHg, respectively. A Valsalva maneuver should be discouraged in all trainees, especially those with cardiovascular problems.

Without lifting or moving an actual object, motivational problems may occur for some athletes. It is also difficult for a coach to evaluate whether the trainees are performing the isometric actions at the desired intensity. Visual feedback of the force being developed, especially during unfamiliar movements, serves as positive feedback and encourages greater force production during isometric actions (Graves and James 1990). For such feedback, a force transducer and a monitoring system are required. This equipment may not be practical in many training situations. However, if isometric actions are to be used optimally in training, the use of a feedback-monitoring system is warranted.

DYNAMIC CONSTANT EXTERNAL RESISTANCE TRAINING

Isotonics is traditionally defined as a muscular contraction in which the muscle exerts a constant tension. The execution of free-weight exercises and exercises on various weight training machines, though usually considered isotonic, is not isotonic according to this definition. The force exerted by a muscle in the performance of such exercises is not constant, but rather varies with the mechanical advantage of the joint involved in the movement and the length of the muscle at a particular point in the movement. A more workable term for resistance training exercise in which the external resistance or weight does not change and both a lifting (concentric) and a lowering (eccentric) phase occur during each repetition is *dynamic constant external resistance (DCER) training.* DCER implies that the weight or resistance being lifted is constant and held constant. When using free weights or machines, the external resistance or weight lifted is chosen. Thus, DCER better describes this type of resistance training than the old term isotonic.

Number of Sets and Repetitions

The optimal number of sets and repetitions of DCER exercises to achieve maximal gains in strength has received a great deal of attention. This line of inquiry assumes that an optimal number of sets and repetitions actually exists, that once found it will work for all individuals and exercises or muscle groups, and that it will promote maximal increases in strength for an indefinite period of time. These assumptions may not be correct.

In reviewing the research concerning DCER, the majority of studies have used novice, college-aged individuals as trainees and a relatively short duration of training (8-12 wk, with several lasting 20-24 wk). Pretraining status and the duration of the study may affect the results. Also common to the vast majority of studies using DCER is the use of an RM resistance at some point in the training program.

Some studies in the 1960s focused on bench press and back squat exercises, trained subjects with RMs, and used 1 RM as the testing criterion. This research indicated that the optimal number of sets and repetitions for the bench press and the back squat was three and six, respectively (Berger 1962b, 1962c). In a later study, Berger trained groups using six sets at 2 RM, three sets at 6 RM, and three sets at 10 RM (Berger 1963a). All groups gained significantly according to the 1-RM testing criterion, but no significant difference was demonstrated between the training groups. This demonstrates that various combinations of sets and repetitions cause similar gains in strength during an initial short period of training, especially in untrained individuals. This point is well supported by several research studies. Using numbers of sets ranging from 1 to 6 and numbers of repetitions per set ranging from 1 to 20, increases in strength have been reported (Dudley et al. 1991; Graves et al. 1988; Häkkinen 1985; Sale et al. 1990; Staron et al. 1989).

Other researchers have substantiated the conclusion that there is no one optimal combination of sets and repetitions. No significant difference in increases of 1 RM were found when training consisted of three sets of six repetitions at 6 RM and two sets of nine at 9 RM (Henderson 1970), when training consisted of five sets of three at 3 RM, four sets of five at 5 RM, or three sets of seven at 7 RM (Withers 1970), or when training consisted of three sets of two to three, five to six, or nine to ten at the same respective RM (O'Shea 1966).

Increases in maximal strength have been reported when doing one set of an exercise per training session (Alén et al. 1988; Berger 1962a; Graves et al. 1988; Luthi et al. 1986; Marcinik et al. 1991; Rasch and Morehouse 1957). It has been recommended for general fitness of healthy adults that a "minimum" of one set of at least one exercise for all major muscle groups be included in a training session (American College of Sports Medicine 1990). This recommendation is for healthy adults desiring minimal fitness and not for athletes because multiple sets do result in greater strength gains than single-set programs. Although one set per exercise per training session may be appropriate as a short-term in-season program for some athletes, it is not recommended as a long-term program for athletes (see chapter 5). Over the course of a training year or career, even small, superior gains in strength by performing multiple sets per training session as compared to one set, will make the difference between winning and losing for many athletes. In addition, a one-set-per-training-session program does not result in increases of short-term, high-intensity endurance as large as those of a multiple-set program or a periodized program (McGee et al. 1992).

Tables 2.3 and 2.4 demonstrate that DCER exercise can result in substantial increases in bench press and leg press strength. These tables and the aforementioned studies indicate that, for a program that is not periodized, the optimal number of repetitions for strength improvement is somewhere between 2 and 10 RM and the optimal number of sets is between two and five.

Maximal Voluntary Muscle Actions

The majority of training studies and training programs used by athletes incorporate maximal voluntary muscle actions (MVMAs) at some point in the training. This does not mean that a 1 RM has to be performed, rather that a set is performed to momentary concentric failure or an RM set is performed. In some exercises such as power cleans or snatch pulls, if the exercise is performed as quickly as possible, an MVMA may be performed on every repetition. If the lifter attempts to lift the bar as fast as possible at points in the motion where he or she is strong, the bar will accelerate (force = mass × acceleration). At points in the motion where the lifter is weaker the bar will decelerate. An MVMA will be performed in either case, the only difference being the velocity of movement.

To produce optimal gains in strength, Berger and Hardage's study (1967) demonstrated a need for MVMA. Two groups underwent a training program of one set of 10 repetitions. Both groups trained three times per week for 8 wk. For group 1 the initial repetition was at the 1-RM level, and each following repetition was adjusted so that a maximal effort was required; group 2 trained with one full set at 10 RM. Both groups made significant gains in strength, but group 1 improved significantly more than group 2. This study indicates that multiple MVMAs are needed to achieve optimal strength improvement.

Frequency of Training

The frequency of DCER training has been the subject of several studies. Studies indicate either that three is superior to two sessions per week (Henderson 1970) or that two is superior to three sessions per week (Berger 1965) in causing increases in strength. Another study demonstrated that five and three sessions per week bring about significantly greater increases in strength than two sessions per week and found no difference between five and three training sessions per week (Barham 1960). A study involving Division I college football players as subjects indicated that four and five training days per week are superior to three and six training days per week over 10 wk of training (J.R. Hoffman et al. 1990).

Table 2.2 presents two studies concerning frequency of training. One of these studies (Gilliam 1981) compared from one to five training sessions per week. The study showed five training sessions to be superior in causing increases in a 1-RM bench press and three training sessions per week to be superior to two. A study comparing four and three training sessions per week using male and female subjects reported significantly greater gains in both genders with more frequent training sessions (Hunter 1985). Interestingly, the four-sessions-per-week subjects trained two consecutive days twice a week (i.e., Monday, Tuesday, Thursday, and Friday), while the three-sessions-per-week groups trained in the traditional alternate-day method (i.e., Monday, Wednesday, Friday).

The aforementioned studies have certain shortcomings: The majority of studies used beginning resistance exercisers (novice subjects); they examined short time periods (up to 12 wk); and most of them did not equate the total number of sets and repetitions performed by the different training groups. A tentative conclusion that arises from all these studies is that more frequent training sessions cause greater increases in strength. However, the majority of research indicates that three training sessions per muscle group per week is the minimum frequency that causes near maximum gains in strength in novice subjects over an initial, short training period.

Two Training Sessions in One Day

Two or more resistance training sessions on the same day are becoming common. Some trainees may have started this practice because of time and schedule constraints. Others may include more than one session per day in an attempt to accumulate a greater training volume in their training pro-

TABLE 2.2								
Effect of Frequency of Training on 1-RM Bench Press								
Reference	Gender	Days per week of training and percentage improvement						
Gilliam 1981	Male	Days	1	2	3	4	5	
		% improvement	19	24	32	29	41	
Hunter 1985	Male	Days	3	4				
		% improvement	12	17				
Hunter 1985	Female	Days	3	4				
		% improvement	20	33				

TABLE 2.3
Changes in Bench Press Strength From Training

Reference	Gender of subjects	Type of training	Length of training (wk)	Days of training/ week	Sets and repetitions	% increase for equipment trained on	Comparative test Type of equipment	% increase
Brown and Wilmore 1974	F	DCER	24	3	8 wk = 1 × 10, 8, 7, 6, 5, 4 16 wk = 1 × 10, 6, 5, 4, 3	38	—	—
Mayhew and Gross 1974	F	DCER	9	3	2 × 20	26	—	—
Wilmore 1974	F	DCER	10	2	2 × 7-16	29	—	—
Wilmore et al. 1978	F	DCER	10	3	40%-55% 1 RM for 30 s	20	—	—
Berger 1962b	M	DCER	12	3	3 × 6	30	—	—
Fahey and Brown 1973	M	DCER	9	3	5 × 5	12	—	—
Wilmore 1974	M	DCER	10	2	2 × 7-16	16	—	—
Allen, Byrd, and Smith 1976	M	DCER	12	3	2 × 8, 1 × exhaustion	44	—	—
Ariel 1977	M	DCER	20	5	4 × 8-3	14	—	—
Wilmore et al. 1978	M	DCER	10	3	40%-55% 1 RM for 30 s	8	—	—
Gettman et al. 1978	M	DCER	20	3	50% 1 RM, 6 wk = 2 × 10-20, 14 wk = 2 × 15	32	IK (12/s)	27
Marcinik et al. 1991	M	DCER	12	3	1 × 8-12 RM	20	—	—
Stone, Nelson et al. 1983	M	DCER	6	3	3 × 6 RM	7	—	—
Hoffman et al. 1990	M college football	DCER	10	3	4 wk = 4 × 8 RM 4 wk = 5 × 6 RM 2 wk = 1 × 10, 8, 6, 4, 2 RM	2	—	—
Hoffman et al. 1990	M college football	DCER	10	4	Same as 3/wk	4	—	—
Hoffman et al. 1990	M college football	DCER	10	5	Same as 3/wk	3	—	—

(continued)

TABLE 2.3
(continued)

Reference	Gender of subjects	Type of training	Length of training (wk)	Days of training/week	Sets and repetitions	% increase for equipment trained on	Comparative test Type of equipment	% increase
Hoffman et al. 1990	M college football	DCER	10	6	Same as 3/wk	4	—	—
Brazell-Roberts and Thomas 1989	F	DCER	12	2	3 × 10 (75% 1 RM)	37	—	—
Brazell-Roberts and Thomas 1989	F	DCER	12	3	3 × 10 (75% 1 RM)	37	—	—
Coleman 1977	M	DCER	10	3	2 × 8-10 RM	12	—	—
Coleman 1977	M	VR	10	3	1 × 10-12 RM	—	DCER[a]	12
Ariel 1977	M	VR	20	5	4 × 8-3	—	DCER	29
Stanforth, Painter, and Wilmore 1992	M & F	VR	12	3	3 × 8-12 RM	11	IK	17
Gettman and Ayres 1978	M	IK (60°/s)	10	3	3 × 10-15	—	DCER	11
Gettman and Ayres 1978	M	IK (120°/s)	10	3	3 × 10-15	—	DCER	9
Gettman et al. 1979	M	IK	8	3	4 wk = 1 × 10 at 60°/s, 4 wk = 1 × 15 at 90°/s	22	DCER	11
Stanforth, Painter, and Wilmore 1992	M & F	IK (1.5 s/ contraction)	12	3	3 × 8-12 RM	20	VR	11

DCER = dynamic constant external resistance

VR = variable resistance

IK = isokinetic

RM = repetition maximum

[a] = values for average training weights

TABLE 2.4

Changes in Leg Press Strength From Training

Reference	Gender of subjects	Type of training	Length of training (wk)	Days of training/ week	Sets and repetitions	% increase for equipment trained on	Comparative test Type of equipment	% increase
Mayhew and Gross 1974	F	DCER	9	3	2 × 10	48[a]	—	—
Brown and Wilmore 1974	F	DCER	24	3	8 wk = 1 × 10, 8, 7, 6, 5, 4 16 wk = 1 ×10, 6, 5, 4, 3	29	—	—
Wilmore et al. 1978	F	DCER	10	3	40%-55% 1 RM for 30 s	27	—	—
Allen, Byrd, and Smith 1976	M	DCER	12	3	2 × 8 1 × exhaustion	71[b]	—	—
Wilmore et al. 1978	M	DCER	10	3	40%-55% 1 RM for 30 s	7	—	—
Gettman et al. 1978	M	DCER	20	3	50% 1 RM, 6 wk = 2 ×10-20 14 wk = 2 ×15	—	IK	43.0
Coleman 1977	M	DCER	10	3	2 × 8-10 RM	17	—	—
Dudley et al. 1991	M	DCER	19	2	4-5 × 6-12 RM	26	—	—
Sale et al. 1990	M & F	DCER	11 (3 wk off) 11 more total 22	3	6 × 15-20 RM (one-legged training)	30		
Tatro, Dudley, and Convertino 1992	M	DCER	19	2	7 wk × 4 × 10-12 RM 6 wk = 5 × 8-10 RM 6 wk = 5 × 6-8 RM	25 (3 RM)	—	—

(continued)

TABLE 2.4
(continued)

Reference	Gender of subjects	Type of training	Length of training (wk)	Days of training/ week	Sets and repetitions	% increase for equipment trained on	Comparative test Type of equipment	% increase
Pipes 1978	M	DCER	10	3	3 × 8	29	VR	7.5
Coleman 1977	M	VR	10	3	1 × 10-12 RM	—	DCER	18.0
Pipes 1978	M	VR	10	3	3 × 8	27	DCER	7.5
Gettman, Culter, and Strathman 1980	M	VR	20	3	3 × 8	18[c]	IK	17.0
Smith and Melton 1981	M	VR	6	4	3 × 10	—	VR[d]	10.5
Gettman et al. 1979	M	IK	8	3	4 wk = 1 × 10 at 60°/s 4 wk = 1 × 15 at 90°/s	38	DCER	18.0
Gettman, Culter, and Strathman 1980	M	IK	20	3	2 × 12 at 60°/s	42	VR	10.0
Smith and Melton 1981	M	IK	6	4	sets to 50% fatigue at 30, 60, & 90°/s	—	VR	9.8
Smith and Melton 1981	M	IK	6	4	sets to 50% fatigue at 180, 240, & 300°/s	—	VR	6.7

DCER = dynamic constant external resistance
VR = variable resistance
IK = isokinetic
RM = repetition maximum
[a] = values for 10 RM
[b] = values for average training weights
[c] = values for number of weight plates
[d] = different type of VR equipment

gram. For whatever reason, two training sessions per day with a relatively high volume is not recommended for the beginning trainee. As with all physical training, time must be allowed for the trainee to adapt to increases in intensity or volume.

When elite Olympic-style weight lifters perform a training session in the morning and one in the afternoon on the same day, strength measures decrease after the first training session but recover by the second session (Häkkinen 1992; Häkkinen et al. 1988c). Strength measures of Olympic-style weight lifters also recover between training sessions when two training sessions per day are performed on four out of seven days (Häkkinen et al. 1988a). Thus, it appears that well-conditioned, resistance-trained athletes can tolerate two training sessions per day, at least for short periods of time.

When two training sessions are performed on the same day by elite Olympic-style weight lifters for 2 d, no significant change in maximal snatch ability occurs (Kauhanen and Häkkinen 1989). However, the angular velocity of the knee in the drop under the bar decreases, and the barbell is pulled to a slightly lower height. After 1 d of rest, knee angular velocity increases, and the maximal height of the pull returns to normal. After 1 wk of two training sessions per day, maximal isometric force production is unchanged in Olympic-style weight lifters (Kauhanen and Häkkinen 1989). However, the time needed to reach maximal isometric force is increased. After 2 wk of two to three training sessions per day, vertical jump ability is decreased in junior elite Olympic-style weight lifters (Warren et al. 1992). Collectively this information indicates that elite strength-trained athletes can tolerate two training sessions per day at least for short periods of time, but that changes in exercise technique and decreased power output can occur. Possible indications that an athlete cannot tolerate two training sessions per day may be small changes in exercise or sport technique and decreases in power-oriented tasks such as a vertical jump.

One reason for performing two training sessions on the same day is to increase the total training volume. Another reason may be to allow almost complete recovery after performing half of the training. This can be accomplished by performing one half of the normal training volume of a one-training-session-per-day program in the morning and one half in the afternoon. This schedule has been investigated, and the results indicate that when total training volume is equal, two half-volume training sessions per day are advantageous (Häkkinen and Pakarinen 1991). In a 2-wk period

trained body builders and power lifters performed one training session per day. In another 2-wk period they performed the same training exercises with the same volume but divided the training volume into two training sessions on the same day. Thus, total training volume was equal in the 2-wk periods; the only difference was the number of training sessions per day. Each 2-wk training period was followed by 1 wk at a reduced training volume. Isometric force during a squat-type movement was unchanged after each 2-wk training period. Isometric force was also unchanged after the week of reduced training volume following the one-training-session-per-day period. However, isometric force increased after the week of reduced training volume following the two-training-session-per-day period. This indicates that dividing the total training volume into two sessions a day may result in greater strength increases after a short recovery period.

Motor Performance

DCER exercise has been proven to increase motor performance. Many studies show significant increases in motor performance tests such as the vertical jump (K. Adams et al. 1992; R.C. Campbell 1962; Stone, Johnson, and Carter 1979; Stone, O'Bryant, and Garhammer 1981), the standing long jump (Capen 1950; Chu 1950), the shuttle run (R.C. Campbell 1962; Kusintz and Kenney 1958), a short sprint (Capen 1950; Schultz 1967), baseball throwing velocity (Thompson and Martin 1965), and the shot put (Chu 1950; Schultz 1967). Statistically insignificant changes in short sprint time (Chu 1950; J.R. Hoffman et al. 1990) and in vertical jump ability (J.R. Hoffman et al. 1990; Stone, Nelson, Nader, and Carter 1983) and decreases in standing long jump ability (Schultz 1967) have also been demonstrated. Like strength increases, changes in motor performance tests will be smaller the better the physical condition of the individual at the start of the program.

Training using over- and underweight balls increases overhand baseball throwing velocity (DeRenne, Ho, and Blitzblau 1990). However, overhead baseball throwing ability for speed and accuracy is not significantly affected by DCER training with weighted-ball or pulley-type exercises, according to two studies (Brose and Hanson 1967; Straub 1968). Maximal forehand, backhand, and serve velocities in female collegiate tennis players has also been found to increase from DCER training (Kraemer in press). Although conflicting results emerge from this research, as a whole it demonstrates that DCER exercise can significantly improve motor performance ability.

Significant increases in vertical jump and shot put ability occur in college-age individuals after training only the toe and finger flexors over a 12-wk period (Kokkonen et al. 1988). Thus, the training of smaller muscle groups involved in a motor performance task is also important if an increase in performance is desired.

Direct practice, alone or combined with resistance or sprint training, increases standing long jump ability to a significantly greater extent than resistance training alone (Schultz 1967). This result indicates that direct practice of the skill and resistance training should be combined in the training program if a major goal is to optimally improve motor performance.

Strength Changes

Increases in strength for both women and men from DCER training are well documented. Tables 2.2, 2.3, and 2.4 present changes in a 1-RM bench press and leg press from short-term DCER training. Women experience substantial increases in 1-RM leg press strength; one project demonstrated a 48% increase in only 9 wk of training (Mayhew and Gross 1974). Increases in 1-RM leg press strength for men range from 71% in 12 wk (Allen, Byrd, and Smith 1976) to 7% in 10 wk (Wilmore et al. 1978). Using a 1-RM bench press as the testing criterion, women have reportedly increased strength by 38% in 24 wk of training (C.H. Brown and Wilmore 1974) and 37% in 12 wk of training (Brazell-Roberts and Thomas 1989). Similarly, men experienced strength increases ranging from 44% in 12 wk (Allen, Byrd, and Smith 1976) to 8% in 10 wk (Wilmore et al. 1978). The wide range of increases in strength is probably caused by differences in the subjects' pretraining status, familiarity with the exercise tests, and training programs.

Body Composition Changes

The normal changes in body composition from short-term DCER exercise in both males and females are small increases in lean body mass and small decreases in percent body fat (table 7.6). These two changes occur simultaneously, thus the end result is little or no change in total body weight.

Safety Considerations

If DCER exercise is performed using free weights, appropriate spotting should be used. For machine DCER exercises, spotters are not normally needed. More time will be needed to learn proper exercise technique for some free-weight exercises than with machines.

VARIABLE RESISTANCE TRAINING

Variable resistance equipment operates through a lever arm, cam, or pulley arrangement. Its purpose is to alter the resistance in an attempt to match the increases and decreases in strength (strength curve) throughout the exercise's range of motion. Proponents of variable resistance machines believe that by increasing and decreasing the resistance to match the exercise's strength curve, the muscle is forced to contract near maximally throughout the range of motion, resulting in maximal gains in strength.

There are three major types of strength curves: ascending, descending, and bell-shaped (figure 2.3). In an exercise with an ascending strength curve, it is possible to lift more weight if only the last half or last quarter of a repetition is performed than if the complete range of motion of a repetition is performed. For example, an exercise with an ascending strength curve is the squat. If an exercise has a descending strength curve, it is possible to lift more weight if only the first half or first quarter of a repetition is performed. Such an exercise is upright rowing. An exercise in which it is possible to lift more resistance if only the middle portion of the range of motion is performed has a bell-shaped strength curve. Elbow curls have a bell-shaped strength curve. To match the three major types of strength curves, a variable resistance machine must be able to vary the resistance in three major patterns. To date this has not been accomplished. Additionally, because of variations in limb length, in the point of attachment of the muscle's tendons to the bones, and in body size, it is hard to conceive of one mechanical arrangement that would match all individuals' strength curves for a particular exercise.

Biomechanical research indicates that one type of variable resistance cam equipment does not match the strength curves of the elbow curl, fly, knee-extension, knee-flexion, and pullover exercises (Harman 1983; Pizzimenti 1992). A second type of cam equipment has been reported to match the strength curves of females fairly well (J.H. Johnson, Colodny, and Jackson 1990). However, for females the cam resulted in too great a resistance near the end of the knee-extension exercise. The

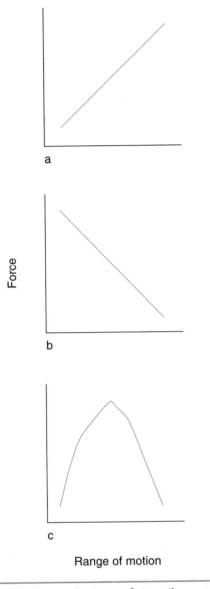

Fig. 2.3 The three major types of strength curves are a. ascending, b. descending, and c. bell-shaped.

cam also provided too much resistance during the first half and too little during the second half of the elbow-flexion and -extension exercises. The knee-flexion machine matched the females' strength curves well throughout the range of motion.

Sets and Repetitions

Significant strength gains from short-term (4 to 16 wk) variable resistance training have been demonstrated with various combinations of sets and repetitions. Significant increases in strength have been shown with (sets × repetitions) 1 × 7-10 RM (Braith et al. 1993; Graves et al. 1989), 1 × 8-12 RM (Hurley, Seals, Ehasani, et al. 1984), 1 × 10-12 RM

(Peterson 1975), 1 × 12-15 RM (Stone, Johnson, and Carter 1979), 2 × 12 at 50% of 1 RM (Gettman, Culter, and Strathman 1980), 2 × 10-12 RM (Coleman 1977), 6 × 15-20 RM (Sale et al. 1990), and four sets with increasing resistance and repetitions decreasing from eight to three in a half-pyramidal program (Ariel 1977). One of these studies reports a substantial strength increase for male trainees of 50% in upper-body exercises and 33% in lower-body exercises after 16 wk of training (Hurley, Seals, Ehasani, et al. 1984). It appears that various combinations of sets and repetitions can cause significant increases in strength using variable resistance equipment.

Strength Increases

Increases in bench press and leg press strength from variable resistance training are depicted in tables 2.3 and 2.4, respectively. It is apparent that this type of training can cause substantial increases in strength when tested using variable resistance equipment and other types of muscle actions.

Motor Performance

Peterson (1975) studied a group of football players who participated in a combined program of in-season football training and variable resistance strength training. The control group participated only in the in-season football training program. The resistance training program consisted of a series of 20 exercises designed to increase the strength of all the major muscle groups. A training session consisted of 2 × 8-12 RM for all 20 exercises. The resistance training group showed a mean decrease of 0.05 s in the 40-yd (36.6-m) sprint and a mean increase of 3.2 cm (1.3 in.) in a vertical jump test. The control group demonstrated a mean decrease of 0.03 s in the 40-yd (36.6-m) sprint and a mean increase of 0.7 cm (0.3 in.) in the vertical jump. Whether the changes were statistically significant or whether a significant difference existed between the two groups was not addressed. Thus, this study offers little concrete evidence concerning the relationship between motor performance and variable resistance training.

Another study (Sylvester et al. 1984) looked at two groups that trained on different variable resistance equipment: Group 1 trained on a cam-type variable resistance machine, and group 2 trained on an increasing lever arm–type variable resistance machine. Group 1 trained 3 d/wk for 6 wk followed by 2 d/wk for 5 wk. This protocol was recommended by the manufacturers of the cam-type machine. Participants did knee extensions immediately followed by leg presses and performed each exercise for one set of 12 repetitions to failure. Group 2 trained 3 d/wk for the entire 11 wk on a leg-press machine using one set of 7 to 10 repetitions followed by one set to failure. No difference in static leg strength was demonstrated between the two groups. Group 1 and group 2 increased their mean vertical jumps by 0.69 cm (0.3 in.) and 2.91 cm (1.1 in.), respectively. The increase in vertical jump of group 2 was significantly greater than that of group 1. The data indicate that motor performance can increase from variable resistance training and that the increase depends in part on training protocol or equipment used.

Body Composition

Increases in lean body mass and decreases in percent body fat occur with variable resistance training. These changes in body composition are depicted in table 7.6 and are of the same magnitude as the changes that occur from DCER training.

Safety Considerations

Without proper instruction and supervision it is possible to overstretch a muscle or joint on some variable resistance machines. However, overall safety is not a major concern with this type of training, and a spotter is not normally necessary. Care must be taken to ensure that the variable resistance machine fits the trainee properly and that the trainee is properly positioned on the machine. Without proper fit and positioning, movement may become jerky, especially when using heavy resistances, and movement of the resistance may actually stop for brief periods of time. The jerky movement may also be caused in part by the strength curve not being closely matched. Jerky movement may increase the possibility of muscle strain and joint discomfort.

ISOKINETICS

Isokinetics refers to a muscular action performed at constant angular limb velocity. Unlike other types of resistance training, there is no specified resistance to meet; rather, the velocity of movement is controlled. The resistance offered by the isokinetic machine cannot be accelerated; any force applied against the equipment results in an equal reaction force. The reaction force mirrors the force applied to the equipment throughout the range of movement of an exercise, making it theoretically possible for the muscle(s) to exert a continual, maximal force through the movement's full range of motion. The majority of equipment found in resistance training facilities allows concentric-only actions. Thus, the effects of concentric-only isokinetic training will be reviewed here. Advocates of isokinetic training believe that the ability to exert maximal force throughout the range of motion leads to optimal strength increases. Other advantages are minimal muscle and joint soreness, making difficult training sessions more tolerable.

Strength Changes

The vast majority of studies examining concentric-only isokinetic training have been of short duration (3-16 wk) and have tested for strength gains using isometric, constant, external resistance and concentric-only isokinetic tests. Concentric-only isokinetic training has also been shown to increase eccentric isokinetic strength (Tomberline et al. 1991). As shown in table 2.5, programs of 1 to 15 sets at various velocities of movement and with various numbers of repetitions cause significant increases in strength.

Gains in strength have also been achieved by performing as many repetitions as possible in a fixed period of time: one set for 6 or 30 s at 180°/s (one for 6 s at 180°/s, one for 30 s at 180°/s) (Lesmes et al. 1978); two sets for 20 s at 180°/s (S.R. Petersen et al. 1987; Bell et al. 1992); two sets for 30 s at 60°/s (Bell et al. 1991a); two sets for 30 s at 120°/s or at 300°/s (Bell et al. 1989); and one set for 60 s at 36°/s or at 108°/s (Seaborne and Taylor 1984). Increases in strength have also been achieved by performing a set of voluntary maximal actions until a given percentage of peak force could no longer be generated. One set continued until at least 60%, 75%, or 90% of peak force could no longer be generated at each velocity of 30°/s, 60°/s, and 90°/s (Fleck 1979) and until 50% of peak force could no longer be maintained during slow-speed training (one set each at a velocity of 30°/s, 60°/s, and 90°/s) or fast-speed training (one set each at a velocity of 180°/s, 240°/s, and 300°/s) (Smith and Melton 1981). All these training regimens resulted in significant increases in strength.

Tables 2.3 and 2.4 include changes in strength in the bench press and leg press, respectively, from isokinetic training. It is apparent that many combinations of sets and repetitions of concentric-only isokinetic training can cause increases in strength.

Number of Sets and Repetitions

Despite the vast quantity of research concerning the effects of concentric-only isokinetic training, few studies have investigated the optimal number of

TABLE 2.5
Isokinetic Training and Combinations of Sets and Repetitions Causing Significant Gains in Strength

Reference	Sets × reps at degrees per second
Jenkins, Thackaberry, and Killian 1984	1 × 15 at 60 1 × 15 at 240
Lacerte et al. 1992	1 × 20 at 60 1 × 20 at 180
Moffroid et al. 1969	1 × 30 at 22.5
Knapik, Mawdsley, and Ramos 1983	1 × 50 at 30
D.R. Pearson and Costill 1988	1 × 65 at 120
Gettman, Culter, and Strathman 1980	2 × 12 at 60
Gettman et al. 1979	2 × 10 at 60 followed by 2 × 15 at 90
Ewing et al. 1990	3 × 8 at 60 3 × 20 at 240
Tomberline et al. 1991	3 × 10 at 100
Gettman and Ayers 1978	3 × 15 at 90 3 × 15 at 60
Kanehisa and Miyashita 1983a	group 1: 1 × 10 at 60; group 2: 1 × 30 at 179; group 3: 1 × 50 at 299
Colliander and Tesch 1990a	4-5 × 12 at 60
Coyle et al. 1981	5 × 6 at 60 5 × 12 at 300
Coyle et al. 1981	(6 sets total) 3 × 6 at 60 and 3 × 12 at 300
Petersen et al. 1990	5 × 10 at 120
Mannion, Jakeman, and Willan 1992	6 × 25 at 240 5 × 15 at 60
Housh et al. 1992	6 × 10 at 120
Narici et al. 1989	6 × 10 at 120
Ciriello, Holden, and Evans 1983	5 × 5 at 60 15 × 10 at 60

sets and repetitions. One study (Lesmes et al. 1978) shows no difference in gains of peak torque between 10 sets of 6-s duration with as many repetitions as possible (approximately 3), and 2 sets of 30-s duration with as many repetitions as possible (approximately 10). Both groups trained at 180°/s four times a week for 7 wk. Another study compared all combinations of 5, 10, and 15 repetitions at slow, intermediate, and fast velocities of movement. After training 3 d/wk for 9 wk no significant differences existed in strength among any of the groups (A.H. Davies 1977). Five sets of 5 repetitions and 15 sets of 10 repetitions have also been compared (Ciriello, Holden, and Evans 1983). In this study both groups trained at 60°/s three times per week for 16 wk. Peak torque was tested at eight velocities ranging from 0°/s to 300°/s. Both groups improved significantly at all test velocities; only one significant difference existed between the two groups: At 30°/s the 15-set group showed greater gains than the 5-set group. All three of these studies agree on at least one point: The number of repetitions performed appears to have little impact on increases in peak torque. (Note that the minimal number of repetitions performed per set in these studies was three.)

Training Velocity

Previously cited studies firmly support the idea that isokinetic training can result in increased strength. Two questions inherent to isokinetic training have yet eluded unequivocal answers: What is the optimal training speed—fast or slow? Do strength increases obtained at a particular training speed carry over to speeds above and below the training speed?

Several studies have investigated the first of these questions. However, no conclusive answer has emerged. A velocity of training that is superior to another would result in greater strength gains not just at one velocity, but over a greater range of movement velocities. Moffroid and Whipple (1970) compared training at 36°/s and 108°/s and determined that training at 108°/s was superior to training at 36°/s. Alternatively, slow-speed training—4 s to complete one leg press repetition—has been shown to result in greater strength increases than fast-speed training—2 s to complete one leg press repetition (Oteghen 1975).

Several studies, however, do provide some insight into the fast-versus-slow-velocity question. Kanehisa and Miyashita (1983a) trained three groups at specified velocities of 60°/s, 179°/s, and 300°/s six times per week for 8 wk. The 60°/s training was 10 voluntary maximal actions per session. The 179°/s and 300°/s training used 30 and 50 repetitions per training session, respectively. All were tested for peak torque at 60°/s, 119°/s, 179°/s, 239°/s, and 300°/s both before and after the training program. Training at 60°/s and 179°/s increased average power of a repetition significantly at all test speeds. Training at 300°/s increased average power of a repetition significantly only at the fastest test speeds (i.e., 239°/s and 300°/s). In addition, training at 179°/s and 300°/s resulted in a significantly greater increase in the average power of a repetition at the test speeds of 239°/s and 300°/s than did training at 60°/s. The fact that this study varied the number of repetitions limits general conclusions. However, from the results it appears that an intermediate speed (approximately 179°/s) is the most advantageous for gains in average power across velocities of movement.

A second study trained groups at 60°/s and 240°/s three times per week for 6 wk (Jenkins, Thackaberry, and Killian 1984). Both groups trained with one set of 15 repetitions per training session. Peak torque test results showed that the 60°/s group improved at all but the 30°/s and 300°/s velocities, whereas the 240°/s group improved significantly at all test velocities from 30°/s to 300°/s (figure 2.4). No significant differences between improvement between the two training groups

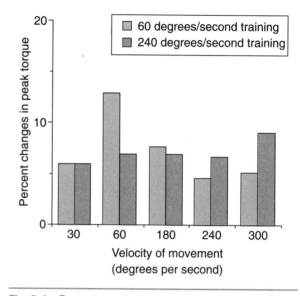

Fig. 2.4 Percentage change in peak torque with training at 60°/s and 240°/s.

Adapted, by permission, from W.L. Jenkins, M. Thackaberry, and C. Killian, "Speed-specific isokinetic training," *Journal of Orthopaedic and Sports Physical Therapy* 6:182.

were shown. However, because of the nonsignificant improvement at the 30°/s and 300°/s test velocities by the 60°/s group, it appears that the 240°/s training resulted in better overall gains in strength.

Another study utilized three groups that trained at different velocities (Coyle et al. 1981). A slow-speed group trained at 60°/s with five sets of 6 maximal actions. A fast-speed group trained at 300°/s with five sets of 12 maximal actions. A third group trained using a combination of slow and fast speeds, with two or three sets of 6 repetitions at 60°/s and two or three sets of 12 repetitions at 300°/s. Peak torque test results are presented in table 2.6. It is evident that each group showed its greatest gains at its specific training velocity, indicating that the velocity of training is dictated by the velocity of desired peak torque increases. However, substantial carry-over to other velocities is also shown. This is especially apparent for velocities slower than the training velocity.

Some research suggests that there is no evidence to favor a particular speed when considering gains in peak torque. Training at 60°/s or 180°/s results in equal gains in peak torque at 60°/s, 120°/s, 180°/s, and 240°/s (Bell et al. 1989, Lacerte et al. 1992). Training at 60°/s or 240°/s results in equal gains in isometric strength (Mannion, Jakeman, and Willan 1992). All of these projects covered a short training duration of no more than 16 wk, making conclusions concerning long-term training difficult. Because the majority of these studies experimented with relatively slow speeds in general, any com-

TABLE 2.6

Percentage Increases in Peak Torque From Isokinetic Training at Specific Velocities

Degrees of peak torque	% peak torque increases		
PT/0	[Fast 23.6	Slow 20.3	Mixed] 18.9
PT/60	[Slow 31.8	Mixed 23.6	Fast] 15.1
PT/180	[Fast 16.8	Slow 9.2	Mixed] 7.9
PT/300	[Fast 18.5	Mixed] 16.1	Slow 0.9

PT/0-PT/300 = peak torque at 0 to 300°/s

Fast = training at 300°/s; Slow = training at 60°/s; Mixed = training at both 300°/s and 60°/s

Bracketed groups exhibit no statistically significant difference in peak torque.

Adapted, by permission, from E.F. Coyle et al., 1981, "Specificity of power improvements through slow and fast isokinetic training," *Journal of Applied Physiology: Respiratory, Environmental and Exercise Physiology* 51:1440.

parison between slow and fast speeds is artificial. During many physical activities angular limb velocities of greater than 300°/s are easily achieved. A conclusion favoring either a slow or a fast speed of training using isokinetic devices (which presently offer velocities up to only 400°/s) therefore has little practical application for most athletes.

Collectively, these studies indicate that if gains in strength over a wide range of velocities are desired, training should be at a velocity of somewhere between 180°/s and 240°/s. However, if the goal of training is to maximally increase strength at a specific velocity, training should be performed at that velocity.

Velocity and Strength Carry-Over

The second question concerning concentric-only isokinetic training is, To what magnitude do increases in torque carry over to velocities other than the training velocity? Moffroid and Whipple (1970) compared 36°/s and 108°/s and found that increases in peak torque carried over only to speeds of movement below the training velocity (see figure 2.5). The study reported in figure 2.5 also lends support to this finding, but it should be noted that the slow group (60°/s) demonstrated some increases at speeds greater than its training velocity. Another study testing at 60°/s to 240°/s (Ewing et al. 1990) suggests that there is carry-over of peak

torque gains at velocities above and below the training velocity. The carry-over may be as great as 210°/s below the training velocity and up to 180°/s above the training velocity. Studies using training velocities of 60°/s or 180°/s indicate that significant gains in peak torque are made at all velocities from 60°/s to 240°/s (Bell et al. 1989; Lacerte et al. 1992).

Collectively these studies indicate that gains in peak torque may occur above and below the training velocity except when the training velocity is

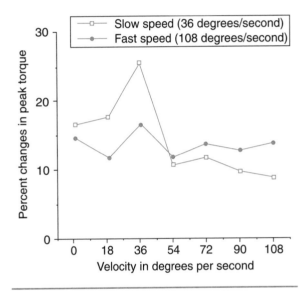

Fig. 2.5   Percentage change in peak torque due to slow- and fast-speed, concentric-only isokinetic training.

Reprinted from *Physical Therapy.* Moffroid M.T. and Whipple R.H. Specificity of speed of exercise. 1970:50:1695 with the permission of the APTA.

very slow (30°/s). These studies all determined peak torque irrespective of the joint angle at which peak torque occurred. It might be questioned whether the torque actually increased at a specific joint angle and therefore at a specific muscle length, an indication that the mechanisms controlling muscle tension at that length have been altered.

Peak torque of the knee extensors irrespective of joint angle at velocities from 30°/s to 300°/s is slightly higher than joint angle specific torque at a knee angle 30° from full extension (Yates and Kamon 1983). When subjects are grouped according to whether they have more or less than 50% Type II muscle fibers, the two groups show no significant difference in the torque velocity curves for peak torque. For angle-specific torque, however, the torque velocity curves are significantly different between the two groups (Yates and Kamon 1983). These data suggest that torque at a specific angle is influenced to a greater extent than peak torque by muscle fiber–type composition. Thus, comparisons of peak torque and angle-specific torque must be viewed with caution.

A study that determined torque at a specific joint angle trained groups at 96°/s and 239°/s (Caiozzo, Perrine, and Edgerton 1981). Figure 2.6 depicts the improvement (in percentages) that occurred at the testing velocities. The 96°/s group showed significant increases in torque above and below the training speed. The 239°/s group showed significant increases at the two testing speeds immediately below the training speed and insignificant increases at all other testing speeds. This study indicates that when the test criterion is angle-specific torque, training at a slow velocity (96°/s) causes significant increases in torque at faster velocities, whereas training at a faster velocity (239°/s) does not.

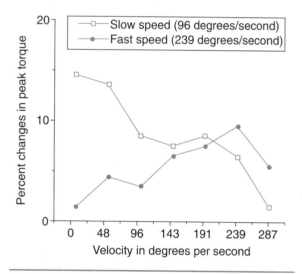

Fig. 2.6 Percent changes in peak torque at a specific joint angle due to slow- and fast-speed, concentric-only isokinetic training.

Adapted, by permission, from V.J. Caiozzo, J.J. Perrine, and V.R. Edgerton, 1981, "Training-induced alterations of the in vivo force-velocity relationship of human muscle," *Journal of Applied Physiology: Respiratory, Environmental and Exercise Physiology* 51:752.

The results of research concerning velocity and carry-over using peak torque and angle-specific torque are not necessarily contradictory (see figures 2.4, 2.5, and 2.6). All studies demonstrate that fast-velocity training (108°/s up to 240°/s) causes significant increases in torque below the training velocity and in some cases above the training velocity. Differences in the amount (significant or insignificant) of carry-over to other velocities may in part be attributed to the velocities that were defined as fast (108°/s up to 240°/s). All studies also indicate that slow-velocity training (36°/s up to

96°/s) causes significant carry-over in torque below and above the training velocity.

A previously cited study (Kanehisa and Miyashita 1983a) demonstrated that an intermediate training velocity (179°/s) caused the greatest carry-over of average power to a wider range of velocities both above and below the training velocity. The studies examining changes in peak torque previously discussed indicate that training velocities in the range of 180°/s to 240°/s result in carry-over to velocities above and below the training velocity, but that the amount of carry-over may decrease as the difference between the training and test velocities increases. Training velocities below 180°/s also result in gains in strength above and below the training velocity, but again the amount of carry-over may decrease as the difference between the training and testing velocities increases.

Body Composition

No significant change (Colliander and Tesch 1990a; Costill et al. 1979; Cote et al. 1988) and significant increases (Coyle et al. 1981; Ewing et al. 1990) in muscle fiber area have been reported due to concentric-only isokinetic training. Increases in muscle cross-sectional area determined by computerized tomography or magnetic resonance imaging have been demonstrated as a result of concentric-only isokinetic training (Bell et al. 1992; Housh et al. 1992; Narici et al. 1989). Increases have also been shown in cross-sectional areas in one muscle group (quadriceps) and not another (hamstrings) from the same training program (Petersen et al. 1990). Thus, concentric-only isokinetic training can result in increased muscle fiber and muscle cross-sectional areas resulting in increased lean body mass.

Changes in body composition as a result of isokinetic training are included in table 7.6. These changes include increases in lean body mass and decreases in percent fat and are of the same magnitude as those induced by other types of training.

Motor Performance

Improved motor performance, specifically significant increases in the vertical jump (Blattner and Noble 1979; Perrine and Edgerton 1975; Smith and Melton 1981; Oteghen 1975), in the standing broad jump (Smith and Melton 1981), and in a 40-yd (36.6-m) sprint (Smith and Melton 1981), occurs with isokinetic training. Ball velocity of a tennis serve is improved with concentric-only isokinetic training (Ellenbecker, Davies, and Rowinski 1988). Power output during 6-s and 30-s maximal sprint cycling is also improved with isokinetic training (Bell et al. 1989; Mannion, Jakeman, and Willan 1992).

Motor performance may be increased by fast-speed training more than by slow-speed training (Smith and Melton 1981). Training in this study consisted of one set to 50% fatigue in peak torque at each velocity of 180°/s, 240°/s, and 300°/s for the fast-speed group and one set to 50% fatigue in peak torque at each velocity of 30°/s, 60°/s, and 90°/s for the slow-speed group. Each group trained three times weekly for 6 wk. The fast-speed and slow-speed groups improved, respectively, 5.4% and 3.9% in a vertical jump test, 9.1% and 0.4% in the standing long jump, and –10.1% and +4.1% in the 40-yd (36.6-m) dash. However, increases in sprint cycling power output are not significantly different when isokinetic training is performed at 60°/s versus 180°/s or 240°/s (Bell et al. 1989; Mannion, Jakeman, and Willan 1992). Thus, fast-speed isokinetic training may be more effective than slow-speed training in increasing some but not all motor performance tasks.

Other Considerations

There are other factors to examine when considering isokinetic training. Training isokinetically has been reported to cause minimal muscular soreness (Atha 1981). Because neither a free weight nor a weight stack has to be lifted in isokinetic training, the possibility of injury is minimal and no spotter is required.

It is difficult to judge an individual's effort unless the machine has an accurate feedback system of either force generated or actual work performed. Furthermore, motivation is a problem with some trainees, because most equipment lacks visible movement of a weight or weight stack. Some equipment does have a monitor that displays such information as force for each repetition, but at present this type of equipment is not widely available.

ECCENTRIC TRAINING

Eccentric training (also called negative resistance training) refers to a muscular action in which the muscle lengthens in a controlled manner. This type of muscle action occurs in daily activities such as walking. Walking down a flight of stairs requires the thigh muscles to perform eccentric muscle actions. During normal DCER training, when the weight is being lifted, the muscles shorten or perform a concentric action. When the weight is lowered, the same muscles that lifted the weight are active and lengthen in a controlled manner, or perform an eccentric action. If the muscles did not perform an eccentric action when the weight was lowered, the weight would fall.

Eccentric training can be achieved on many resistance training machines by lifting resistances greater than 1 RM with both arms or legs and lowering the resistance with only one arm or leg. Some isokinetic machines also have an eccentric mode. Resistances heavier than 1 RM may also be achieved with free weights by having spotters add more weight after the weight is lifted or by having a spotter help with the lifting of a resistance heavier than 1 RM and then lowering the resistance. It is now also possible to use commercially available weight release hooks to achieve a resistance heavier than 1 RM or electronically controlled machines that provide greater eccentric force than concentric force. For added safety when performing eccentric training with some free-weight exercises, such as the bench and squat, it is possible to set the pins of a power rack so that they will catch the weight at the lowest position of the exercise. Care must be used when performing eccentric training, especially when using free weights or nonisokinetic machines, because it is easy to use more weight than can be lowered in a controlled and safe manner.

Strength Changes

Normal DCER training of the legs with both a concentric and an eccentric action causes greater concentric and eccentric strength increases than performing concentric-only resistance training for the same number of repetitions (Dudley et al. 1991). Performing 50% or 75% of the repetitions in an eccentric manner over 12 wk of training results in greater increases in squat, but not bench press, ability than performing the same training program in a concentric-only manner (Häkkinen, Komi, and Tesch 1981). Thus, an eccentric component during DCER training appears to be important, especially for the leg musculature.

Isokinetic training with eccentric and concentric actions results in greater increases in eccentric and concentric force across a range of velocities from isometric (0°/s) to 240°/s than does concentric-only isokinetic training (Lacerte et al. 1992; Colliander and Tesch 1990a). However, concentric-only isokinetic training also results in increases in concentric and eccentric force.

The foregoing discussion indicates that eccentric contractions are needed to optimally increase strength. However, the real question for most practitioners is, When performing DCER training, do eccentric contractions using a concentric resistance greater than 1 RM result in greater or faster gains in strength than normal resistance training?

Eccentric force output is greater than concentric force output (Rizzardo, Bay, and Wessel 1988; Tesch et al. 1990). Advocates of eccentric training believe that, because greater resistances can be used during eccentric training, greater increases in strength occur in eccentric training than in concentric-only or normal DCER training. Short-term (8- to 12-wk) eccentric training can result in significant increases in isometric, concentric, eccentric, and DCER force output (Atha 1981; Clarke 1973; Fleck and Schutt 1985). Six eccentric actions performed four times per week for 7 wk resulted in slightly, although not significantly, greater percentage increases in maximal eccentric, concentric, and isometric force than the same program using only concentric actions. It has also been shown that eccentric training results in no increase in maximal isometric force (Bonde-Petersen 1960) and that isokinetic eccentric training results in a significant increase in maximal isokinetic concentric but not eccentric force (Ellenbecker, Davies, and Rowinski 1988). However, the majority of evidence indicates that eccentric training results in no greater gains in isometric, eccentric, and concentric strength than normal DCER training (Atha 1981; Clarke 1973; Fleck and Schutt 1985).

Optimal Eccentric Resistance Training

The optimal resistance to be used for eccentric training has received little study. Jones (1973) believes the optimal resistance to be one that the trainee can lower slowly and stop at will. Using this definition others claim a resistance of 120% of the DCER 1 RM is the optimal eccentric resistance (Johnson et al. 1976).

During a 12-wk training period Olympic weight lifters who performed 25% of their training with 100% to 130% of the DCER 1 RM improved in the clean and jerk significantly more than a group of Olympic weight lifters performing the same training program in a normal fashion, without an emphasis on the eccentric training component (Häkkinen and Komi 1981). The snatch ability of the weight lifters performing the eccentric training did not improve to any greater extent than that of the weight lifters performing the normal train-

ing. Thus, some eccentric training may be important when high strength levels are required.

Motor Performance and Body Composition

Few studies have examined the effects of eccentric training on motor performance and lean body mass. It has been suggested that eccentric strength of the leg musculature may be related to alpine skiing performance (Abe et al. 1992). Vertical jumping ability increased (Bonde-Petersen and Knuttgen 1971) or showed no change (Stone, Johnson, and Carter 1979) with eccentric-only training. Velocity of serving in tennis showed no change as a result of 6 wk of eccentric training of the shoulder and arm musculature (Ellenbecker, Davies, and Rowinski 1988). Thus, the impact of eccentric training on motor performance is unclear.

Upper-arm circumference showed significant increases with eccentric-only training, but the increase did not differ significantly from increases caused by concentric training (Komi and Buskirk 1972). Increases in limb circumference and muscle cross-sectional area are usually associated with muscular hypertrophy. Cross-sectional area of the quadriceps increased 5% with eccentric-only training, but this increase was not greater than concentric-only training (Jones and Rutherford 1987).

Postexercise Soreness

A disadvantage of eccentric training with greater than 1-RM concentric strength is the development of greater postexercise soreness than that which accompanies isometric, DCER exercise or concentric-only isokinetic training (Carpinelli and Gutin 1991; Fleck and Schutt 1985; Talag 1973). The soreness peaks 2 to 3 d after eccentric exercise (Clarkson, Nosaka, and Braun 1992). After eccentric exercise, strength is decreased for up to 10 d (Clarkson, Nosaka, and Braun 1992). However, one bout of eccentric exercise appears to result in protection from excessive soreness from another eccentric training session for a period of up to 5 or 6 wk in untrained or novice weight-trained individuals (Clarkson, Nosaka, and Braun 1992; Ebbling and Clarkson 1990; Golden and Dudley 1992; Newham, Jones, and Clarkson 1987; Nosaka et al. 1991). It appears that for excessive soreness to develop the eccentric actions must be performed with a resistance greater than the concentric 1 RM (Donnelly, Clarkson, and Maughan 1992) and that performance of some eccentric actions prior to complete recovery from an eccentric exercise bout does not aid or hinder recovery from the initial eccentric exercise (Donnelly, Clarkson, and Maughan 1992). After 1 to 2 wk of eccentric training the soreness appears to be no greater than that which follows isometric training (Komi and Buskirk 1972).

The exact explanation of why there is more soreness after eccentric training than after normal DCER or concentric-only training is unclear. One possible explanation is that the integrated electromyographic activity is less during an eccentric action than during a concentric action (Komi, Kaneko, and Aura 1987; Tesch et al. 1990). This indicates that fewer muscle fibers are active to develop force during an eccentric action than during a concentric action and that the force is distributed over fewer muscle fibers than during a concentric action. This could lead to muscle soreness. Damage to muscle fibers has been observed after eccentric training (Clarkson, Nosaka, and Braun 1992; Lieber and Friden 1993; Lieber, Woodburn, and Friden 1991; Stauber et al. 1990). However, the damage does not follow the same time course as the postexercise pain associated with eccentric training (Clarkson, Nosaka, and Braun 1992; Newham 1988). Thus, muscle damage in itself may not be the cause of the postexercise pain. Other factors, such as edema, swelling, or inflammation, may be related to the postexercise pain (Clarkson, Nosaka, and Braun 1992; Newham 1988; Stauber et al. 1990).

Motivational Considerations

Several other factors should be considered with regard to eccentric training. It is necessary to have a partner or some kind of equipment to assist in lifting the heavier resistance encountered in eccentric training. Some individuals derive great satisfaction from training with very heavy resistance. Eccentric training for these individuals will be a positive motivational factor.

Other Considerations

If one aim of the training program is to increase 1-RM bench press and squat, the incorporation of eccentric training is appropriate. One factor that separates great from good power lifters in the bench press and squat is the speed at which the eccentric portion of the lift is performed. Lifters who can lift greater weights lower the resistance more slowly (Madsen and McLaughlin 1984; McLaughlin,

Dillman, and Lardner 1977). This suggests that eccentric training may facilitate both the slowness of lowering the resistance and proper form while the resistance is being lowered.

PLYOMETRICS

The term *stretch-shortening cycle exercise* is starting to replace the term *plyometrics* and describes this type of resistance exercise more accurately. The stretch-shortening cycle refers to a natural part of most movements. As an example, during walking every time a foot hits the ground, the quadriceps go through a stretch-shortening cycle. When the foot hits the ground, the quadriceps first go through an eccentric action, then an isometric action, and finally a concentric action. If the reversal of the eccentric action to an isometric and then a concentric action is performed quickly, the resultant concentric action is more powerful than if no eccentric action was performed. This entire sequence of eccentric, isometric, and concentric actions is called the stretch-shortening cycle.

When the sequence of eccentric to concentric actions is performed quickly, the muscle is stretched slightly prior to the concentric action. Thus, the term *stretch-shortening cycle* describes what happens: The muscle is stretched slightly and then shortens. The slight stretching stores elastic energy. The addition of the elastic energy to the force of a normal concentric action is one of the reasons commonly given to explain why a more forcible concentric action results after a stretch-shortening cycle. The other common explanation for the more forcible concentric action is a reflex that results in quicker recruitment of muscle fibers or recruitment of more muscle fibers involved in the movement.

That a stretch-shortening cycle results in a more powerful concentric action is easy to demonstrate. During a normal vertical jump (a countermovement jump) the jumper bends at the knees and hips (eccentric action of the extensors), quickly reverses directions, and jumps (isometric followed by concentric action). A countermovement jump involves a stretch-shortening cycle. A jump performed by bending at the knees and hips, stopping for 3 to 5 s in the bent-knee and -hip position, and then jumping is termed a noncountermovement jump, does not involve a stretch-shortening cycle, and will result in a lower jump than a countermovement jump (a jump involving a stretch-shortening cycle). It is also possible to demonstrate the effect of a stretch-shortening cycle by throwing a ball for distance. Throwing a ball with a normal overhand throwing motion, which involves a stretch-shortening cycle, will result in a longer throw than throwing a ball without a windup, starting from the end of the windup position (no stretch-shortening cycle).

Stretch-shortening cycle exercises can be performed with both the upper and lower body. Many medicine ball exercises for the upper body involve a stretch-shortening cycle. In-depth jumps (dropping from a bench and immediately jumping) are the exercise perhaps associated most frequently with the stretch-shortening cycle, but virtually all jumping exercises involve a stretch-shortening cycle.

Elastic Energy and Reflexes

The ability to use stored elastic energy and reflexes are the most frequently cited explanations of why stretch-shortening cycle training increases force output. There is evidence to support the idea of the use of stored elastic energy during a stretch-shortening cycle (Bosco et al. 1987; Bosco, Tarkka, and Komi 1982; Farley et al. 1991). In fact, it has been estimated that elastic energy may account for 20% to 30% of the difference between a counter- and noncountermovement jump (Bosco et al. 1987). Elastic energy could be stored in tendons and other connective tissue. Whether a structural adaptation in connective tissue takes place with training to allow storage and therefore use of more elastic energy is possible but unproven. If elastic energy were stored during prestretch by the muscles' contractile protein (actin and myosin), it would be lost as soon as the crossbridges detached from an active site. The average attachment time of a crossbridge to an active site is 30 ms. The enhancement of force from a prestretch lasts longer than this; therefore the ability of elastic energy to be stored and used by this mechanism is in doubt.

Reflex recruitment of additional motor units or an increased rate of firing by already recruited motor units may result in increased force as a result of a stretch-shortening cycle. However, myoelectric activity does not change significantly in muscle that performs an isometric action and is then stretched (D.B. Thompson and Chapman 1988). This indicates that reflex activity does not account for the increased force caused by a stretch-shortening cycle. It is apparent that some type of potentiation of force is caused by a stretch-shortening cycle. However, the mechanism responsible is not completely understood.

Number of Jumps

Significant and nonsignificant increases in the vertical jump ability of untrained individuals of 2.0 to 10.2 cm (0.8 to 4.0 in.) have occurred when they trained with in-depth jumps from heights ranging from 25 to 100 cm (9.8 to 39.4 in.) (Bartholomeu 1985; Miller 1982; Scoles 1978; Steben and Steben 1981). One to three training sessions per week were performed for a period of 7 or 8 wk during these training programs. The in-depth jumps were performed in sets of approximately 10 jumps, and the total number of jumps per training session ranged from 25 to 62. Some of these programs gradually increased the number of jumps per training session during the training period (Bartholomeu 1985).

Significant and nonsignificant increases in vertical jump ability of 1.7 to 9.4 cm (0.7 to 3.7 in.) have also occurred when in-depth jumps were performed from heights ranging from 50 to 114 cm (19.7 to 44.9 in.) in conjunction with other types of stretch-shortening cycle exercises such as jump squats, bench jumps, bench hops, and split squats (K. Adams et al. 1992; Bartholomeu 1985; Bosco and Pittera 1982; Ford et al. 1983). Training during these programs was performed two to three times per week and lasted 7 to 10 wk. The number of jumps per training session ranged from 23 to 170. Increases in vertical jump ability of 1.7 and 10.7 cm (0.7 and 4.2 in.) have also occurred with other types of stretch-shortening cycle exercises instead of in-depth jumps (Bartholomeu 1985; Bauer, Thayer, and Baras 1990).

It appears that a wide variety in number of jumps and in height from which in-depth jumps are performed can result in increased vertical jump ability in previously untrained individuals. However, no clear pattern arises of the optimal number of jumps or the height of in-depth jumps to use with untrained individuals (Bobbert 1990).

Height of Drop

Increases in jumping ability as a result of the performance of in-depth jumps from a wide range of heights have been shown. However, the determination of an optimal height has received little attention from the sport science community. It has been stated that in-depth jumps from a height greater than 110 cm (43.3 in.) are counterproductive because the change from eccentric to concentric action takes place too slowly (Verhsoshanski 1967). It has also been suggested that the height should not be so great that the athlete cannot prevent his or her heels from touching the ground

(Schmidtbleicher and Gollhofer 1982). This is in part because an increased chance of injury from the high impact forces is encountered if the heels do touch the ground.

After 8 wk of training with in-depth jumps only no significant difference in increased vertical jump ability has been shown between training from 50 or 80 cm (19.7 to 31.5 in.) (Bartholomeu 1985). After 16 wk of performing an identical resistance training program with and without in-depth jump training from 75 or 110 cm (29.5 or 43.3 in.) no significant difference was shown in increased vertical jump ability, 1-RM squat strength, or isometric knee-extension strength (Clutch et al. 1983). Presently there is insufficient information to substantiate the optimal height from which to perform in-depth jumps.

Weighted Exercises

The wearing of a weighted vest or belt of up to 12% of body weight while performing stretch-shortening cycle exercises has also resulted in increased vertical jump ability. Increases in vertical jump ability of 5.2 and 8.1 cm (2.1 and 3.2 in.) in untrained individuals over 6 and 8 wk of training have been reported with this type of training (Blattner and Noble 1979; Polhemus et al. 1981). However, a decrease in vertical jump ability of 2.6 cm (1.0 in.) in skilled jumpers has also been shown (Bosco and Pittera 1982). The use of a 1.36-kg (3-lb) weighted jump rope while performing rope jumping exercises has been shown to increase vertical jump ability and power output during a 30-s stationary bicycle maximal sprint, but not to decrease 50-yd (45.7-m) sprint time (Masterson and Brown 1993). The training in this project was performed three times per week for a period of 10 wk. These few studies do not allow any firm conclusions concerning the value of this type of training.

Concurrent Strength Training

Performance of both strength and stretch-shortening cycle exercises two to three times per week during 4 to 10 wk of training results in increased vertical jump ability (K. Adams et al. 1992; Bauer, Thayer, and Baras 1990; Clutch et al. 1983). Increases in vertical jump ability have ranged from 3.0 to 10.7 cm (1.2 to 4.2 in.) with this type of training. This type of training has also been shown to significantly increase standing long jump ability in males but not females and to significantly decrease 40-yd (36.6-m) sprint time (Polhemus et al. 1981). In general, the positive changes in motor performance

tests with concurrent strength and stretch-shortening cycle training are greater than with either training type alone (K. Adams et al. 1992; Bauer, Thayer, and Baras 1990; Polhemus et al. 1981), indicating that both types of training should be included in a resistance training program when gains in motor performance are desired.

Strength

The effect of stretch-shortening cycle training on strength has received a limited amount of study. Isometric force of the knee extensors but not the knee flexors is significantly increased by stretch-shortening cycle–only jump training for 10 wk, three times per week (Bauer, Thayer, and Baras 1990). Rope jump training with a weighted rope for 10 wk, three times per week, results in a significant gain in 1-RM leg press and bench press strength (Masterson and Brown 1993). It appears that stretch-shortening cycle training can increase strength, but that the increases may be muscle-group specific, depending on the type of training exercises performed.

Body Composition

The performance of only jump-type stretch-shortening cycle training in females for 10 wk, three times per week, results in no significant change in percent body fat or lean body mass (Bauer, Thayer, and Baras 1990). Performance of stretch-shortening cycle jump-type training and some normal resistance training (8 wk, three sessions per week; 8 wk, one session per week) for 16 wk results in no significant Type I or II muscle fiber hypertrophy or change in percent body fat or lean body mass (Häkkinen et al. 1990). Thus, it appears that stretch-shortening cycle training does not result in a significant amount of muscle hypertrophy or change in body composition.

Injury Potential

The concern that stretch-shortening cycle training will result in injury is expressed by some strength and conditioning professionals. As with all types of physical training there is an inherent risk of injury, and anecdotal evidence indicates that injuries have occurred as a result of stretch-shortening cycle training. However, these injuries appear to be related to such factors as performing in-depth jumps from too great a height or improper flooring or landing areas. In fact several authors of stretch-shortening cycle training studies explicitly state that no injuries occurred from performance of the training (Polhemus et al. 1981), even in untrained individuals who had no preparatory resistance training prior to performing the stretch-shortening cycle training (Bartholomeu 1985; Blattner and Noble 1979). As an injury-prevention measure, it has been suggested any individual performing stretch-shortening cycle exercises should first be able to perform a back squat with at least 1.5 to 2 times body weight. This appears to be merely a suggestion, as no data are readily available to support this concept. However, because of the stresses encountered during this type of training, it is important to introduce stretch-shortening cycle training slowly into the program and to keep the volume of training relatively low.

Other Considerations

Many athletes enjoy stretch-shortening cycle training and may contend that if they perform stretch-shortening cycle exercises, there is no need for normal resistance training. As with all types of resistance training, stretch-shortening cycle exercises should not be the only type of resistance training in the program, although they should be a part of a well-designed program for many sports and activities. The major contribution of stretch-shortening cycle exercises is developing the ability to generate maximal power in a movement; this type of resistance training does not result in body composition changes and may not increase strength in all muscle groups involved in a given stretch-shortening cycle exercise.

The body weight and body composition of an individual may be a consideration in the stretch-shortening cycle exercise prescription. The majority of these type of exercises, especially lower-body exercises, use body weight as the resistance to be overcome. An individual with a higher percentage of body fat must perform the exercises at a greater resistance (body weight) with a smaller relative muscle mass (lean body mass). Thus, a heavy individual may need to use a smaller training volume (i.e., number of jumps) than a light individual.

COMPARISON OF TRAINING TYPES

Studies comparing the various types of resistance training are rare, and there are several problems in identifying the most beneficial type of training for strength gains. A major issue is specificity of training. When training and testing are performed using the same type of resistive equipment, a large increase in strength is demonstrated. If training and testing are performed on two different types of equipment, however, the increase in strength is substantially less and sometimes nonexistent. Problems in comparison also arise in equating total training volume (i.e., sets and repetitions), total work (i.e., total repetitions times resistance), and total training time. These discrepancies make it difficult to prove the superiority of one type of resistance training over another. Training studies may have to be longer than the 10 to 20 wk often used in an attempt to demonstrate differences between types of resistance training. Several of these problems are illustrated in one particular study (Leighton et al. 1967). Subjects trained twice a week for 8 wk using several isometric and dynamic constant resistance training (DCER) regimens. Two particular regimens were an isometric program consisting of one 6-s maximal voluntary muscle action and a Delorme DCER program. The Delorme program uses three sets of 10 repetitions progressing in resistance from 50% to 75% and finally to 100% of 10-RM resistance. Each of the training groups exercised three muscle groups. The isometric and Delorme programs produced increases in strength of 9.8% and 8.3%, respectively. According to these results isometric training proved to be superior to DCER training. Another DCER program, however, resulted in a 38% increase in strength. The overall results are therefore ambiguous: Isometric training is both inferior and superior to DCER training. This study demonstrates that the result of comparing two types of training in part depends on the effectiveness of the training programs used for each type of training.

Isometric Versus Dynamic Constant External Resistance Training

Comparisons of strength gains between isometric training and DCER training for the most part follow a pattern of test specificity. When isometric testing procedures are used, isometric training is superior (Amusa and Obajuluwa 1986; Berger 1962a; Berger 1963b; Moffroid et al. 1969), and when DCER testing (1 RM) is used, DCER training is superior (Berger 1962a; Berger 1963c). However, it has also been shown that DCER training results in greater increases in isometric force than does isometric training (Rasch and Morehouse 1957). Isokinetic testing for increases in strength are inconclusive. When isokinetically tested at 22.5°/s, both isometric and DCER training improved peak torque 3% (Moffroid et al. 1969). A second study demonstrated a 13% increase in peak torque for isometric training and a 28% increase for DCER training (the velocity of isokinetic testing was not given) (Thistle et al. 1967). A review of the literature indicates that well-designed DCER programs are more effective than standard isometric programs for increasing strength (Atha 1981). Comparisons of an optimal isometric program versus a well-designed DCER program have yet to be performed. It is clear that motor performance is improved to a greater extent by DCER training than by isometric training at only one joint angle (B.S. Brown et al. 1988; R.C. Campbell 1962; Chu 1950).

Isometric Versus Variable Resistance Training

The authors are aware of no studies that directly compare isometric and variable resistance training. Because various studies report no improvement in motor performance with isometric training (Clarke 1973; Fleck and Schutt 1985) along with some improvement in motor performance with variable resistance training (Peterson 1975; Silvester et al. 1984), it can be speculated that variable resistance training may be superior to isometric training in this parameter. Thus, if an increase in motor performance is desired, variable resistance training would be a better choice than isometric training.

Isometric Versus Isokinetic Resistance Training

Comparisons of isometric and isokinetic training for the most part follow a pattern of test specificity. However, comparisons to date have used only relatively slow velocity isokinetic training (up to 30°/s). Isometric is superior to isokinetic training at 22.5°/s in increasing isometric strength (Moffroid et al. 1969). Isometric force of the knee extensors at knee angles of 90° and 45° increased 17% and 14%, respectively, with isometric training and 14% and 24%, respectively, with isokinetic training. Likewise, knee-flexor strength at knee angles of 90° and 45° increased 26% and 24%, respectively, with isometric training and 11% and 19%, respectively, with isokinetic training. The isometrically trained group demonstrated superior isometric force improvements over the isokinetically trained group in three of these four tests. However, isokinetic training of the elbow extensors at 30°/s results in greater increases of isometric force than does isometric training (Knapik, Mawdsley, and Ramos 1983).

Isokinetic training is superior to isometric training in the development of isokinetic torque (Moffroid et al. 1969; Thistle et al. 1967). For example, knee-extensor strength for isokinetically and isometrically trained groups increased 47% and 13%, respectively (Thistle et al. 1967). Another project reported that isokinetically and isometrically trained groups increased 11% and 3%, respectively, in knee-extension peak torque at 22.5°/s. For knee flexion the increases in peak toque were 15% and 3%, respectively, at 22.5°/s (Moffroid et al. 1969). Thus, the phenomenon of test specificity is evident in the strength increases for both isometric and isokinetic training.

The issue of improved motor performance has not been addressed in comparisons between isometric and isokinetic training. Isometric programs lead to no improvement in motor performance (Clarke 1973; Fleck and Schutt 1985), whereas some improvement has been achieved with isokinetic training (Bell et al. 1989; Blattner and Noble 1979; Mannion, Jakeman, and Willan 1992). The evidence suggests that isokinetic training is superior in this parameter.

Isometric Versus Eccentric Resistance Training

The comparisons made in this section are between isometric training and eccentric training with free weights or normal resistance training machines, not isokinetic eccentric training. Measured isometrically there is no difference in the strength gains derived from isometric and eccentric training. Bonde-Petersen (1960) trained the elbow flexors and knee extensors of both males and females for 36 training sessions in 60 d. The participants trained either only isometrically or eccentrically. All trainees performed 10 maximal 5-s actions per day. The isometrically trained individuals experienced the following improvements in isometric strength: elbow flexion, 13.8% for males and 1% for females; knee extension, 10% for males and 8.3% for females. The eccentrically trained individuals exhibited the following improvements in isometric strength: elbow flexion, 8.5% for males and 5% for females; knee extension, 14.6% for males and 11.2% for females. Thus, it appears that there is no significant difference between these two types of training with regard to isometric strength.

Laycoe and Marteniuk (1971) reached the same conclusion after training subjects' knee extensors three times per week for 6 wk. The isometric and eccentric groups improved 17.4% and 17%, respectively, in isometric knee-extension force. Other studies also report no difference in strength gains between these two training methods (Atha 1981).

Reviews conclude that isometric training does not result in increased motor performance (Clarke 1973; Fleck and Schutt 1985) and that the effect of eccentric training on motor performance is unclear, with increases (Bonde-Petersen and Knuttgen 1971) and no change (Ellenbecker, Davies, and Rowinski 1988; Stone, Johnson, and Carter 1979) in motor performance shown. Thus, the superiority of one of these training types over the other in terms of motor performance increases is unclear.

Dynamic Constant External Resistance Versus Variable Resistance Training

Comparisons of strength increases as a result of DCER and variable resistance training are equivocal. After 20 wk of training, variable resistance training demonstrated a clear superiority over DCER training in a 1-RM free-weight bench press (Ariel 1977). DCER and variable resistance training produced gains of 14% and 29.5%, respectively. Further information concerning this study is presented in table 2.3.

Leg press strength illustrates the phenomenon of test specificity for these two types of training (Pipes 1978). After 10 wk of training a variable resistance group increased 27% when tested with variable resistance methods and 7.5% when tested with DCER methods. Conversely, a group trained with DCER improved 7.5% when tested by variable resistance methods and 28.9% when tested with DCER methods. More information concerning this study is presented in table 2.4. Three other exercises tested and trained for in this study demonstrated a similar test-specificity pattern.

In a 5-wk program of three training sessions per week, DCER training was found to be superior to variable resistance training in producing strength gains determined by DCER testing (Stone, Johnson, and Carter 1979). No difference between the two types of training was shown when tested for variable resistance strength improvements.

After 10 wk of training two to three times per week, cam-type variable resistance training and DCER training resulted in no difference in isometric knee-extension strength (Manning et al. 1990). Isometric force was tested throughout the range of motion starting at 9° and ending at 110° of full knee extension. Both types of training consisted of one set of 8 to 12 repetitions at 8 to 12 RM. An earlier study (Silvester et al. 1984) supports the conclu-

sion that these two training types result in the same gains in isometric strength. Collectively this information indicates no clear superiority of either training type over the other.

It has been shown (Silvester et al. 1984) that both the DCER (free weight) and increasing lever-arm training result in significantly greater increases in vertical jump ability than does cam-type variable resistance training. Thus, the superiority of either training type over the other may depend on the type of variable resistance or the training program used.

Table 7.6 indicates that body composition changes from these two types of training are of the same magnitude. A 10-wk comparative study noted no significant difference between DCER and variable resistance training with regard to changes of percent fat, body mass, and total body weight (Pipes 1978).

Concentric Versus Eccentric Resistance Training

Concentric and eccentric training can both be performed isokinetically or using DCER equipment. A review of comparative studies indicates that there is no significant difference between gains in strength from concentric and eccentric training when the training is performed using DCER equipment (Atha 1981).

No significant difference has been reported between concentric and eccentric training when using DCER training methods. Strength tested with DCER elbow curls, arm presses, knee flexions, and knee extensions after 6 wk of training three times per week is not significantly different between these two types of training (Johnson et al. 1976). Concentric training consisted of two sets of 10 repetitions at 80% of 1 RM. Eccentric training consisted of two sets of 6 repetitions at 120% of 1 RM.

Häkkinen and Komi (1981) compared three groups training with DCER exercise for 12 wk. A concentric-only group performed the concentric portion of a squat exercise. A concentric-eccentric group performed primarily the concentric portion with some of the eccentric portions of a squat exercise. An eccentric-concentric group trained primarily with the eccentric portion and some concentric portions of a squat exercise. The groups that trained with both eccentric and concentric actions made significantly greater gains in 1 RM squat ability (about 29%) than the group that trained with concentric actions only (about 23%). This suggests that both eccentric and concentric actions may be necessary to bring about maximal gains in strength. However, a direct comparison of concentric-only to eccentric-only training cannot be made from this study.

Concentric and eccentric resistance training have also been compared using isokinetic muscle actions. After a 7-wk program of training four times per week with six muscle actions of the elbow flexors per training session, no significant difference in maximal isometric, eccentric, or concentric tension was demonstrated between concentric and eccentric training (Komi and Buskirk 1972). The exact training velocities are not given, but the muscle actions were isokinetic. Testing specificity has also been shown when training with isokinetic concentric and eccentric actions (Tomberline et al. 1991). Concentric and eccentric training consisted of three sets of 10 maximal repetitions of the knee extensors three times per week for 6 wk. All training and testing was performed at 100°/s. The concentric training increased concentric and eccentric strength (peak torque) significantly. Eccentric training significantly increased eccentric but not concentric strength. In addition, the concentric training increased concentric strength significantly more than did the eccentric training. No significant difference between the two types of training in eccentric strength gains was found.

The effect isokinetic concentric and eccentric training have on shoulder internal and external rotation indicates that concentric but not eccentric training increases tennis serve velocity (Ellenbecker, Davies, and Rowinski 1988). Training in this study was performed two times per week for 6 wk. Concentric and eccentric training consisted of six sets of 10 repetitions at each of the velocities of 60°/s, 180°/s, 210°/s, 210°/s, 180°/s, and 60°/s. Testing was performed at the velocities of 60°/s, 180°/s, and 210°/s. Both types of actions significantly increased concentric strength (peak torque) of the shoulder internal and external rotators at all three testing velocities. No significant difference was shown between the two types of training in concentric strength at any of the testing velocities. Concentric training significantly increased eccentric strength of the shoulder internal and external rotators at two and one of the testing velocities, respectively. Eccentric training increased eccentric strength of the shoulder internal rotators at one testing velocity and showed no change in eccentric strength of the shoulder external rotators at any of the testing velocities. This study does not indicate testing specificity for strength but does indicate that isokinetic concentric training may improve

motor performance in some skills to a greater extent than does isokinetic eccentric training.

Eccentric-only training does, however, produce more muscular soreness than concentric-only training, especially during the first few weeks of the program (Atha 1981; Carpinelli and Gutin 1991).

Dynamic Constant External Resistance Versus Isokinetic Resistance Training

Studies comparing DCER and concentric isokinetic resistance training indicate no clear superiority of either type over the other. After 8 wk of training the isokinetic torque of the knee extensors of an isokinetically trained group increased 47.2%, whereas that of a DCER group increased 28.6% (Thistle et al. 1967). Daily training of the knee extensors and flexors for 4 wk showed that isokinetic training (22.5°/s) is superior to DCER training in isokinetic and isometric strength increases (Moffroid et al. 1969). The isokinetic and DCER groups exhibited increases of 24% and 13%, respectively, in isometric knee-extension force and 19% and 1%, respectively, in isometric knee-flexion force. Isokinetic peak torque at 22.5°/s of the isokinetic and DCER groups increased 11% and 3%, respectively, in knee extension and 16% and 1%, respectively, in knee flexion.

DCER training has been demonstrated to increase isokinetic torque at a medium and a fast velocity to a significantly greater extent than isokinetic training at a medium and a fast (but not at a slow) velocity (Davies 1977). No significant difference in isokinetic torque at any velocity was shown between the DCER and slow isokinetic training in this comparison. DCER and isokinetic training have also shown testing specificity (Pearson and Costill 1988). After 8 wk DCER and isokinetic training showed 32% and 4% increases, respectively, in 1-RM strength tested in a DCER fashion. The DCER and isokinetic training resulted in 8% and 12% increases, respectively, in isokinetic force at 60°/s and 1% and 10% increases, respectively, at 240°/s, indicating testing specificity.

A biomechanical examination of free-weight and isokinetic bench pressing has been performed (Lander et al. 1985). Subjects performed a free-weight bench press at 90% and 75% of their 1 RM. The same subjects also performed maximal isokinetic bench presses at a speed corresponding to the individual subject's movement speed during a 90% and 75% free-weight bench press. No significant difference in maximal force existed between the isokinetic bench press and the 90% or the 75% of 1 RM free-weight bench press. The study indicates that free weights may affect muscles in a manner similar to isokinetic devices, at least in the context of force production during the major portion of a movement.

Body composition changes from DCER and isokinetic training are of the same magnitude. See table 7.6 for information concerning comparative changes in percent fat, body mass, and total body weight.

Isokinetic Versus Variable Resistance Training

Comparisons of isokinetic and variable resistance training demonstrate a test-specificity phenomenon. Slow- and fast-speed isokinetic training have been compared with variable resistance training (Smith and Melton 1981). Slow-speed isokinetic training consisted of one set until peak torque declined to 50% at the velocities of 30°/s, 60°/s, and 90°/s. Fast-speed isokinetic training followed the same format as slow-speed training, except the training velocities were 180°/s, 240°/s, and 300°/s. Variable resistance training initially consisted of three sets of 10 repetitions at 80% of 10 RM; once all sets could be completed, more resistance was added. All groups performed knee extensions and flexions only. Tables 2.7 and 2.8 present the results

TABLE 2.8
Isokinetic Versus Variable Resistance Training: Motor Performance Changes

Test	Group (% change)		
	VR	SIK	FIK
Leg press	+10.5	+9.8	+6.7
Vertical jump	+1.6	+3.9	+5.4
Standing long jump	+0.3	+0.4	+9.1
40-yd dash	-1.4	+1.1	-10.1

VR = variable resistance
SIK = slow-speed isokinetic
FIK = fast-speed isokinetic
- indicates better 40-yd time
Adapted, by permission, from M.J. Smith and P. Melton, 1981, "Isokinetic versus isotonic variable resistance training," *American Journal of Sports Medicine* 9 (4):277.

of this study. In measures of strength the isokinetic groups demonstrated a relatively consistent pattern of test speed specificity. The variable resistance group demonstrated consistent increases in knee flexion, irrelevant of the test criterion, but knee extension showed large increases in isometric force only. Another study involving changes in leg press strength illustrates more clearly a test-specificity phenomenon between these two types of training (Gettman, Culter, and Strathman 1980). See table 2.4 for information concerning this study.

Table 2.8 compares the benefits of isokinetic and variable resistance training for motor performance. Fast-speed isokinetic training demonstrated increases in three of four motor performance tests, which surpassed improvement brought about by the slow-speed isokinetic or variable resistance training. The training protocols used by all three groups were described previously (Smith and Melton 1981). These results indicate that fast-speed isokinetic training may be superior to slow-speed isokinetic and variable resistance training in the context of motor performance improvement.

TABLE 2.7
Isokinetic Versus Variable Resistance Training: Strength Changes

Test and group	Test (% improvement)		
	Isometric	60°/s	240°/s
Knee extension			
VR	14.6	3.1	2.2
SIK	0.5	21.3	24.7
FIK	6.7	3.4	60.9
Knee flexion			
VR	10.9	14.5	13.6
SIK	15.5	17.4	10.3
FIK	9.0	8.6	51.3

VR = variable resistance
SIK = slow-speed isokinetic
FIK = fast-speed isokinetic
Adapted, by, permission, from M.J. Smith and P. Melton, 1981, "Isokinetic versus isotonic variable resistance training," *American Journal of Sports Medicine* 9 (4):276.

Stretch-Shortening Cycle Versus Dynamic Constant External Resistance Training

Training 2 d/wk for 7 wk resulted in no significant difference in increasing vertical jump ability between stretch-shortening cycle and DCER training methods (K. Adams et al. 1992). DCER training consisted of a periodized program of back squats progressing from four sets of eight repetitions at 80% of 1 RM in week 1 to two sets of two repetitions at 100% of 1 RM in week 6. Plyometric training consisted of a periodized program of in-depth jumps, double leg hops, and split jumps. In-depth jumps progressed from three sets of 10 repetitions from a height of 51 cm (20.1 in.) during week 1 to two sets of 6 repetitions from a height of 114 cm (44.9 in.) during week 6. Double leg hops and split jumps progressed from three sets of 15 repetitions during week 1 to two sets of 15 repetitions of double leg hops and three sets of 6 repetitions of split jumps during week 6. The squat and stretch-shortening cycle training resulted in increases of vertical jump ability of 3.3 and 3.8 cm (1.3 and 1.5 in.), respectively.

Body composition is not changed as a result of stretch-shortening cycle training but is changed as a result of DCER exercise (table 7.6). Therefore, lean body mass is increased and percent body fat decreased to a greater extent by DCER exercise than by stretch-shortening cycle exercise.

Stretch-Shortening Cycle Versus Eccentric and Isometric Training

Direct comparisons of these training types have not been performed. However, stretch-shortening cycle exercise does not result in body composition changes, whereas both isometric and eccentric exercise do result in body composition changes (table 7.6). Therefore, isometric and eccentric exercise result in greater increases in lean body mass and greater decreases in percent body fat than stretch-shortening cycle exercise.

Stretch-Shortening Cycle Versus Isokinetic Training

Eight weeks of training three times per week resulted in no significant difference in increases of vertical jump ability between stretch-shortening cycle and isokinetic training (Blattner and Noble 1979). Isokinetic training consisted of three sets of 10 repetitions of leg presses per training session. Stretch-shortening cycle training consisted of three sets of 10 repetitions of in-depth jumps from a height of 86.9 cm (34.2 in.) per training session. Beginning with training weeks 3, 5, and 7, respectively, a 4.5-kg, 6.8-kg, and 9.1-kg (9.9-lb, 15-lb, and 20-lb) weighted vest was worn during the in-depth jumps. The stretch-shortening cycle and isokinetic training resulted in increased vertical jump ability of 4.8 and 5.1 cm (1.9 and 2.0 in.) respectively.

Isokinetic training can result in body composition changes, whereas stretch-shortening cycle training does not (table 7.6). Therefore, isokinetic training increases lean body mass and decreases percent body fat to a greater extent than stretch-shortening cycle training.

SUMMARY

The information presented in this chapter concerning types of resistance training and changes in strength, body composition, motor performance, and test specificity should be considered in the design of all resistance training programs. The next chapter discusses the process involved in developing a resistance training program. Several decisions have to be made regarding the program design to satisfy the needs analysis and to meet the goals of the individuals performing the program.

SELECTED READINGS

Fleck, S.J., and Schutt, R.C. 1985. Types of strength training. *Clinics in Sports Medicine* 4:150-69.

Häkkinen, K. 1985. Factors affecting trainability of muscular strength during short-term and prolonged training. *National Strength and Conditioning Association Journal* 7:32-37.

Lacerte, M.; deLateur, B.J.; Alquist, A.D.; and Questad, K.A. 1992. Concentric versus combined concentric-eccentric isokinetic training programs: Effect on peak torque of human quadriceps femoris muscle. *Archives of Physical Medicine and Rehabilitation* 73:1059-62.

Manning, R.J.; Graves, J.E.; Carpenter, D.M.; Leggett, S.H.; and Pollock, M.L. 1990. Constant vs. variable resistance knee extension training. *Medicine and Science in Sports and Exercise* 22:397-401.

McDonagh, M.J.N., and Davies, C.T.M. 1984. Adaptive response of mammalian skeletal muscle to exercise with high loads. *European Journal of Applied Physiology* 52:139-55.

Petersen, S.; Wessel, J.; Bagnall, K.; Wilkens, H.; Quinney, A.; and Wenger, H.A. 1990. Influence of concentric resistance training on concentric and eccentric strength. *Archives of Physical Medicine and Rehabilitation* 71:101-5.

Pizzimenti, M.A. 1992. Mechanical analysis of the Nautilus leg curl machine. *Canadian Journal of Sport Science* 17:41-48.

Potteiger, J.A.; Williford, H.N., Jr.; Blessing, D.L.; and Smidt, J. 1992. Effect of two training methods on improving baseball performance variables. *Journal of Applied Sport Science Research* 6:2-6.

Tomberline, J.P.; Basford, J.R.; Schwen, E.E.; Orte, P.A.; Scott, S.C.; Laughman, R.K.; and Ilstrud, D.M. 1991. Comparative study of isokinetic eccentric and concentric quadriceps training. *Journal of Orthopaedic and Sports Physical Therapy* 14:31-36.

CHAPTER 3

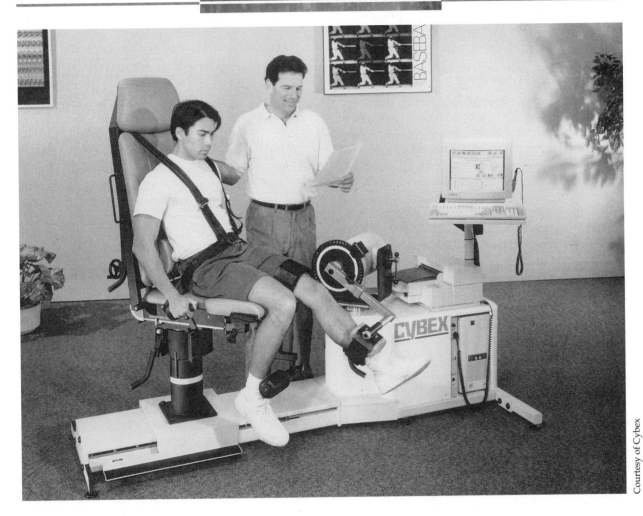

Muscle Physiology

T he ultimate goal of a resistance training program is to improve the physiological function of muscle. A basic understanding of how muscle functions to produce force is vital for the practitioner, as it allows insights into potential adaptations and program design. Force production is a product of neural stimulus, muscle activation, and available energy. In this chapter these areas are examined to provide the basis for discussion of training adaptations. Understanding how muscle functions allows for scientifically sound resistance training program design.

THE NEUROMUSCULAR UNIT

In order for a muscle to be activated, neural innervation is necessary. The muscle and its nerves are considered a neuromuscular unit. Muscle function is controlled by the nervous system. An alpha motor neuron and the muscle fibers it innervates are called a motor unit. The motor unit is the basic functional component of the neuromuscular system and will be discussed later in the chapter in much greater detail. Understanding how to enhance motor unit recruitment is paramount to the specificity of resistance training.

Nerve Cell Anatomy

The central nervous system consists of more than 100 billion nerve cells. Figure 3.1 is a schematic of an alpha motor nerve cell, or neuron. A neuron consists of three basic components: dendrites, cell body, and axon. Neurons come in all sizes and shapes. The dendrites receive information via impulses from other neurons. This information is carried in the form of an impulse, or action potential, to the cell body of the neuron. In the cell body this information is processed and sometimes modified or inhibited by other neurons. If an impulse is to be carried down the axon, an action potential is again developed. The terminal ending of a motor neuron's axon on a skeletal muscle fiber is termed the *motor end plate* or *neuromuscular junction.*

Axons can be covered with a white substance high in lipid (fat) content, called the myelin sheath. The myelin sheath is sometimes even thicker than the axon itself and is composed of multiple layers of this lipid substance. Nerve fibers possessing a myelin sheath are referred to as myelinated nerve fibers; those lacking a myelin sheath are called unmyelinated nerve fibers. The myelin sheath is created and maintained by Schwann cells. In a typical nerve there are about twice as many unmyelinated

fibers as myelinated fibers. The smaller unmyelinated fibers typically are found between myelinated fibers. The myelin helps to electrically insulate the nerve impulse as it travels down the axon. This helps prevent impulses from being transferred to neighboring axons. The myelin sheath does not run continuously along the length of the axon, but is segmented, with small spaces about every 1 to 2 mm along the length of the axon. These small spaces, about 2 to 3 μm in length are called the nodes of Ranvier (see figure 3.1).

Conduction of Nerve Cell Impulses

A nerve impulse is conducted in the form of electrical energy. When no impulse is being conducted, the inside of the neuron has a net negative charge as compared to the outside of the neuron, which has a net positive charge. This arrangement of the positive and negative charges is termed the *resting membrane potential.* It is attributed to the distribution of molecules with electrical charges, or ions, and the impermeability of the resting cell membrane to these ions. Sodium (Na^+) and potassium (K^+) ions are the major molecules responsible for the membrane potential. Na^+ ions are located predominantly outside the neuron's cell membrane. K^+ ions are located mainly inside the neuron. There are, however, more Na^+ ions on the outside of the neuron than K^+ on the inside, giving the inside a less positive, or net negative, charge as compared to the outside of the neuron.

When an impulse is being conducted down a dendrite or an axon, the cell membrane of the neuron becomes permeable to both Na^+ and K^+ ions.

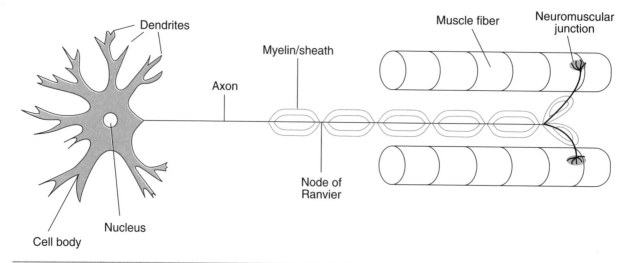

Fig. 3.1   A motor neuron and the muscle fibers it innervates are called a motor unit.

Ions tend to move down a concentration gradient from areas where they are highly concentrated to areas where they are less concentrated, so Na⁺ ions move into the neuron and K⁺ ions move out of the neuron. This gives the inside a positive charge compared to the outside of the neuron. This is termed *depolarization,* and such a reversal of electrical potential is called the action potential. The action potential lasts for only a brief period of time (milliseconds). The membrane quickly becomes impermeable to the ions again. An energy-dependent pumping system, called the *Na⁺-K⁺ pump,* restores the resting membrane potential. This pump actively moves Na⁺ ions from the inside back to the outside of the neuron and moves K⁺ ions from outside back to the inside of the neuron. This quickly restores the neuron to its original resting membrane potential with a net negative charge on the inside. The process is repeated each time a nerve impulse or action potential is conducted by a neuron.

The type of nervous system conduction is related to whether the nerve is myelinated or unmyelinated. Myelinated nerves conduct their impulses using what is called *saltatory conduction,* and unmyelinated nerves use a conduction process called *local conduction.* The movement of the ions to produce an action potential with either type of conduction is the same as described in the preceding paragraph. However, as depicted in figure 3.2, the nodes of Ranvier allow the action potential to jump from node to node (thus the term *saltatory,* meaning *to jump*). Ions cannot move in significant numbers through the thick myelin sheath but can easily move through the membrane at the nodes of Ranvier because of low resistance to ionic current at the nodes of Ranvier. Saltatory conduction has two advantages. First, it allows the action potential to make jumps down the axon, thereby increasing the velocity of nerve transmission as much as 5- to 50-fold. Second, it conserves energy, as only the nodes depolarize, and this reduces the energy needed to reestablish the resting membrane potential. Saltatory conduction results in the action potentials moving along at a velocity of 60 to 100 m/s. In addition, the velocity of an impulse increases with the nerve fiber diameter in myelinated nerves. In other words, larger nerve fibers can conduct an impulse at faster velocities than smaller fibers.

Conversely, unmyelinated nerve fibers use a local circuit of ionic current flow to conduct the action potential along the entire length of the nerve fiber (see figure 3.2). Thus, a small part of the nerve fiber membrane depolarizes, the continuation of local-circuit ionic current flow causes nerve mem-

Saltatory conduction

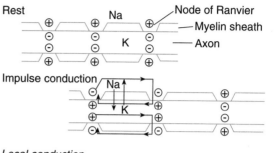

Local conduction

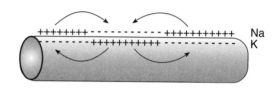

Fig. 3.2   Conduction events for both saltatory conduction in myelinated nerve fibers (*top*) and local conduction flow (*bottom*). At rest K⁺ is concentrated inside the axon and Na⁺ outside the axon, giving the interior of the axon a net negative charge as compared with its exterior. During impulse conduction, movement of the K⁺ and Na⁺ ions results in the interior of the axon having a net positive charge compared with its exterior. This takes place either at the nodes of Ranvier, in saltatory conduction, or along the entire nerve cell membrane, in local conduction.

brane depolarization to continue, and the action potential travels down the entire length of the nerve fiber. The velocity of this type of nerve impulse conduction is slower than in myelinated nerve fibers, ranging from 0.5 to 10 m/s.

Diameter of Neurons

As previously noted, the neuron's diameter determines in part the impulse conduction velocity. In general, the greater the diameter of a nerve fiber, the greater the velocity of conduction. In myelinated nerve fibers the impulse velocity increases approximately with the increase in the fiber diameter. In unmyelinated nerve fibers the velocity of the impulse increases with the square root of the fiber diameter. The faster velocities of the larger myelinated fibers, such as the ones that innervate skeletal muscle, produce more rapid stimulation of muscle actions but have higher thresholds for recruitment. Typically Type II (fast-twitch) skeletal muscle fibers are innervated by larger diameter axons than Type I (slow-twitch) muscle fibers. Thus, motor units made up of a high percentage of Type I fibers are typically recruited first due to the lower recruitment thresholds of their neurons. Motor units made up of a high percentage of Type II fibers are recruited after the Type I fibers because their larger axons have higher recruitment thresholds. This is termed the *size principle of recruitment* and will be discussed in more detail later in this chapter.

Sensory and Motor Neurons

Sensory neurons convey impulses from receptor sites to the central nervous system (brain and spinal cord). Examples of sensory neurons are those excited by sound, pain, and light.

Motor and sensory neurons' cell bodies are located in the spinal cord. A motor neuron has relatively short dendrites and a long axon that carries impulses from the central nervous system to the neuromuscular junction. Conversely, a sensory neuron has relatively long dendrites that carry information from the periphery to the central nervous system and a relatively short axon.

Sensory neurons vary a great deal in diameter (0.5 to 20 μm) and can be myelinated or unmyelinated. Therefore, the conduction velocity of sensory neurons can vary from very slow (0.5 m/s) to among the fastest (120 m/s).

Neuromuscular Junction

Figure 3.3 is a schematic of the neuromuscular junction, the functional connection between the nerve and the muscle fiber. All neuromuscular junctions have five common features: (1) a Schwann cell that forms a cap over the axon, (2) a nerve terminal that contains the neurotransmitter acetylcholine (ACh)

and other substances needed for metabolic support and structural function (adenosine triphosphate (ATP), mitochondria, lysosomes, glycogen molecules, etc.), (3) a junctional cleft or space, (4) a postjunctional membrane that contains ACh receptors, and (5) a junctional sarcoplasm and cytoskeleton that provides metabolic and structural support.

The interface formed by an axon from a motor neuron and a muscle fiber is called the neuromuscular junction. When an impulse reaches the end of the neuron side of the neuromuscular junction, it causes the release of ACh. ACh is the primary stimulatory neurotransmitter for a motor neuron and is stored within the synaptic vesicles in the terminal ends of the axon. Approximately 50 to 70 ACh-containing vesicles are found per square micrometer of nerve terminal area. As the action potential travels down the axon, calcium channels along the membrane of the nerve terminal open, causing the uptake of calcium ions (Ca^{2+}). The increase in Ca^{2+} causes the release of ACh from the vesicles. The ACh diffuses from the prejunctional membrane across the junctional cleft (about 50 nm wide) between the pre- and postjunctional membranes to the postjunctional membrane.

On the postjunctional side of the neuromuscular junction the ACh attaches to a receptor located on the postjunctional membrane. The postjunctional membrane is a specialized part of the muscle cell's membrane and has junctional folds and ACh receptors. If enough ACh becomes bound to the postjunctional membrane receptors, the permeability of the membrane will increase and

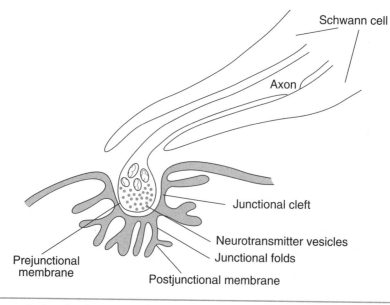

Fig. 3.3   The neuromuscular junction in cross section.

create a conducted ionic current similar to that found within the axon, except Ca^{2+} is the ion predominantly involved. This postjunctional ionic current or electrical impulse is what initiates muscle action (e.g., muscle contraction). The muscle fiber will continue to be activated (e.g., to perform concentric, isometric, or eccentric muscle actions) as long as a sufficient amount of ACh is bound to the postjunctional membrane receptors.

The ACh will eventually be broken down by the enzyme acetylcholinesterase found at the base of the junctional folds of the junctional cleft. Destruction of ACh stops the stimulus needed for muscle fiber activation. The majority of by-products produced by the breakdown of ACh by acetylcholinesterase are taken up by the prejunctional membrane and used to produce new ACh.

Why is ACh needed at the neuromuscular junction? Why can't the ionic current of the neuron simply be conducted to the membrane surrounding the muscle fiber and thus stimulate muscle actions? Because the neuron is very small compared with a muscle fiber, the ionic current it conducts is insufficient to be directly transferred to the muscle fiber's membrane and stimulate the fiber. ACh is needed to cause an ionic current of sufficient strength (threshold) to be conducted by the muscle fiber's membrane and initiate muscle action. Figure 3.4 presents an actual micrograph of motor end plates showing several structural aspects of the neuromuscular junction (Deschenes et al. 1993).

THE MOTOR UNIT

A motor unit consists of an alpha neuron and all the muscle fibers (cells) it innervates. The motor unit is the functional unit of muscular activity under neural control. Each muscle fiber is innervated by at least one alpha motor neuron. The smaller the number of muscle fibers in a motor unit, the smaller the amount of force that can be produced by that motor unit when activated. The number of muscle fibers in a motor unit depends on the amount of fine control required for its function. For example, in muscles that stretch the lens of the eye, motor units may contain only 10 muscle fibers, whereas in the gastrocnemius 1000 muscle fibers may be found in one motor unit. The average for all the muscles in the body is about 100 muscle fibers per motor unit.

The muscle fibers in a motor unit are not all located together, but are spread out in the muscle in what are called microbundles of about 3 to 15 fibers. Thus, two adjacent muscle fibers do not necessarily belong to the same motor unit. The spread of a motor unit's muscle fibers throughout a muscle allows the intact muscle to be activated without exhibiting all the force production potential of the whole muscle. Without such a dispersal of muscle fibers in a motor unit throughout the muscle, the muscle would be activated in segments rather than as a whole muscle.

In humans motor units vary not only in number of muscle fibers, but also in the metabolic characteristics of the muscle fibers innervated. A motor unit is typically made up of both Type I (slow-twitch) or Type II (fast-twitch) muscle fibers. Some individuals may have a greater overall percentage of Type I or Type II fibers in some muscles, and this affects the composition of their motor units. A distance runner may have 80% Type I fibers in the thigh muscles, and thus a larger number of

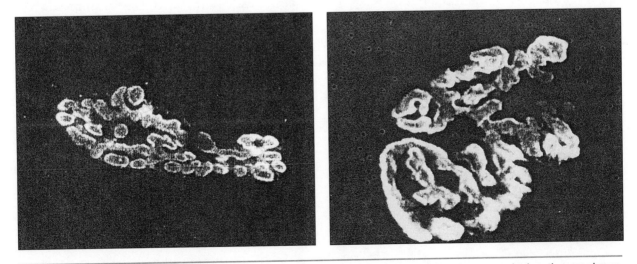

Fig. 3.4   Type I, slow-twitch (*left*), and Type II, fast-twitch (*right*), motor end plates of the neuromuscular junction are shown. Courtesy of Dr. Michael Deschenes's laboratory.

motor units, although containing Type II fibers, would contain predominantly Type I fibers.

Motor Unit Activation

Only the motor units that are recruited in an exercise produce force and will be subject to adaptational changes with exercise training. Thus, motor unit recruitment is of fundamental importance in the prescription of resistance exercise. The demands placed on the muscle dictate the amount of muscle tissue that is activated to perform the movement and thus adapts to the training.

All-or-None Law

The fact that either all the muscle fibers within a motor unit are activated or none of them are activated is referred to as the all-or-none law. While the all-or-none law holds true for individual motor units, whole muscles such as the biceps are not governed by the all-or-none law. As discussed previously, some motor units can be activated in the muscle while others are not. Without this phenomenon, there would be very little control of the amount of force the whole muscle can generate and therefore poor control of body movement.

Gradation of Strength

The fact that motor units follow the all-or-none law makes possible one method by which force variations produced by a muscle can be achieved. The more motor units within a muscle that are stimulated, the greater the amount of force that is developed. In other words, if one motor unit is activated, a very small amount of force is developed. If several motor units are activated, more force is developed. If all the motor units in a muscle are activated, maximal force is produced by the muscle. This method of varying the force produced by a muscle is called multiple motor unit summation. The activation of motor units is based upon the force production needs of the activity. For example, one might activate only a small number of motor units to perform 10 repetitions of an arm curl using 15 lb (6.8 kg), because the resistance may represent only about 10% of the maximal strength. Therefore, a small number of muscle fibers can provide the force to perform the exercise movement. Conversely, a 150-lb (68-kg) arm curl that represents a 1 RM would require all the available motor units to produce maximal force to perform the exercise movement.

Gradations of force can also be achieved by controlling the force produced by one motor unit. This is called wave summation. A motor unit responds to a single nerve impulse by producing a *twitch*. A twitch (figure 3.5) is a brief period of muscle activity producing force that is followed by relaxation of the motor unit. When two impulses conducted by an axon reach the neuromuscular junction close together, the motor unit responds with two twitches. The second twitch, however, occurs before complete relaxation from the first twitch. The second twitch adds to the force of the first twitch, producing more total force than the first. This wave (twitch) summation can continue until the impulses occur frequently enough that the twitches are completely summated. The complete summation is called *tetanus* and is the maximal force a motor unit can develop.

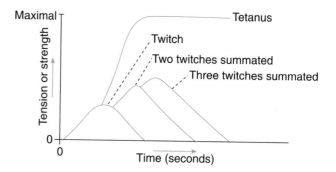

Fig. 3.5   Gradations in force of one motor unit caused by wave summation.

Huxley's Sliding Filament Theory

The major function of skeletal muscle is to provide force to move the joints of the body. The Huxley sliding filament theory is an explanation of how muscle fibers are activated to produce force. Activated muscle can produce force during a shortening of the muscle (concentric action), with no change in the muscle's length (isometric action), or during a lengthening of the muscle (eccentric action).

To understand the sliding filament theory of muscular activation, it is necessary to know the structural arrangement of skeletal muscle. Skeletal muscle is called striated muscle because the arrangement of protein molecules in the muscle give it a striped or striated appearance under a microscope. A sarcomere is the smallest functional unit of the muscle fiber. Muscle fibers are composed of sarcomeres stacked one on top of the other. At rest, there are several distinct light and dark areas creating striations within each sarcomere. These light and dark areas are caused by the arrangement of the actin and myosin filaments, the major proteins

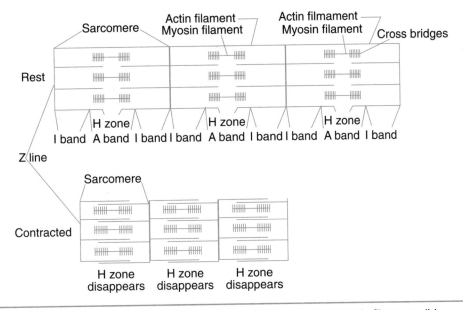

Fig. 3.6 Sarcomeres demonstrating the sliding filament theory. As the actin and myosin filaments slide over one another, the entire sarcomere shortens, but the length of the individual filaments does not change.

involved in the contractile process. In the contracted (fully shortened) state there are still striations of the muscle tissue, but they have a different pattern. This change in the striation pattern occurs from the sliding of the actin over the myosin protein filaments (figure 3.6).

A sarcomere runs from one Z line to the next Z line and is the smallest functional unit that can shorten. At rest there are two distinct light areas in each sarcomere: the H zone, which contains no actin and only a small amount of myosin, and the I bands located at the ends of the sarcomere, which contain only actin filaments. These two areas appear light in comparison with the A band, which contains both actin and myosin filaments.

As the sarcomere shortens, the actin filaments slide over the myosin filaments. This causes the H zone to seem to disappear as actin filaments slide into it and give it a darker appearance. The I bands become shorter as the Z lines come closer to the ends of the myosin filaments. When the sarcomere relaxes and returns to its original length, the H zone and I bands return to their original size and appearance. The striated pattern and other structures of skeletal muscle can be seen in figure 3.7.

Phases of Muscle Action

Since Huxley originally proposed the sliding filament theory over 40 years ago, a great deal more has been discovered about how the protein filaments of muscle interact. The actin filament has active sites on which the myosin crossbridges can

interact with the actin to cause shortening. At rest the projections or crossbridges of the myosin filaments can touch the actin filaments but cannot

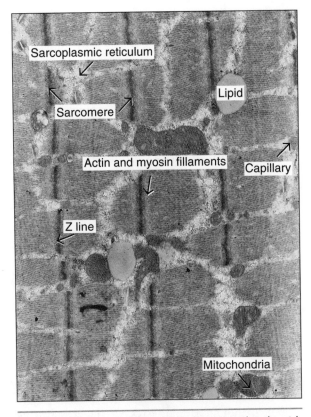

Fig. 3.7 An electron micrograph demonstrating the striated appearance of human skeletal muscle and some structures present in it. Sarcomeres are fully shortened. Courtesy of Dr. William J. Kraemer's laboratory.

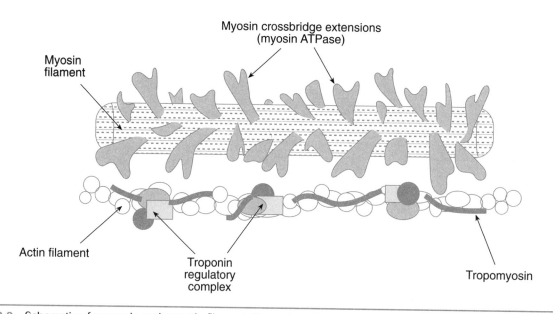

Myosin crossbridge extensions
(myosin ATPase)

Myosin
filament

Actin filament

Troponin
regulatory
complex

Tropomyosin

Fig. 3.8   Schematic of a myosin and an actin filament. The active sites are located on the actin underneath the troponin and tropomyosin molecules.

interact to cause shortening. At rest the active sites are covered by troponin and tropomyosin, two regulatory proteins associated with the actin filament (figure 3.8).

When ACh causes an ionic current within the membrane surrounding the muscle fiber, it triggers the release of calcium ions (Ca^{2+}) from the sarcoplasmic reticulum. The sarcoplasmic reticulum is a membranous structure that surrounds each muscle fiber. The released Ca^{2+} binds to the troponin molecule and triggers a structural change in the troponin and tropomyosin that exposes the active sites on the actin. This is called the *steric blocking model*. With the active site now exposed, the myosin crossbridges make contact with the active sites. This is called the *excitation-coupling* phase of the muscle action process.

Contraction, or shortening of the sarcomere, can now take place. The attachment of the crossbridge head to the active site activates the enzyme myosin ATPase that breaks down an ATP molecule located on the crossbridge head and in so doing releases energy. ATP is an energy source for many cellular activities, including muscle action. The released energy is used to cause the crossbridge to swivel to a new angle (Huxley 1969) or to collapse (R. Davies 1966). The result of either of these two actions is to pull the actin over the myosin, causing the sarcomere to shorten.

For further shortening to occur, the crossbridge must break with the active site with which it is in contact and bind to another active site on the actin filament closer to the Z line. This is accomplished

by reloading the crossbridge with an ATP molecule. Once the crossbridge is reloaded, it breaks the bond with the active site with which it is in contact and binds to a new active site closer to the Z line. The process of breaking contact with one active site and binding to another is termed *recharging*. ATPase breaks down the new ATP, causing the crossbridge head to be cocked and ready for interaction with a new active site. On contact with a new active site the head swivels forward or collapses, causing the actin to slide over the myosin and resulting in shortening of the sarcomere. This cyclical process, called the *ratchet theory*, is repeated until either the sarcomere has shortened as much as possible or relaxation of the muscle takes place.

Relaxation of the muscle occurs when the impulse from the motor axon ends. This triggers the active pumping of Ca^{2+} back into storage within the sarcoplasmic reticulum. This pump mechanism also requires energy from the breakdown of ATP to function. The troponin and tropomyosin assume their original positions covering the active sites. The crossbridges of the myosin filament now have no place at which to contact the actin to pull the actin over the myosin. With relaxation muscle activity stops, and the muscle will remain in the shortened position unless pulled to a lengthened position by gravity or an outside force, because muscle can only shorten and produce force.

Length-Tension (Force) Curve

The length-tension (force) curve (figure 3.9) dem-

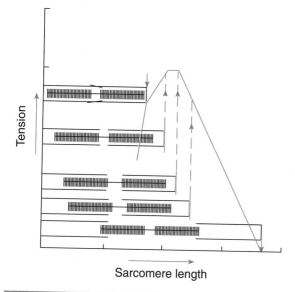

Fig. 3.9 There is an optimal length at which a sarcomere develops maximal tension. At lengths less than or greater than optimal, less tension is developed.

Data from A.M. Gordon, A.F. Huxley, and F.J. Jullian, 1966, "The variation in isometric tension with sarcomere length in vertebrate muscle fibers," *Journal of Physiology* 7: 170-92.

onstrates that there is an optimal length at which muscle fibers generate their maximal force. The total amount of force developed depends on the total number of myosin crossbridges interacting with active sites on the actin. At the optimal length there is potential for maximal crossbridge interaction and thus maximal force. Below this optimal length, less tension is developed during an activation because with excessive shortening there is an overlap of actin filaments so that the actin filaments interfere with each other's ability to contact the myosin crossbridges. Less crossbridge contact with the active sites on the actin results in a smaller potential to develop tension.

At lengths greater than optimal there is less and less overlap of the actin and myosin filaments. This results in less potential for crossbridge contact with the active sites on the actin. Thus, if the sarcomere's length is greater than optimal, less force can be developed.

The length-tension curve indicates that some prestretch of the muscle prior to initiation of an action will increase the amount of force generated. Too much prestretch will, however, actually decrease the total amount of force developed.

Force-Velocity Curve

As the velocity of movement increases, the force a muscle can produce concentrically (while shorten-

ing) decreases (figure 3.10). This is empirically true. If an athlete is asked to bench press the maximal amount of weight possible, the weight will move very slowly. But if he or she is asked to bench press half his or her maximal weight, the bar moves at a faster velocity. Maximal velocity of shortening occurs when no resistance is being moved or lifted. Maximal velocity is determined by the maximal rate at which crossbridge connections can be formed and broken with the actin active sites. The force-velocity curve is important when examining forms of weight training, such as isokinetic training, in which the velocity of the movement and not the resistance (as in free weights or variable resistance) is controlled.

Conversely, as the velocity of movement increases, the force that a muscle can develop eccentrically (lengthening) actually increases (figure 3.10). This is thought to be caused in part by the elastic component of the muscle. However, the actual explanation for such a response remains unclear. It is interesting to note that eccentric force at even low velocities is higher than the highest concentric or isometric force. Such high force development when using maximal eccentric muscle actions has been related to muscle damage in untrained individuals. However, it has been demonstrated that muscle exposed to repeated eccentric actions can adapt and the damage per training session reduced (Clarkson and Tremblay 1988). It is interesting to note that eccentric force is not maximal at percentages of 1 RM normally

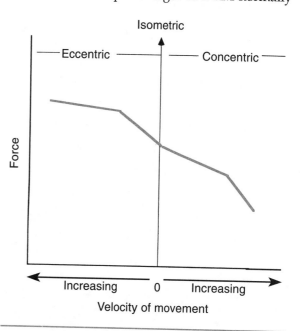

Fig. 3.10 Force-velocity relationship in eccentric and concentric muscle action of elbow flexors.

used for resistance training. Thus, it is possible that with normal weight training the eccentric portion of the repetition is not optimal in terms of strength gains.

BIOENERGETICS

Bioenergetics concerns the sources of energy for muscle activity. Such words as *aerobic* (energy production with oxygen) and *anaerobic* (energy production without oxygen) training have become popular among coaches and athletes. There are two major sources that produce anaerobic energy (the adenosine triphosphate-phosphocreatine system and glycolysis) and one source to produce aerobic energy (oxidative phosphorylation). Knowledge of these energy sources and their interactions with each other is necessary to successfully plan a resistance training program that will optimally condition an individual for a particular sport or activity.

ATP: The Energy Molecule

The source of energy for muscle action is the adenosine triphosphate (ATP) molecule. The main functional components of ATP are a sugar molecule called adenosine and three phosphate groups. When ATP is broken down to adenosine diphosphate (ADP; two phosphates) and a free phosphate molecule, energy is released (figure 3.11). This energy is used by the crossbridges to pull the actin filaments across the myosin filaments and cause shortening of the muscle.

Although ATP is the immediate source of energy for muscular actions, there are three major

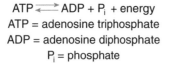

$$ATP \rightleftharpoons ADP + P_i + energy$$

ATP = adenosine triphosphate
ADP = adenosine diphosphate
P_i = phosphate

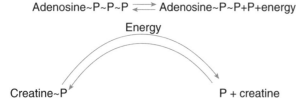

$$Adenosine{\sim}P{\sim}P{\sim}P \rightleftharpoons Adenosine{\sim}P{\sim}P + P + energy$$

Energy

Creatine~P   P + creatine

i designates inorganic
P designates a phosphate group

Fig. 3.11 When ATP breaks down to ADP, the derived energy can be used to perform muscular actions. When PC breaks down to P_i and C, the energy released is used to rebuild ATP.

sources of ATP in the cell. Two of these sources, the adenosine triphosphate–phosphocreatine (ATP-PC) source and the formation of lactic acid (HLa), require no oxygen to provide ATP and are called anaerobic. The third source requires oxygen to provide ATP and is referred to as aerobic.

Phosphocreatine System

Stored within muscle and ready for immediate use to supply energy to the cell are two compounds. One of these compounds is ATP. The other compound, phosphocreatine (PC), is similar to ATP in that it also has a phosphate group and a high-energy bond. In PC the phosphate group is bound to a creatine molecule.

When ATP is broken down to ADP and inorganic phosphate (P_i), energy is released. This energy is used to cause muscular actions. However, when PC is broken down to creatine and P_i, the resulting energy is used to recombine ADP and P_i back into ATP (see figure 3.11). The rebuilt ATP can then be broken down again to ADP and P_i, and the energy released used to perform more muscular actions. The energy released from the breakdown of PC cannot be used to cause muscle shortening because PC does not have a receptor on the crossbridges.

Only a limited amount of ATP and PC are stored within the muscle; this limits the amount of energy that the ATP-PC source can produce. In fact, in an all-out exercise bout the energy available from the ATP-PC source will be exhausted in 30 s or less (Larson and Davies 1970; Meyer and Terjung 1979). One advantage of this energy source is that the energy is immediately available for use. A second advantage is that the ATP-PC source has a large power capacity; this source is capable of giving the muscle a large amount of energy per second.

Because of the characteristics of the ATP-PC energy source, it is the primary source of energy for short-duration, high-power events. It supplies the major portion of energy to the muscles for such activities as a maximal lift, the shot put, the high jump, and the 40-yd (36.6-m) dash. One of the reasons for continued heavy breathing after the completion of an intense, short-duration exercise bout is that the muscular stores of ATP and PC must be replenished aerobically if the ATP-PC energy source is to be used again at a later time.

Glycolysis

Glycogen, a carbohydrate, is stored within the muscle. Glycogen is a long chain of glucose (a type of sugar) molecules. The energy necessary to make ATP is derived by splitting glucose molecules in half, yielding two pyruvate molecules and releasing energy. The energy released from splitting each glucose molecule produces a net gain of two ATP molecules. The pyruvate is then transformed into lactic acid. No oxygen is required for this process to take place, so this energy system is anaerobic.

The extreme fatigue, the needles-and-pins feeling in the fingers and toes, and a nauseous feeling after several squat sets using a 10-RM resistance are caused in part by the buildup of lactic acid. The breakdown of lactic acid in the muscle to lactate and its associated hydrogen ions causes these compound concentrations to increase in the muscle and blood. Lactate itself can contribute to fatigue by reducing the force the muscle is capable of producing (Hogan et al. 1995). Lactic acid breakdown causes the acid level of the body to build up and pH to decrease. With severe exercise blood pH can go from a resting level of 7.4 to as low as 6.9 (S.E. Gordon et al. 1994). This decrease in pH, increased H^+ concentration, and increased lactate concentration are thought to be a major contributor to fatigue (S.E. Gordon, Kraemer, and Pedro 1991).

The buildup of lactate in the muscle and blood has several side effects. One of these effects occurs when the lactate and hydrogen ion concentrations are high enough to affect nerve endings, causing pain. As the concentration of lactate increases, the interior of the muscle cells becomes more acidic. This can interfere with the chemical processes of the cell, including the processes of producing more ATP (Trivedi and Danforth 1966) and the binding of Ca^{2+} to troponin (Nakamura and Schwartz 1972). The amount of energy that can be obtained from the lactic acid source is therefore limited due to the side effects of lactate and decreased pH.

Despite the side effects of lactate accumulation, this energy source can produce a greater amount of energy than the adenosine triphosphate-phosphocreatine system. Glycolysis, however, cannot supply the muscle with as much energy per second as the adenosine triphosphate-phosphocreatine system and therefore is not as powerful.

The lactic acid energy source is a major supplier of ATP in all-out exercise bouts lasting from approximately 1 to 3 min (Kraemer, Patton, et al. 1989). Such exercise bouts may include high-intensity sets at 10 to 12 RM with very short rest periods (30 to 60 s) and the 400-m sprint. Heavy breathing continues after completion of these types of exercise bouts. This is caused in part by the need to remove the accumulated lactate from the body.

Oxygen Energy Source

The oxygen energy source has received a lot of attention for many years. The major goal of jogging, swimming, and aerobic dancing is to improve cardiovascular fitness, which is analogous to improving oxidative phosphorylation. This energy source utilizes oxygen in the production of ATP and is therefore an aerobic energy source.

The oxidative phosphorylation system can metabolize carbohydrates (sugar) and fats. Significant amounts of protein are normally not metabolized. However, during long exercise bouts up to 10% of the needed ATP can be obtained from metabolizing protein. (Dohm et al. 1982; Lemon and Mullin 1980; Tarnopolsky, MacDougall, and Atkinson 1988). At rest the body normally derives one third of the needed ATP from metabolizing carbohydrates and two thirds from fats. During physical exercise there is a gradual change to metabolizing more and more carbohydrates and less and less fat as the intensity of the exercise increases. During maximal physical exercise the muscle metabolizes nearly 100% carbohydrates if sufficient carbohydrates are available (Maresh et al. 1989; Maresh et al. 1992).

Aerobic metabolism of the carbohydrate glycogen begins in the same manner as it does in anaerobic glycolysis. In aerobic metabolism, however, because of the presence of sufficient oxygen, the pyruvate is not converted into lactic acid but enters into two long series of chemical reactions called *Krebs cycle* and *electron transport*. These series of reactions eventually produce carbon dioxide, which is expired at the lungs, and water. The water is produced by combining hydrogen molecules with the oxygen that was originally taken into the body through the lungs. Thirty-seven ATP molecules can be produced by aerobically metabolizing one glycogen molecule. The aerobic metabolism of fats does not start with glycolysis. Fats go through a series of reactions called *beta oxidation* and then enter directly into Krebs cycle. The end products of fat metabolism are similarly water, carbon dioxide, and ATP.

The maximal amount of energy that can be produced via aerobic metabolism depends on how much oxygen the body can obtain and utilize. Maximal aerobic power ($\dot{V}O_2max$) is the maximal amount of oxygen the body can obtain and utilize per unit of time. It is usually expressed either in absolute terms as liters of oxygen per minute ($L\ O_2 \cdot min^{-1}$) or in relative terms as milliliters of oxygen per kilogram (2.2 lb) of body weight per minute ($ml\ O_2 \cdot kg^{-1} \cdot min^{-1}$). $\dot{V}O_2max$ in $L\ O_2 \cdot min^{-1}$ does not take into account body weight. A heavy individual might be expected to use more oxygen per minute solely because of his or her body size. Expressing $\dot{V}O_2$max in ml $O_2 \cdot kg^{-1} \cdot min^{-1}$ places everyone on a scale relative to body weight. In this manner comparisons can be made between individuals of different body weights.

Compared with the two anaerobic energy sources, the oxidative phosphorylation source is the least powerful. The aerobic energy source cannot produce enough ATP per second to allow the performance of maximal intensity exercise, such as a 1-RM lift or a 40-m sprint. On the other hand, because of the abundance of glycogen and fats and the lack of production of by-products that can inhibit various energy reactions, the aerobic energy source can supply virtually an unlimited amount of ATP over a long period of time. Therefore, it is the predominant energy source for long-duration, low-intensity activities, such as extremely long sets of an exercise with a low resistance and distance running (e.g., the marathon or ultramarathon). In addition, this energy source contributes a moderate to high percentage of the energy during activities composed of high-intensity work interspersed with rest periods and high-intensity activities lasting longer than about 25 s, such as interval run training and wrestling. These activities result in very high blood lactate levels of up to 15 or 22 mmol $\cdot L^{-1}$ (Serresse et al. 1988). In these activities the oxygen and lactate energy sources both will contribute significant amounts of energy.

Restoring the Anaerobic Energy Sources

After an intense exercise bout the anaerobic energy sources must be replenished if they are to be utilized again at a later time. The anaerobic energy sources are replenished by the aerobic energy source. After cessation of an anaerobic activity heavy breathing continues for a period of time, even though physical activity is no longer taking place. The oxygen taken into the body, above the resting value, is used to replenish the two anaerobic energy sources. This extra oxygen has been referred to as an *oxygen debt* or more recently as the *excess postexercise oxygen consumption* (EPOC).

Replenishing the ATP-PC Energy Source

Immediately after an intense exercise bout there is a several-minute period of very heavy, rapid breath-

ing. The oxygen taken into the body above normal resting oxygen consumption is used to aerobically produce ATP in excess of that required during rest. Part of this excess ATP is immediately broken down to ADP and P_i; the energy released is utilized to combine P_i and creatine back into PC. Part of the excess ATP is simply stored as intramuscular ATP. This rebuilding of the ATP and PC stores is accomplished in several minutes (Hultman, Bergstrom, and Anderson 1967; Karlsson et al. 1975; Lemon and Mullin 1980). This part of the oxygen debt has been referred to as the alactacid portion of the oxygen debt.

The half-life of the alactacid portion of the oxygen debt has been estimated to be approximately 20 s (DiPrampero and Margaria 1978; Meyer and Terjung 1979) and as long as 36 to 48 s. Half-life means the time within which half of the alactacid debt is repaid. Within 20 to 48 s 50% of the depleted ATP and PC is replenished, in 40 to 96 s 75% is replenished, and in 60 to 144 s 87% is replenished. Thus, the majority of the depleted ATP and PC intramuscular stores are replenished within approximately 3 to 4 min.

If activity is performed during the alactacid portion of the oxygen debt, the rebuilding of the ATP and PC intramuscular stores will take longer. This is because part of the ATP generated via the aerobic system has to be used to provide energy to perform the activity. An understanding both of the alactacid portion of the oxygen debt and of the building of the ATP-PC energy source is important in the planning of a training program that involves short-duration, high-intensity work, such as heavy sets of an exercise. The ATP-PC energy source is the most powerful energy source and is therefore the major source of energy for maximal lifts and heavy sets. Several minutes of rest must be allowed between heavy sets and maximal lifts to replenish the ATP and PC intramuscular stores; otherwise, they will not be available for use in the next heavy set. If sufficient recovery time is not allowed between heavy sets or maximal lifts, the lift or set either will not be completed or will not be completed with the desired speed or technique.

Replenishing the Lactic Acid Energy Source

The aerobic energy source is also responsible in part for removing accumulated lactate from the body. However, in this case the oxygen taken in above resting values is believed to be used in part to aerobically metabolize the lactate accumulated during activity. This produces energy needed by the tissues and is termed the lactacid portion of the oxygen debt.

The relationship between the lactacid portion of the oxygen debt and lactate removal has been questioned (Roth, Stanley, and Brooks 1988); however, many tissues of the body can aerobically metabolize lactate. Skeletal muscle active during an exercise bout (Hatta et al. 1989), skeletal muscle that was inactive during an exercise bout (Kowalchuk et al. 1988), cardiac muscle (Hatta et al. 1989; Spitzer 1974; Stanley 1991), kidney (Hatta et al. 1989; Yudkin and Cohen 1974), the liver (Rowell et al. 1966; Wasserman, Connolly, and Pagliassotti 1991), and the brain (Nemoto, Hoff, and Sereringhaus 1974) can all metabolize lactate. Sixty percent of the accumulated lactate is aerobically metabolized (Gasser and Brooks 1979). Portions of the remaining 40% are converted to glucose and protein, and a small portion is excreted in the urine and sweat (Ingjer 1969). The half-life of the lactacid portion of the oxygen debt is approximately 25 min (Hermansen et al. 1976). Thus, approximately 95% of the accumulated lactic acid is removed from the blood in 1 hr 15 min.

If light activity (walking, slow jogging, stretching) is performed after a workout, the accumulated lactate is removed more quickly than if complete rest follows the workout (Hermansen et al. 1976; Hildebrandt, Schutze, and Stegemann 1991; McLoughlin, McCaffrey, and Moynihan 1991; Mero 1988). When light activity is performed following the activity, a portion of the accumulated lactate is aerobically metabolized to supply some of the needed ATP to perform the light activity. It also appears that accumulated lactate is removed from the blood more quickly if the light activity is performed by the muscles active during the exercise bout and not with muscles that were inactive during the exercise bout (Hildebrandt, Schutze, and Stegemann 1991). Because of this, it is recommended that, if practical, the rest period between sets (e.g., in short-rest-period programs or circuit weight training) in which lactate accumulation occurs consist of light activity of the muscles used during the activity rather than complete rest.

Interaction of the Energy Sources

Although one energy source may be predominant for a particular activity (e.g., ATP-PC for a maximal lift, aerobic for running a marathon), all three sources supply a portion of the ATP needed by the body at all times. Thus, the ATP-PC energy source is operating even when the body is at rest, and the aerobic energy source is operating during a maxi-

mal lift. Even at rest some lactate is being released by muscles into the blood (G.A. Brooks et al. 1991). During a marathon, even though the majority of energy is supplied by the oxygen energy source, some of the needed energy is supplied by the ATP-PC and lactic acid energy sources.

Although all three energy sources supply some portion of the ATP necessary for any activity, as the duration and intensity of activity changes, the predominant energy source also changes. At one end of the spectrum are activities such as a maximal lift, the shot put, and the 40-yd (36.6-m) sprint. The ATP-PC energy source supplies the vast majority of energy for these activities. The lactic acid energy source supplies the majority of the necessary energy for activities such as sets of 20 to 25 repetitions, three sets of 10 RM with 1-min rest periods, and sprints of 440 yd (402.3 m). The aerobic energy source supplies the majority of the needed ATP for extremely long sets and 5-mi (8-km) runs. However, all three energy sources are still producing some energy at all times.

There is no exact point at which one energy source provides the majority of ATP for an activity. Rather, the percentage contribution from each particular energy source gradually shifts based on the intensity and duration of the activity. It is also possible that the energy contribution of an energy source during an activity changes in response to different energy needs. For example, as a marathon runner climbs a hill and lactate accumulates in the body, the lactic acid source contributes more energy to the performance of the activity. The contribution of all three energy sources to an activity is dynamic and changes as the intensity and duration of the activity changes.

MUSCLE FIBER TYPES

Over the past 20 years a great deal of interest has been generated about muscle fiber types, changes that occur in the muscle fiber with training, and changes from resistance training. Because muscle tissue is one of the most obvious places in which adaptations occur from resistance training, a great deal of interest about muscle fiber types has developed. It is therefore important to understand what is meant by a muscle fiber type. Greater understanding of muscle fiber typing will allow better interpretation of the many popular and scientific articles now being published and discussed in the area of resistance training and muscle.

Skeletal muscle is a heterogeneous mixture of several types of muscle fibers. Quantification of

TABLE 3.1
Some Primary Muscle Fiber–Type Classification Systems

Classification system	Theoretical basis
Red and white fibers	Fiber color; the more myoglobin (oxygen carrier in a fiber), the darker or redder the color.
Fast twitch and slow twitch	The speed and shape of the muscle twitch with stimulation. Fast-twitch fibers have higher rates of force development and a greater fatigue rate.
Slow oxidative, fast oxidative glycolytic, fast glycolytic	Metabolic staining and characteristics of oxidative and glycolytic enzymes.
Type I and Type II	Stability of the enzyme myosin ATPase. Under different pH conditions, the enzyme myosin ATPase has different forms; some forms result in quicker enzymatic reactions for ATP breakdown and thus higher cycling rates for that fiber's actin-myosin interactions.

different biochemical and physical characteristics of the different muscle fibers has led to the development of several muscle fiber classification systems (Pette and Staron 1990). Although these classification systems appear similar, they are different. Table 3.1 reviews some of the basic muscle fiber–type classification schemes. The characteristics of Type I and Type II muscle fibers are shown in table 3.2.

Figure 3.12 shows classification of muscle fiber types according to a popular myosin ATPase histochemical staining method. The head of the crossbridge is made up of myosin ATPase, an enzyme that is intimately involved in the cleaving of ATP to produce ADP, P_i, and energy. This classification system is possible because there are different types of myosin ATPase in the different muscle fiber types. The histochemical assay uses different

TABLE 3.2
Characteristics of Type I and Type II Muscle Fibers

Characteristic	Type I	Type II
Force per cross-sectional area	Low	High
Myofibrillar ATPase activity (pH 10.4)	Low	High
Intramuscular ATP stores	Low	High
Intramuscular PC stores	Low	High
Contraction speed	Slow	Fast
Relaxation time	Slow	Fast
Glycolytic enzyme activity	Low	High
Endurance	High	Low
Intramuscular glycogen stores	No difference	No difference
Intramuscular triglyceride stores	High	Low
Myoglobin content	High	Low
Aerobic enzyme activity	High	Low
Capillary density	High	Low
Mitochondrial density	High	Low

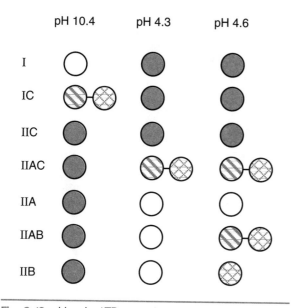

pH 10.4   pH 4.3   pH 4.6

I
IC
IIC
IIAC
IIA
IIAB
IIB

Fig. 3.12 Myosin ATPase stain nomenclature for determination of Type I and Type II muscle fiber types. Hatching indicates intermediate staining between dark and light. Courtesy of Dr. Robert S. Staron.

pH conditions that result in the different muscle fiber types staining at different intensities. Myosin ATPase is an enzyme very specific to the cycling speed of myosin's head on the actin active sites, thus it provides a functional classification of a muscle fiber without the actual determination of twitch speed.

The most common method of obtaining a muscle sample in humans is a muscle biopsy technique (figure 3.13). A hollow needle is used to obtain about 200 to 400 mg of muscle tissue (typically a thigh, calf, or arm muscle). This sample is processed and frozen. The muscle sample is then cut (sectioned) into consecutive (serial) sections and placed on cover slips for histochemical assay (a series of biochemical treatments involving different pH conditions) to determine the various muscle fiber types. Other factors such as glycogen content of the fibers can also be analyzed from a section of a biopsy.

It is very important in the histochemical muscle fiber–typing procedure that serial sections from the same muscle are placed into each of the preincubation baths, which consist of an alkaline (pH 10.4) and two acid baths (pH 4.6 and 4.3), prior to the rest of the histochemical assay. Ultimately, after the assay is completed a muscle fiber is typed by comparing the fiber's color under each of the pH conditions using a microscope (see figure 3.12).

In the classification system presented in figure 3.12 muscle fibers are classified as Type I or Type

II. In addition, various muscle fiber subtypes (e.g., Type IIA) can also be determined in both the general categories Type I and Type II. The Type I fiber is the most oxidative muscle fiber. Starting at the top and progressing toward the bottom of figure 3.12, each succeeding fiber type becomes less oxidative. In figure 3.14 the various fiber subtypes can be seen in the muscle fibers after staining. Fiber subtypes are highly related to the type of myosin heavy chain contained in the muscle structure (Staron et al. 1991; Fry, Allemeier, and Staron 1994) and therefore to the rate at which the crossbridges can be cycled and to twitch speed of the fiber.

Functional abilities have been associated with the classifications of fiber types. Type II (white, fast-twitch, fast oxidative glycolytic, fast glycolytic) and Type I (red, slow-twitch, slow oxidative) fibers have different metabolic and contractile properties. Type II fibers (fast-twitch) are better adapted to perform anaerobic work, whereas Type I fibers (slow-twitch) are better adapted to perform aerobic exercise (see table 3.2).

Type II fibers are suited to the performance of high-intensity, short-duration work bouts as evidenced by their biochemical and physical characteristics (see table 3.2). Such exercise bouts include the 40-m sprint, a 1-RM lift, and sets with heavy resistance (e.g., two 4-RM repetitions). These fiber types have high activity of myofibrillar ATPase, the enzyme that breaks down ATP and releases the energy to cause fiber shortening. Type II fibers are able to shorten with a high velocity and have a fast relaxation time. Possessing these characteristics allows these fibers to develop force in a short period of time and to have a high power output. Type II fibers rely predominantly on anaerobic sources to supply the energy necessary for muscle action. This is evidenced by their large ATP and PC intramuscular stores, as well as their high glycolytic enzyme activity. Type II fibers have a low aerobic capability as evidenced by their low intramuscular stores of triglyceride, low capillary density, low mitochondrial density, and low aerobic enzyme activity. The fact that Type II fibers rely predominantly on anaerobic sources of ATP and have a poor capability to supply ATP aerobically makes them highly susceptible to fatigue. Type II fibers are suited to perform short-duration activities in which a large power output is necessary.

Type I fibers are more suited to the performance of endurance (aerobic) activities. Type I fibers' characteristics include high levels of aerobic enzyme activity, high capillary density, high mitochondrial density, large intramuscular triglyceride stores, and low fatigability. Type I fibers are ideal for the

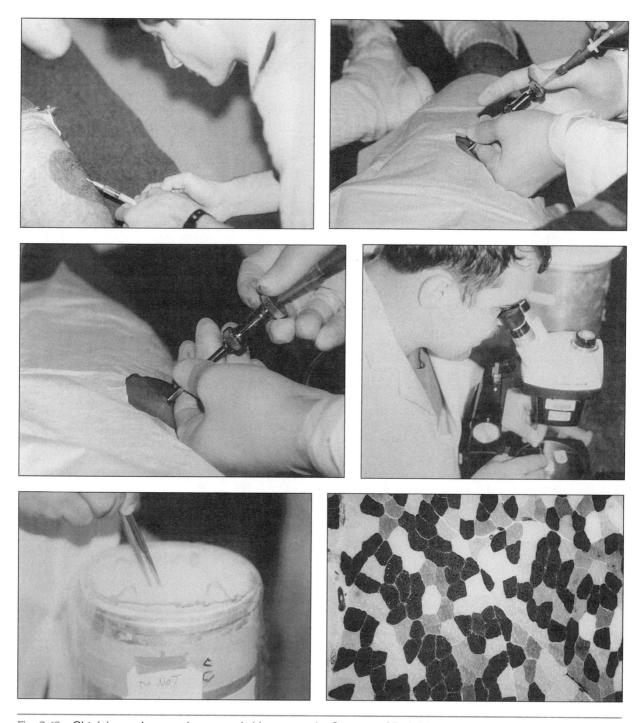

Fig. 3.13   Obtaining and processing a muscle biopsy sample. Courtesy of Dr. William Kraemer's laboratory.

performance of low-intensity, long-duration (endurance) activities, such as long-distance running and swimming and long sets of an exercise (20 repetitions or more).

As discussed previously, several subtypes of Type I and Type II fibers have been discovered. Type IIA fibers possess good aerobic and anaero-

bic characteristics, whereas Type IIB fibers possess good anaerobic characteristics but poor aerobic characteristics (Essen et al. 1975; Staron, Hikida, and Hagerman 1983). It now appears that the Type IIB fibers may in fact be just a pool of unused fibers (with low oxidative ability) that on recruitment start a transformation process to the Type IIA fiber type

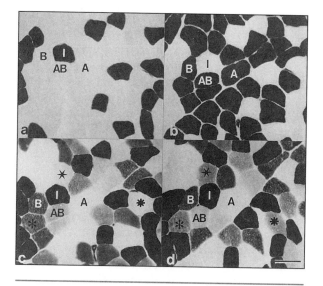

Fig. 3.14 Myosin ATPase–stained muscle fibers demonstrating Types I, IIA, IIAB, and IIB fibers: a. pH 4.3; b. pH 10.4; c. and d. pH 4.6. Courtesy of Dr. Robert S. Staron's laboratory.

(G.R. Adams et al. 1993; Staron et al. 1991; Staron et al. 1994). Dramatic reductions in Type IIB fibers occur with heavy resistance training, a fact that supports such a theory. Type IIC fibers are very few in number in humans (0% to 5% of the fibers) and are more oxidative than Types IIA and IIB in several biochemical characteristics. Type IIAB fibers represent a combination of both Types IIA and IIB and is a transitional or intermediate fiber type. Thus, a fiber might be transformed from Type IIB to Type IIAB to Type IIA with exercise training.

The subtypes of the Type I fiber are Type I and Type IC. There are few Type IC fibers, and they are a less oxidative (aerobic) form of the Type I fiber. With resistance training or anaerobic training Type IC fibers may increase in number because of the lack of oxidative stress from the training modality.

The subtypes of the Type II fibers represent a continuum in aerobic and anaerobic capabilities. Some studies suggest that physical training may play a role in fiber-type transformation among Type II fiber subtypes (Ingjer 1969; Staron, Hikida, and Hagerman 1983; Staron et al. 1991; Staron et al. 1994). Although a number of studies suggest that there might be a fiber transformation between the Type I and Type II fibers (Haggmark, Jansson, and Eriksson 1982; Howald 1982), it now appears that the changes occur only within the subtypes of Type I or Type II fibers. For example, anaerobic training may cause Type IIB fibers to transform into Type

IIA fibers or Type I to Type IC fibers. Thus, adaptations may occur along a continuum of fiber subtypes based on the demands of the exercise.

Muscle Fiber–Type Recruitment

Muscle fibers found within a motor unit vary in size and metabolic characteristics (Roy and Edgerton 1992). However, muscle fibers within a motor unit are more similar to each other than to muscle fibers in other motor units in the same region of a muscle. The order in which motor units are recruited in most cases is relatively constant (Desmedt and Godaux 1977).

According to the *size principle* for recruitment of motor neurons, the smaller, or *low-threshold* (low stimuli level needed for activation), motor units are recruited first. Low-threshold motor units are composed predominantly of Type I fibers. After low-threshold motor units, progressively higher-threshold motor units are recruited based on the increasing demands of the activity. The higher-threshold motor units are composed predominantly of Type II fibers. Heavier resistances (e.g., 3 to 5 RM) require the recruitment of higher-threshold motor units than lighter resistances (e.g., 12 to 15 RM). However, according to the size principle, lifting heavier resistances will start with the recruitment of low-threshold motor units (Type I). The high-threshold motor units (Type II) needed to produce greater force will be recruited as the force required increases. This concept is shown in figure 3.15.

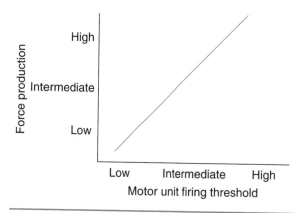

Fig. 3.15 Schematic representation of the size-principle order of recruitment. Low- and intermediate-threshold motor units are recruited before high-threshold motor units. Exceptions to the size principle involve the recruitment of high-threshold motor units first by active inhibition of lower-threshold motor units. This may have importance for high power or rapid, quick motions in training and sports.

Exceptions to recruitment order by size are thought to be related to very high velocity and high-power outputs using trained movement patterns. Throwing a fast ball might be the type of sport skill that may have the potential for recruitment patterns to enhance power production that do not adhere to the size principle. Thus, rather than low-threshold motor units, high-threshold motor units are recruited first. This means that the low-threshold motor units are not recruited in the activity. They are skipped over so that the high-threshold motor units are recruited first. In fact, the low-threshold motor units may be inhibited to facilitate power production. It is possible that novice lifters may not be able to activate the highest-threshold motor units in the early phase of training (Sale 1992). With training, the ability of the motor nerves to activate the highest-threshold motor units becomes possible and is part of the training effect.

The factor that determines whether to recruit high- or low-threshold motor units is the total amount of force necessary to perform the muscular action. If a large amount of force is necessary either to move a heavy weight slowly or to move a light weight at a fast velocity, high-threshold motor units will be recruited. The higher-threshold motor units have a larger number of Type II muscle fibers in them. Thus, their recruitment results in high power production. The size-principle order of recruitment ensures that low-threshold motor units are recruited predominantly to perform low-intensity, long-duration (endurance) activities and that higher-threshold motor units are used only to produce higher levels of force or speed. The order of recruitment holds the high-threshold motor units, made up primarily of fatigable Type II muscle fibers, in reserve until the low-threshold motor units can no longer perform the particular muscular action because of its higher force production requirements.

Recruitment order is important for several reasons from a practical standpoint. First, in order to recruit the Type II fibers and so to attain a training effect in these fibers, the exercise must be intense. Second, the order of recruitment is fixed for a specific movement (Desmedt and Godaux 1977). If the body position is changed, the order of recruitment can also change (Grimby and Hannerz 1977). The order of recruitment can also change for multifunctional muscles from one movement or exercise to another (Grimby and Hannerz 1977; Harr Romeny, Denier Van Der Gon, and Gielen 1982). Recruitment order in the quadriceps for the performance of a knee extension is different from that for a squat.

Variation in the recruitment order may be one of the factors responsible for the specificity of strength gains to a particular exercise. The variation in recruitment order provides some evidence to support the belief held by many strength coaches that to completely develop a particular muscle it must be exercised with several different movements or exercises.

PROPRIOCEPTORS

Length and tension within muscles and tendons are continually monitored by specialized sensory receptors located within the muscles and tendons, called *proprioceptors*. The length and tension of the muscles acting at a joint determine the joint's position. Thus, if the lengths of the muscles acting on a joint are known, the joint's position is also known, and changes in the joint's position can be monitored. The information that proprioceptors gather is constantly relayed to conscious and subconscious portions of the brain and is important for motor learning (Hutton and Atwater 1992). Proprioceptors keep the brain constantly informed about the progress of a movement or series of movements.

Muscle Spindles

The two functions of muscle spindles are to monitor the stretch or length of the muscle in which they are embedded and to initiate a contraction to reduce the stretch in the muscle. The knee-jerk or stretch reflex is attributed to the response of muscle spindles.

Spindles are located in modified muscle fibers that are arranged parallel to the normal muscle fibers. The modified muscle fibers containing spindles are called intrafusal fibers. These intrafusal fibers are composed of a stretch-sensitive central area, or sensory area, embedded in a muscle fiber capable of contracting. If a muscle is stretched, as in tapping the patellar tendon to initiate the knee-jerk reflex or adding an external weight, the spindles are also stretched. The sensory nerve of the spindle carries an impulse to the spinal cord; here the sensory neuron synapses with alpha motor neurons. The alpha motor neurons carry a nerve impulse that causes activation of the stretched muscle and its agonist muscles. In addition, other neurons inhibit activation of the antagonistic muscles of the stretched muscle. The stretched muscle shortens, and the stretch on the spindle is relieved. Strength training exercises with prestretch take advantage of this stretch reflex. This reflex is one explanation for greater force output from a prestretch.

Gamma motor neurons innervate the end portions of the intrafusal fibers, which are capable of shortening. Stimulation of these end portions by the brain regulates the length of the spindles and therefore their sensitivity to changes in the extrafusal fibers' length. Adjustments of the spindles in this fashion enable the spindles to more accurately monitor the length of the muscles in which they are embedded.

Golgi Tendon Organs

Golgi tendon organs' main functions are to respond to tension within the tendon and to relieve the tension if it becomes excessive. These proprioceptors are located within the tendons of muscles and are consequently in a good location to monitor tension developed by a muscle.

The sensory neuron of a Golgi tendon organ travels to the spinal cord. In the spinal cord it synapses with the alpha motor neurons both of the muscle whose tension it is monitoring and of the antagonistic muscles. As an activated muscle develops tension, the tension within the muscle's tendon increases and is monitored by the tendon organs. If the tension becomes great enough that damage to the muscle or tendon is possible, inhibition of the activated muscle occurs and activation of the antagonist muscle(s) is initiated. The tension within the muscle is alleviated and damage to the muscle or tendon avoided.

This protective function is not foolproof. It may be possible through resistance training to learn to disinhibit the effects of the Golgi tendon organs. The ability to disinhibit this protective function may in part be responsible for some injuries that occur in maximal lifts by highly resistance trained athletes.

SUMMARY

Basic physiological knowledge about how the muscular and nervous systems work together to control muscle action assists in designing scientifically based resistance training programs. Knowledge of the neuromuscular system is also important when developing programs involving integration of the various fitness components covered in the next chapter.

SELECTED READINGS

Armstrong, R.B.; Marum, P.; Saubert, C.W.; Seeherman, J.J.; and Taylor, C.R. 1977. Muscle fiber activity as a function of speed and gait. *Journal of Applied Physiology: Respiratory, Environmental and Exercise Physiology* 43:672-77.

Billeter, R., and Hoppler, H. 1992. Muscular basis of strength. In *Strength and power in sport*, ed. P.V. Komi, 39-63. Oxford: Blackwell Scientific.

Boyd, I.A. 1981. The muscle spindle controversy. *Scientific Progress* (Oxford) 47:205-21.

Donaldson, S.K.B., and Hermansen, L. 1986. Differential, direct effects of H+ on CA++ activated force of skinned fibers from the soleus, cardiac and adductor magnus muscles of rabbits. *Pflugers Archives* 376:55-65.

Edgerton, V.R.; Roy, R.R.; Gregor, R.J.; Hager, C.L.; and Wickiewicz, T. 1983. Muscle fiber activation and recruitment. In *Biochemistry of exercise*, eds. H.G. Knuttgen, J.A. Vogel, and S. Poortmans, 31-49. Champaign, IL: Human Kinetics.

Garett, W.E.; Mumma, M.; and Lucaveche, C.L. 1985. Ultrastructural differences in human skeletal muscle fiber types. In *Clinics in sports medicine*, ed. G.G. Weiker, vol. 4, 189-201. Philadelphia: W.B. Saunders.

Gordon, A.M.; Huxley, A.F.; and Julian, F.J. 1966. Variation in isometric tension with sarcomere length in vertebrate muscle fibers. *Journal of Physiology* (London) 184:170-92.

Murray, J., and Weber, A. 1974. The cooperative action of muscle proteins. *Scientific American* 230:58-71.

Noth, J. 1992. Motor units. In *Strength and power in sport*, ed. P.V. Komi, 21-28. Oxford: Blackwell Scientific.

Sullivan, T.E., and Armstrong, R.B. 1978. Rat locomotor muscle fiber activity during trotting and galloping. *Journal of Applied Physiology: Respiratory, Environmental and Exercise Physiology* 4:358-63.

Urbova, G. 1979. Influence of activity on some characteristic properties of slow and fast mammalian muscles. In *Exercise and sport science reviews*, eds. R.J. Hutton and D.I. Miller, 181-212. New York: Franklin Institute.

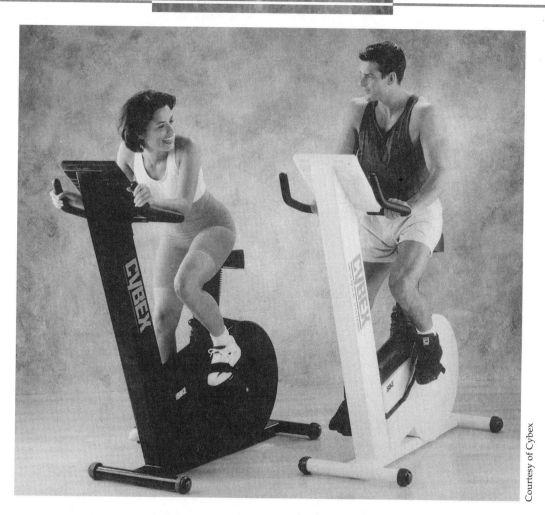

CHAPTER 4

Courtesy of Cybex

Integrating Other Fitness Components

Resistance training is one method of addressing the conditioning needs of the body. Its effectiveness as a training tool varies with the specific fitness component one wishes to enhance (figure 4.1). For example, resistance training normally increases the strength component to a greater extent than it does cardiovascular endurance (see chapter 7). Resistance training can make a significant contribution to increasing physical fitness. The level of fitness desired for each component depends on the specific needs and goals of the individual or the sport. The impact and importance of fitness on health has been well documented (Blair et al. 1989; American College of Sports Medicine 1990). Resistance training is just one conditioning modality within a total program. It is interesting to note that over the past five years the importance of resistance training as a vital contributor to both health and functional abilities has been realized by the scientific and medical communities. In this chapter we review the basic guidelines for

Fitness Components

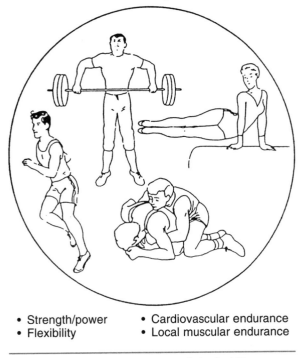

- Strength/power
- Flexibility
- Cardiovascular endurance
- Local muscular endurance

Fig. 4.1 The major components of physical fitness.

exercise prescription in other training modalities and how resistance training interacts with other exercise stimuli. Resistance training programs should be designed to meet the specific needs of the individual within a total conditioning program.

ENDURANCE TRAINING

A great deal of information exists regarding the effects and prescription of endurance exercise. The knowledge base spans cardiac rehabilitation to elite distance running (Froelicher 1983; American College of Sports Medicine 1991). The ability to prescribe aerobic exercise is necessary to address the cardiovascular endurance requirements of a conditioning program. Such aerobic endurance programs can be either continuous or intermittent.

According to the American College of Sports Medicine (1990), "persons of any age may significantly increase their habitual levels of physical activity safely if there are no contraindications to exercise and a rational program is developed." It is very important that each individual is prescribed the proper intensity, duration, and frequency of exercise in a progressive manner. Before starting a vigorous total conditioning program a medical evaluation is useful. According to Wilmore and

Costill (1994) a medical exam can have the following positive benefits:

- Some people either should not be exercising or are considered at high risk and should be restricted to exercising only under close medical supervision. A comprehensive medical evaluation will help identify these high-risk individuals.
- The information obtained in a medical evaluation can be used to develop the exercise prescription.
- The values obtained for certain clinical measures such as blood pressure, body fat content, and blood lipid levels can be used to motivate the person to adhere to the exercise program.
- A comprehensive medical evaluation, particularly of healthy people, can provide a baseline against which any subsequent changes in health status can be compared.
- Children and adults should establish a habit of periodic medical evaluations because many illnesses and diseases, such as cancer and cardiovascular diseases, can be identified in their earliest stages when the chances of successful treatment are much higher.

The prescription of aerobic exercise intensity should be individualized based on a stress test if possible. This is especially important for older adults or when the functional capacity of an individual is in doubt. It can also provide very specific training data for elite athletes. Treadmill or cycle ergometry testing is a direct method of individualizing exercise prescription for endurance training (figure 4.2). From this information the intensity of the exercise can be related to a heart-rate value. A training heart-rate zone for the aerobic exercise stimulus is typically prescribed. An individual then performs steady-state exercise within the training zone. Energy demands are expressed in metabolic equivalents (METs) or as an amount of oxygen. One MET is equivalent to resting oxygen consumption, which is approximately $3.5 \text{ ml} \cdot \text{kg}^{-1} \cdot \text{min}^{-1}$. For example, 10 METs represents an exercise intensity approximately 10 times the resting metabolic rate. An individual with a 10-MET functional capacity would have a maximal oxygen consumption value of approximately $35 \text{ ml} \cdot \text{kg}^{-1} \cdot \text{min}^{-1}$ (10 METs $\times$ 3.5 $\text{ml} \cdot \text{kg}^{-1} \cdot \text{min}^{-1}$). High MET values, which reflect high maximal oxygen consumption values, are as-

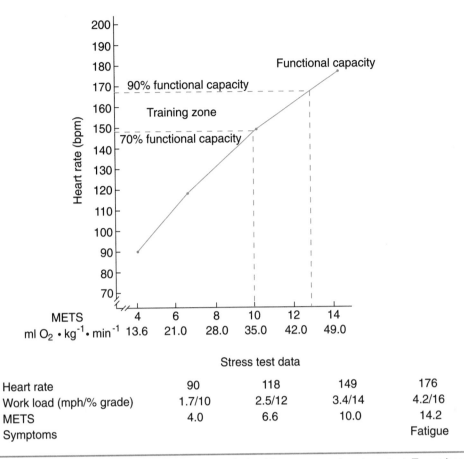

Stress test data				
Heart rate	90	118	149	176
Work load (mph/% grade)	1.7/10	2.5/12	3.4/14	4.2/16
METS	4.0	6.6	10.0	14.2
Symptoms				Fatigue

Fig. 4.2   Training zone of 70% to 90% of maximal capacity, derived from an exercise stress test. Target heart rate is 148 bpm, with a training zone of 148 to 167 bpm.

sociated with the functional capacities of individuals who possess good cardiovascular endurance. In healthy individuals functional capacity is the end point of the test (e.g., voluntary exhaustion). The upper limit of functional capacity could also be the point of the test at which abnormal response(s) (e.g., abnormal ECG responses) are observed, as is the case with cardiac patients.

Many individuals do not have the resources

available to obtain laboratory stress tests, most notably coaches who are prescribing exercise for hundreds of athletes. Yet an individual prescription for exercise should be given. Thus, for healthy individuals a training zone can be calculated using a percentage of predicted maximal heart rate (see table 4.1). Coaches and individuals must realize that for basic aerobic fitness, endurance training doesn't have to hurt to be effective. This is quite

TABLE 4.1
Training Zone Based on Maximal Heart Rate

220 − 20 yr. = 200 bpm predicted max. HR*

70% max. HR = 70% × 200 = 140 bpm

90% max. HR = 90% × 200 = 180 bpm

Target HR = 140 bpm   Training zone = 140 to 180 bpm

*A conservative estimate of maximal heart rate can be calculated as 200 − age (yr.) = maximal heart rate in beats per minute (bpm).

TABLE 4.2
Basic Guidelines for Intensity, Frequency, and Duration of Endurance Exercise

Fitness level	Intensity	Frequency	Duration
Endurance athletes	85%-90%	5-7 d	1-2 hr
Healthy individuals	70%-90%	3-5 d	15-60 min

Adapted from P.S. Fardy, 1977, "Training for aerobic power," *Toward an understanding of human performance*, ed. E.J. Burke, (Ithaca: Movement Press), 10-14.

different from the competitive endurance athlete who has to use a much higher training intensity to prepare for a race.

The duration and frequency of exercise also need to be progressively increased as the individual becomes more tolerant of exercise stress. For basic cardiovascular endurance fitness, the duration of exercise should be 15 to 60 min and should be performed 3 to 5 d/wk (Pollock, Wilmore, and Fox 1978; Wilmore and Costill 1994). Running, bicycling, cross-country skiing, and swimming are the best cardiovascular conditioners. Table 4.2 gives a basic summary of endurance training ranges. Im-

provement of aerobic capacity can be accomplished through interval training. Because the intensity is higher, interval training should be used only by individuals who already have a good endurance base (Fardy 1977).

An endurance exercise training session has a warm-up, a training period, and a cool-down (figure 4.3). The heart rate is checked and the pace of the exercise adjusted so that an individual is exercising within his or her training zone. The heart rate can be manipulated by the pace at which one exercises. A 10-s pulse rate can be taken after a steady-state exercise duration is achieved (usually

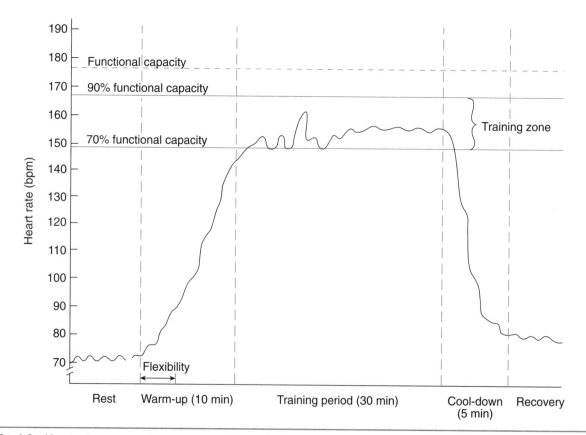

Fig. 4.3   Heart-rate response to warm-up, training period, and cool-down during endurance training session.

Adapted, by permission, from B.J. Sharkey, 1984, *Physiology of fitness,* 1st ed. (Champaign, IL: Human Kinetics Publishers), 45.

3 to 5 min). One should conduct a pace test over a number of training sessions. When running or bicycling, the pace tests should be performed on flat terrain. Also, as fitness levels improve, it is important to check the pace against the heart-rate response. In figure 4.4 a 1-mi (1.6-km) run is used to illustrate the pace–heart rate relationship, but shorter distances can also be used to evaluate this relationship. A less-conditioned individual usually requires shorter pace distances to evaluate a training pace. It is important to ensure that steady-state exercise is achieved at the selected distance (3-5 min of exercise after warm-up).

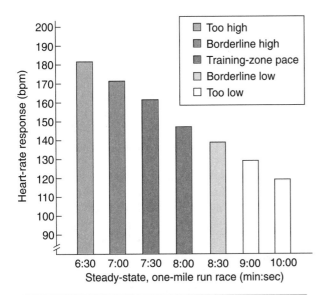

Fig. 4.4 An individual's response to different paces of steady-state endurance exercise. Target training zone is 148 to 167 bpm; training zone pace is 7:30 to 8:00 (min:sec) per mile.

Concurrent Strength and Endurance Training

Training is specific. The body attempts to adapt to the imposed demands. The understanding of exercise training compatibility has focused on both aerobic endurance training and strength training performed together (Chromiak and Mulvaney 1990; Dudley and Fleck 1987). Studies examining concurrent training using high levels of training for endurance and strength present the following conclusions.

- Strength can be compromised, especially in high-velocity muscle actions, by the performance of high-intensity endurance training.
- Power capabilities may be compromised by

the performance of both strength and endurance training.

- Anaerobic performance may be negatively affected by high-intensity endurance training.
- Development of maximal oxygen consumption is not compromised when concurrent strength and endurance training are performed.
- Endurance capabilities are not negatively affected by concurrent strength and endurance training.

The topic of exercise compatibility came to the attention of the sport science community when Hickson (1980) compared three groups: One group underwent both resistance and aerobic training, the second group only resistance training, and the third group only aerobic training. He observed decrements in leg strength in the group training simultaneously for strength (5 RM) and high-intensity aerobic fitness during the last 2 wk of an 8-wk conditioning program, as compared with the group that trained only for strength. This study demonstrates that the development of dynamic strength may be compromised by performance of both resistance training and high-intensity endurance training. This study lasted 8 wk, so whether the reduction of strength development would continue over a longer training period is unknown. Because no periodization of either the resistance or the endurance training was used and a relatively high training volume was performed, the possibility exists that overtraining occurred in the group that performed both types of training simultaneously. Conversely, in the group training for strength and endurance, improvement in aerobic capacity was not compromised compared with the group performing only endurance training.

Five years later Dudley and Djamil (1985) used a more conventional frequency of training and found decrements only in the magnitude of increase in angle-specific peak torque at fast velocities of movement (160°/s-278°/s) in a group simultaneously trained for strength and endurance as compared with a group trained only for strength. No decrements in angle-specific peak torque were observed at slow velocities of movement (48°/s-96°/s) in the group that simultaneously trained for strength and endurance. This study was the first investigation to suggest that it may in fact be power output that is affected by concurrent training, even over a short training period. Again, aerobic power of the combination-training group was not compromised compared with a group trained for endurance only. These conclusions are supported by Hunter, Demment, and Miller (1987), who examined simultaneous resistance and endurance training over 12 wk of training. Barbell squats were emphasized in this training program. An increase in strength of 39% was observed in the strength-only group, while the combined group's strength increased by 24%. No impairment of maximal oxygen consumption was observed in the combined group, but strength at high velocities of movement was compromised in an endurance-only training group.

These early studies started an interest in the physiological compatibility of simultaneous strength and endurance training. Using various experimental protocols to explore adaptational responses to concurrent strength and endurance training, studies have shown that strength can be either compromised (Hennessy and Watson 1994; G.A. Nelson et al. 1990) or increased (Bell et al. 1991b; Hortobágyi, Katch, and LaChance 1991; Sale et al. 1990), while observed endurance capabilities are not affected. Other studies report that both strength and endurance capabilities can be attenuated, especially over longer periods of concurrent training or in trained athletes (Hennessy and Watson 1994; Nelson et al. 1990). Hennessy and Watson (1994) clearly demonstrated that strength, power, and speed performance are susceptible to "incompatibility" because of the high intensity and volume of training performed by highly trained athletes.

Recently, McCarthy et al. (1995) examined the effect of simultaneous strength and endurance training using a more realistic and typical 3 d/wk routine for both training methods. The strength training program consisted of four sets of five to seven repetitions of eight exercises, and the endurance protocol consisted of 50 min of cycle exercise at 70% of the heart-rate reserve. A strength-only, an endurance-only, and a combined group trained for 10 wk. Subjects who performed the strength-only training or both types of training increased their 1-RM squat, bench press, vertical jump, maximal isometric knee-extension strength, and fat-free mass. The endurance group demonstrated no changes in these variables but did increase peak oxygen consumption, as did the combined-training group. The results of this study demonstrate that conventional training frequencies and programs are in fact compatible and further indicate that overtraining may be the ultimate cause of exercise incompatibility. Thus, the compatibility of concurrent strength and endurance training may depend on many factors, such as training status, training intensity, and training volume.

Almost all the studies have used men as subjects, and only a limited amount of data are available on this issue for women. But in a study by Volpe and colleagues (1993) previously sedentary college-age women used conventional strength training (periodized program) and endurance training (75% of predicted maximal heart rate) programs for 3 d/wk over 9 wk; no incompatibility was observed for strength or endurance performances. One interpretation of these results is that training status does affect whether concurrent strength and endurance training are incompatible.

Cellular Changes

Few cellular data are available to provide insights into changes at the muscle fiber level with concurrent strength and endurance training (G.A. Nelson et al. 1990; Sale et al. 1990). The muscle fiber is faced with the dilemma of trying to adapt to the oxidative stimulus to improve its aerobic function and to the stimulus from the heavy resistance training program to improve its force production ability. So what happens in the muscle fiber population? Kraemer and colleagues (1995) examined changes in muscle fiber morphology over a 3-mo training program in physically fit males. Training took place 4 d/wk for 3 mo. Both high-intensity strength and endurance training programs were varied throughout the week to provide a periodized training program to enhance recovery from a high-volume exercise program and so prevent overtraining (i.e., a decrease in performance). The weight training program used two "heavy" days (i.e., 5 RM) and two "moderate" days (10 RM) per week, and the endurance training program utilized two "interval training" days and two "long-duration" run days per week. Five subject groups were used to evaluate muscle fiber changes in the vastus lateralis muscle, with training as follows: The strength (S) group performed a total-body strength training program, the combined (C) group performed the same total-body strength training program but also performed a high-intensity endurance training program, the upper-body (UB) group performed only an upper-body strength training program and the high-intensity endurance training program, the endurance (E) group performed only the high-intensity endurance training, and a control group performed no training.

The data from the muscle fiber profile is depicted in figure 4.5 and presented in table 4.3. All training groups had a shift of muscle fiber types from Type IIB to Type IIA. It is doubtful that the remaining Type IIB fibers were true Type IIB fibers, because no Type IIAB subtype fibers were analyzed. Ploutz and colleagues (1994) have shown that if Type IIAB fibers are not detected after high-intensity resistance training, the remaining Type IIB fibers have a high concentration of aerobic enzymes and therefore may not be true IIB fibers. In this study the number of Type IIB muscle fibers was lower after high-intensity strength training (group S) than after high-intensity endurance training including interval training (group E). This may have been caused by the greater recruitment of high-threshold motor units with heavy resistance training.

From an aerobic perspective it is interesting to note the small but significant changes in the Type IIC population of muscle fibers. Also, the use of just upper-body strength training appears to mitigate the decreases in Type I muscle fiber size in the legs with endurance training (UB group). This may be caused by the isometric muscle actions of the legs needed to support the upper body during resistance exercise. Changes in muscle fiber cross-sectional areas occurred differentially across the continuum of exercise training modalities and were dictated by the type or combination of training stimuli to which the muscle was exposed. It is interesting to note that the muscle fiber adaptations observed in the C group were different from those of either the S or the E groups. This indicates that the adaptive response at the level of the muscle fiber when two high-intensity training programs are used, with one focusing on high-intensity endurance training and the other on high-intensity strength training, is not the same as when a single

training mode is used. In this study lower-body power was compromised in the C group, and the rate of strength development tended toward a compromised state in the C group as well. However, the response of the UB group clearly indicated that upper-body strength training is not affected by lower-body endurance training. Thus, training two different muscle groups, one for endurance and one for strength, can be done successfully. Consistent with several other studies, maximum oxygen consumption was not diminished by the performance of both high-intensity strength and endurance training programs (Dudley and Djamil 1985; McCarthy et al. 1995). Thus, the mechanisms of adaptation to resistance exercise depend on the global exercise stimuli presented to the activated musculature. In addition, concurrent training will begin to negatively affect strength increases in 2 to 3 mo. It appears that a differential response to the simultaneous training occurred at the cellular level and that single training modes result in different muscle fiber changes than those observed with concurrent training.

The physiological mechanisms that mediate adaptational responses to concurrent training remain speculative but appear related to alterations in neural recruitment patterns, attenuation of muscle hypertrophy, or both (Dudley and Djamil 1985; Chromiak and Mulvaney 1990; Dudley and Fleck 1987). Such physiological attenuation may in fact result in overtraining (i.e., a decrease in performance) with longer periods of training (Hennessy and Watson 1994; G.A. Nelson et al. 1990). Conversely, if concurrent exercise training is properly designed, it may require only a longer time for the summation of physiological adaptations. It

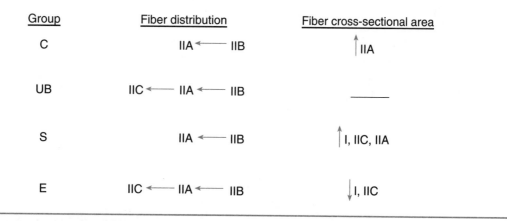

Fig. 4.5 Fiber-type changes with different training combinations.

Adapted, by permission, from W.J. Kraemer, J. Patton, S.E. Gordon, E.A. Harman, M.R. Deschenes, K. Reynolds, R.U. Newton, N.T. Triplett, and J.E. Dziados, 1995, "Compatibility of high intensity strength and endurance training on hormonal and skeletal muscle adaptations," *Journal of Applied Physiology* 78 (3):976-89.

TABLE 4.3
Muscle Fiber Characteristics Pre- and Posttraining

Group		C		S		E		UB		Control	
		Pre	Post	Pre	Post	Pre	Post	Pre	Post	Pre	Post
% Type I		55.6 (±11.1)	57.7 (±11.1)	55.21 (±11.7)	55.44 (±11.5)	54.1 (±5.9)	54.6 (±5.3)	50.6 (±8.0)	51.1 (±7.9)	52.0 (±11.5)	52.8 (±10.8)
	IIC	1.9 (±2.2)	1.8 (±2.7)	2.4 (±1.6)	2.0 (±1.3)	0.9 (±0.6)	2.5* (±2.0)	1.3 (±1.0)	3.0* (±2.2)	1.6 (±0.9)	1.3 (±1.3)
	IIA	28.4 (±15.4)	39.4* (±11.1)	23.3 (±11.5)	40.5* (±10.6)	25.75 (±4.8)	34.1 (±3.9)	25.5 (±4.2)	34.2* (±6.9)	25.6 (±1.6)	26.6 (±4.6)
	IIB	14.11 (±7.2)	1.6* (±0.8)	19.1 (±7.9)	1.9* (±0.8)	19.2 (±3.6)	8.8* (±4.4)	22.6 (±4.9)	11.6* (±5.3)	20.8 (±7.6)	19.2 (±6.4)
Area (µm²)	I	5008 (±874)	4756 (±692)	4883 (±1286)	5460* (±1214)	5437 (±970)	4853* (±966)	5680 (±535)	5376 (±702)	4946 (±1309)	5177 (±1344)
	IIC	4157 (±983)	4658 (±771)	3981.2 (±1535)	5301* (±1956)	2741 (±482)	2402* (±352)	3050 (±930)	2918 (±1086)	3733 (±1285)	4062 (±1094)
	IIA	5862 (±997)	7039* (±1151)	6084 (±1339)	7527* (±1981)	6782 (±1267)	6287 (±385)	6393 (±1109)	6357 (±1140)	6310 (±593)	6407 (±423)
	IIB	5190 (±712)	4886 (±1171)	5795 (±1495)	6078 (±2604)	6325 (±1860)	4953 (±1405)	6052 (±1890)	5855 (±867)	5917 (±896)	6120 (±1089)

Means (±SD)

Note. C = combined, S = strength, E = endurance, UB = upper body combined

* = $p \leq .05$ from corresponding pretraining value

Adapted, by permission, from W.J. Kraemer et al., 1995. "Compatibility of high intensity strength and endurance training on hormonal and skeletal muscle adaptations," *Journal of Applied Physiology* 78 (3):976-89.

appears that one cannot have optimal adaptation to both modes of training, because the programs needed to effectively alter high fitness levels may not be compatible. Thus, priority training programs may be important when several fitness components must be trained at the same time.

A multitude of factors (e.g., exercise prescriptions, pretraining fitness levels, exercise modalities) can affect the exercise stimulus and therefore the subsequent adaptational responses (Chromiak and Mulvaney 1990; Dudley and Fleck 1987; Sale et al. 1990). The majority of studies in the literature have utilized relatively untrained subjects to examine the physiological effects of simultaneous strength and endurance training (Chromiak and Mulvaney 1990; Dudley and Fleck 1987). Few data are available regarding the effects of simultaneous strength and endurance training using previously active or fit individuals who are able to tolerate much higher intensity exercise training programs (Hennessy and Watson 1994). Thus, there is a need for more study

of this topic, especially concerning the effect of concurrent training on trained individuals and females.

Endurance Sports and Concurrent Training

MacDougall and colleagues (1979) demonstrated that mitochondrial volume density in the triceps muscle decreased following a high-intensity strength training program. Because mitochondria are the site of aerobic energy production, any decrease in the volume density of mitochondria could theoretically decrease the oxidative capacity of the muscle. Thus, because of the results of this study, many distance runners do not perform resistance training, fearing it will compromise their endurance capabilities. A decrease in mitochondrial density from resistance training would appear to support this belief. Yet one of the most consistent findings of concurrent training studies has been that even heavy resistance training does not impair endurance performance. However, in a concurrent training study Kraemer and colleagues (1995) observed that the magnitude of gain in maximal oxygen consumption tended to decrease.

Many distance runners have overreacted to the information concerning mitochondrial density by eliminating resistance exercise from their training regimens. They fail to recognize that resistance training offers other benefits, such as injury prevention and the reduction of overuse phenomena. It is obvious that if protein is being removed from a muscle fiber, as was the case in the study by Kraemer and colleagues (1995) for the Type I and IIC muscle fibers with high-intensity endurance running, connective tissue is also lost. Over time, these factors may result in injury and decreased performance. Thus, resistance training programs that use moderate intensities (12-15 RM) and emphasize injury prevention are appropriate for distance runners and do not affect endurance performance. At present, the vast majority of the limited data indicates that resistance training does not compromise development of aerobic power.

It is possible that, in a sport that depends almost exclusively on one of the three energy sources, training of a second energy source may retard the development of the primary energy source. For example, distance runners depend heavily on the oxygen energy source, and training the ATP-PC energy source using resistance training may compromise the development of the oxygen energy source over long training periods (years). For the same reason, weight lifters may not wish to heavily train the oxygen energy source. It is still unknown whether the impairment of one energy source by developing another is caused by overtraining resulting from the high volume and intensity necessary to train simultaneously for endurance and strength or by some underlying physiological mechanism. It should be pointed out that many sports do not depend on only one energy source (Fox and Mathews 1981). The needs analyses of individuals in these sports dictate training multiple energy sources. In this case the compatibility question may be irrelevant, and research should center on the mixture of strength and endurance training that will cause the greatest possible gains in both parameters when simultaneous training must be performed.

Exercise Prescription Guidelines

Exercise prescription must take into consideration the demands of the total program and make sure

the volume of exercise does not become counterproductive to optimal physiological adaptations and performance. This requires the following:

- Prioritizing the training program and the goals of training. High-intensity, high-volume strength and endurance training should not be performed together.
- Allowing for adequate recovery from training sessions by using periodized training programs and planned rest phases.
- Limiting high-intensity aerobic training for strength/power athletes. Strength/power athletes can perform lower-intensity aerobic training, but the high oxidative stress accompanying high-volume or high-intensity endurance training appears to negatively affect power development.

ANAEROBIC SPRINT AND INTERVAL TRAINING

Many sports involve a large anaerobic component. Athletic performance also usually entails a large motor skill component. An individual therefore has to address both the skill and the conditioning components to be successful. We discuss training adaptations associated with resistance exercise in chapter 7. In this chapter we address other anaerobic training guidelines.

In addition to resistance training, other anaerobic training that is sport specific may be necessary. Some examples are sprinting for football and sprint swimming for water polo. This type of training enhances both the motor skill and conditioning component needed for performance in a particular sport. Thus, to improve sport performance, sport-specific movement needs to be performed in addition to resistance training. Anaerobic training adaptations are similar to those observed for resistance training (Burke, Thayer, and Belcamino 1994; Howald 1982) and are discussed in chapter 7.

Interval Training

Conditioning is necessary to enhance speed or anaerobic endurance. Sprint activities of a few seconds require a higher power output than do longer-duration sprints of 1 to 2 min (Wilmore and Costill 1994). Training needs to be related to both the distance and the duration of the activity performed in the particular sport. For a football lineman, 5- to 20-yd sprints (1-3 s) are appropriate, whereas a receiver may need to train using sprint distances ranging from 10 to 60 yd. An 800-m sprinter would need to train at distances and paces equivalent to the distance and pace needed in a race (Wilt 1968). An 800-m training program involves interval training, which emphasizes anaerobic and aerobic conditioning, both of which are needed for success in this activity. It is important to differentiate between quality sprint training for maximal speed versus quantity sprint conditioning for speed endurance.

Sprint Workouts

Sprint workouts should be performed 1 to 5 d/wk depending on the sport and the training cycle (e.g., in-season soccer vs. preseason track sprinting). A sprint workout includes

- warm-up,
- flexibility exercise,
- form running drills,
- start drills,
- a conditioning phase, and
- cool-down.

It is interesting to note from the data of Callister and colleagues (1988) that sprint training performed 3 d/wk (set 1: 3 × 100 yd [91.4 m]; set 2: 3 × 50 yd [45.7 m]) with a rest interval of 4 min 30 s between each sprint and 5 min between sets) resulted in increases in sprint speed but no increase in maximal oxygen consumption over an 8-wk training program. Conversely, when two sets of four 20-s sprint intervals are separated by only 1 min of rest, significant increases in maximal oxygen consumption were observed by the eighth week of a 10-wk training program (Kraemer, Patton, et al. 1989). Thus, the exercise-to-rest ratio

is a vital factor in determining the effects of sprint intervals on increases in maximal oxygen consumption or sprint speed. The old concept of an aerobic base (e.g., the need to develop aerobic capability prior to anaerobic capability) is not necessary, because one can achieve changes in the maximal oxygen consumption with sprint intervals when the exercise-to-rest ratio is low. It is important that the progression is appropriate so the trainees can tolerate the exercise, which is a function of the exercise volume and intensity and the exercise-to-rest ratio used in the sprint interval program.

Shorter sprint training involves all-out exercise intensity. As the duration of the activity increases to longer sprint distances (e.g., 800 m), pace becomes important and can be learned through interval training. Interval training can also be designed to address the aerobic metabolism necessary to perform longer sprints (Fox and Mathews 1981). Figure 4.6 depicts a power-unit workout. The power-unit workout is a symmetrical form of interval training. It consists of long units (distances longer than the race itself), short units (40 to 60 m), and kick units (approximate distances used for the kick in a race). Track coaches use the power-unit workout to promote the development of race speed. The long units develop endurance at the race distance, and the short units help to develop leg speed. This program is typically performed during the preseason and in-season on straightaways. An adequate endurance-conditioning base must be attained before initiating such high-intensity workouts.

The importance of tolerating the high lactate levels associated with different sport activities (e.g., longer-duration sprinting and wrestling) necessitates training that increases lactate production and in turn enhances lactate removal (Brooks and Fahey 1984). Exercise intervals shorter than 20 s do not

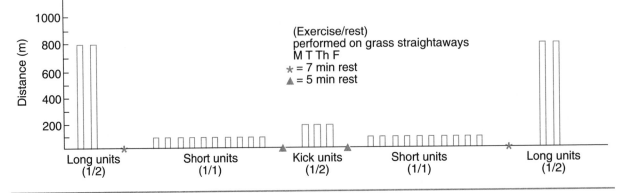

Fig. 4.6 Sample power-unit workout for development of aerobic and anaerobic capabilities.

TABLE 4.4				
General Guidelines for Interval Training				
Exercise duration (min:s)	Intensity (%)	Recovery (min:s)	Number of intervals	Sessions per week
0:05	100	0:05	20-30	2-4
0:10	100	0:10	20-30	2-4
0:20	100	0:15	10-20	2-4
0:30	100	1:00-2:00	8-18	2-4
1:00	95-100	3:00-5:00	5-15	2-4
2:00	90-100	5:00-15:00	4-10	2-4
3:00	80-90	5:00-15:00	3-8	2-4

D.R. Lamb, *Physiology of exercise: Responses and adaptations*, © 1978. All rights reserved. Reprinted by permission of Allyn & Bacon.

result in anaerobic energy source depletion when used with a recovery interval of a similar duration (Lamb 1978). This allows repeating short sprints at a near maximal velocity but requires that recovery time between sprint distances be carefully controlled (table 4.4). For example, a sprint workout to develop anaerobic endurance for basketball might include a 5-s exercise duration. From table 4.4 it is clear that each sprint has to be run at 100% intensity and that only a 5-s recovery period between sprints should be allowed. Twenty to 30 intervals are required two to four times per week.

Another method of determining a training pace for sprint intervals is based on the individual's 2-mi (3.2-k) run time (table 4.5). Using this type of estimation one can determine the pace of the intervals as a function of the current best 2-mi run time. As with any exercise conditioning program it is important that good clinical decisions are made about the progress of a workout, and it is important that athletes listen to their bodies.

FLEXIBILITY TRAINING

Flexibility is an important component of physical fitness and needs to be addressed in a resistance training program. Stretching can be performed in both the warm-up and cool-down phases of a training session. There are four basic types of stretching techniques (Hutton 1992; Moore and Hutton 1980):

- Static stretching
- Dynamic or ballistic stretching
- Slow movements

- Proprioceptive neuromuscular facilitation (PNF) techniques

Deciding which technique to employ in a program depends on the amount of time available for stretching, the effectiveness of the flexibility technique, and the availability of a training partner.

Static Stretching

The most common type of stretching is the static stretching technique. This form of stretching involves a voluntary, complete relaxation of the muscle while it is elongated. This technique has become popular because it is easy to learn, effective, and accompanied by minimal soreness or injury (Moore and Hutton 1980).

Static stretching is still one of the most effective and desirable techniques to use when comfort and limited training time are major factors in the implementation of a stretching program (Moore and Hutton 1980). This technique involves holding the muscle in a static position at the desired length. Many variations of this technique have been proposed with stretch time ranging up to 60 s. Typically a muscle is stretched 10 to 20 s, and the stretch repeated two to three times. An example of this technique is the toe touch. In this exercise a person bends over and tries to touch his or her toes while keeping the knees straight. The movement is held where minimal discomfort is experienced. It is important that stretching be performed progressively. On each repetition the individual tries to reach further to extend the range of movement and holds the stretch at that point in the range of movement

TABLE 4.5
General Guidelines for Initial Pace Speeds

Total 2-mi run time (min)	Time for interval distance (min)		70% $\dot{V}O_2$max
	90%-100% $\dot{V}O_2$max		
	440 yd	880 yd	1 mi
10	1:15	2:30	6:50
11	1:22.5	2:45	7:30
12	1:30	3:00	8:00
13	1:37.5	3:15	8:40
14	1:45	3:30	9:20
15	1:52.5	3:45	10:00
16	2:00	4:00	10:40
17	2:07.5	4:15	11:20
18	2:15	4:30	12:00
19	2:22.5	4:45	12:50
20	2:30	5:00	13:20
21	2:37.5	5:15	14:00
22	2:45	5:30	14:40

Based on 2-mi run time and percentage of the maximal oxygen consumption for distance and interval run programs.

Adapted, by permission, from W.J. Kraemer et al., 1987, "The effects of various physical training programs on short duration high intensity load bearing performance and the Army physical fitness test," *USARIEM Technical Report* 30/87 August.

where only minimal discomfort is experienced. Subsequent stretching continues to improve the range of motion.

Ballistic Stretching

Ballistic stretching involves a bouncing or bobbing movement during the stretch; the final position in the movement is not held. Ballistic stretching is unpopular because of the increased amount of delayed muscle soreness and the possibility of injury during the stretching exercise (DeVries 1980). This type of exercise might be more appropriate to use as part of a dynamic warm-up after a static stretch has been performed. The exact value of ballistic stretching techniques prior to activity remains unclear, and caution must be taken to eliminate delayed muscle soreness and the possibility of injury.

Slow Movements

Slow movements of a muscle or muscles, such as neck rotations, arm rotations, and trunk rotations, are also a type of stretching activity. This type of

stretching technique may be more important in warm-up activities than in achieving increases in flexibility. It might provide a better dynamic technique than ballistic stretching in warm-up activities.

Proprioceptive Neuromuscular Facilitation Techniques

Proprioceptive neuromuscular facilitation (PNF) stretching techniques have increased in popularity over the last 10 years as a method of improving flexibility (Cornelius 1985; Shellock and Prentice 1985; Cornelius et al. 1992). A number of different PNF procedures have been proposed, including contract-relax and contract–relax agonist–contract (Moore and Hutton 1980). The theoretical basis of these techniques is that the voluntary action of the agonist muscle will provide neural activation resulting in reciprocal inhibition of the antagonist muscle, thus allowing greater range of motion. Some studies have shown PNF to be more effective than other types of flexibility training. Etnyre and Lee (1988) made a comparative examination of static stretching and PNF techniques in men and women. After 12 wk of training they found that all groups had improved in flexibility. Women had greater range of motion than men throughout the program, but their comparative increases were not greater than those of the men. PNF techniques were more effective than static stretching for increasing the range of motion for both hip flexion and shoulder extension for both genders. Men showed better results with the contract–relax agonist–contract method, whereas women showed no differences among PNF methods.

There are several variations of PNF techniques, but there are three major types of PNF stretching techniques (Shellock and Prentice 1985):

- Slow reversal–hold
- Contract-relax
- Hold-relax

Using the hamstring stretch as an example, the slow reversal–hold technique is performed as follows. The trainee lies on his or her back with the knee extended and the ankle flexed to 90°; a partner pushes on the leg, passively flexing the hip joint until slight discomfort is felt in the hamstring. The individual then pushes for 10 s against the partner's resistance by activating the hamstring muscle. The hamstring muscles are then relaxed and the antagonist quadriceps muscles are activated, while the partner applies force for 10 s to further stretch the hamstrings. The leg should move so there is increased hip joint flexion. All muscles are then relaxed for 10 s, after which time the stretch is repeated beginning at this new joint angle. This sequence is typically repeated at least three times.

The other two commonly used PNF techniques are similar to the slow reversal–hold method. The contract-relax technique involves a dynamic concentric action prior to the relaxation/stretch phase. The hold-relax technique uses an isometric action prior to the relaxation/stretch phase.

Osternig and colleagues (1990) examined acute changes in 10 high-intensity athletes, 10 endurance athletes, and 10 control subjects and demonstrated that the agonist contract–relax procedure produced 89% to 110% greater hamstring EMG activity and 9% to 13% more knee-joint range of motion than the contract-relax or stretch-relax PNF methods, respectively. Endurance athletes had 58% and 113% greater EMG activity in the hamstrings compared with the high-intensity and control groups, respectively. However, it is interesting to note that the

endurance athletes attained significantly less range of motion than the other two groups in all cases. Short-term, high-intensity activity may necessitate less hamstring resistance to knee extension than long-term endurance training (Osternig et al. 1990). It was also concluded that decreases in muscle activity may not be related to increases in joint range of motion and that factors other than muscle relaxation are important in achieving increased range of motion. The differential effects of different stretch techniques need to be considered for different athletic groups so that any stretch-induced injury can be avoided. Understanding the various stretching techniques is vital to their proper use and application (for review see Etnyre and Lee 1987).

The different PNF techniques have been studied by Moore and Hutton (1980). PNF has not proved to be superior to static stretching in all studies. Each technique is capable of improving flexibility. Individuals must be well motivated and have the time to perform PNF stretching. Except for the hold-relax technique, PNF methods require a partner. Furthermore, a period of time is required for individuals to learn such techniques. Moore and Hutton suggested that, unless an individual is willing to tolerate the greater discomfort associated with PNF training, the use of static stretching is more appropriate.

Flexibility and Resistance Training

Being muscle-bound is often associated in people's minds with resistance training. Some individuals and coaches believe that resistance training results in a decrease in flexibility. Little scientific or empirical evidence supports this contention (Todd 1985). As early as 1956 Massey and Chaudet demonstrated that heavy resistance training does not cause a decrease in flexibility. Thrash and Kelly (1987) examined the effects of weight training on the range of motion of the ankle, trunk, and shoulder joints. Flexibility was determined before and after an 11-wk, three-times-per-week weight training program in which all of the major muscle groups were exercised for three sets of eight repetitions at 8 RM. The results showed significant increases in ankle dorsiflexion and shoulder extension without any additional flexibility training. Thus, the authors concluded that a weight training program to develop muscular strength would not impair flexibility and might enhance certain ranges of motion.

Beedle, Jessee, and Stone (1991) found differences in flexibility related to the type of training program performed (e.g., weight lifting vs. power lifting) among athletes who weight train. Olympic weight lifters and even control subjects had greater flexibility on five flexibility measures than power lifters, indicating that power lifting may result in muscle-size increases that can partially limit range of motion (e.g., chest size so big that one cannot touch elbows in front) (Kraemer and Koziris 1994). Such data support the contention that lifting alone may not promote flexibility. Thus, flexibility training may need to be performed in addition to some type of resistance training program (Hurley 1995). Conversely, it is interesting to note that ballet dancers improved their functional range of voluntary movement, which enhanced the aesthetics of their dance movements, with the addition of a resistance training program (Stalder, Noble, and Wilkerson 1990). Although flexibility training may extend the functional range of motion, control of that range of motion is a function of strength and power development. These two training types appear to be complementary in certain situations.

Heavy resistance training typically results in either an improvement or no change in flexibility (Massey and Chaudet 1956). Competitive weight lifters possess average or above-average flexibility of most joints (Leighton 1955, 1957b; Beedle, Jessee, and Stone 1991). Olympic weight lifters in a descriptive study of several groups of athletes were observed to be second only to gymnasts in a composite flexibility score (Jensen and Fisher 1979) and had better scores than power lifters or control subjects (Beedle, Jessee, and Stone 1991). It appears that resistance training does not have to result in a loss of flexibility but that flexibility training programs may be needed to enhance the range of motion. Furthermore, as muscle hypertrophy becomes extreme, joint-specific range of motion flexibility training might need to be added, and required ranges of motion monitored.

Nevertheless, it must be pointed out that in some cases limited flexibility in range of motion may provide a competitive advantage for certain performances (e.g., power lifters in the bench press) (Kraemer and Koziris 1994). It appears that competitive power lifters have limited flexibility that may be caused by the competitive task, especially in the upper body (e.g., bench press) (Beedle, Jessee, and Stone 1991; Chang, Buschbacker, and Edlich 1988). Typically, however, care should be taken to stress the full range of motion of both the agonist and antagonist muscle groups and to choose exercises that strengthen both the agonists and antagonists of a joint to ensure balanced strength between

both sides of the joint. By following these guidelines, flexibility can be increased or maintained at its present level.

INTEGRATING THE FITNESS COMPONENTS

Muscular strength, flexibility, cardiovascular endurance, and local muscular endurance all play various roles in health fitness and sports performance. Training for sports performance is considerably different from training for health and fitness. Also, better sports performance is not always associated with better health. This is especially true as performances progress toward an elite level and risk of injury is high because of the high training volume and intensity.

Developing an overall conditioning program that addresses each fitness component is necessary. The needs analysis facilitates the determination of the time and effort that needs to be spent on a specific fitness component. Although certain data suggest that some incompatibility exists between different fitness components, proper modification of the exercise program makes it possible to address each component. The shot put champion may not spend a great deal of time performing cardiovascular endurance exercises but may perform cardiovascular conditioning 3 d/wk for 20 to 30 min to assist anaerobic recovery, to maintain remedial aerobic fitness levels, or both. Conversely, the champion cross-country runner may not perform a high volume of resistance training but may work out in the weight room twice a week for 20 to 30 min with exercises for the ankles, quadriceps, hamstrings, shoulders, and back to help prevent injury and improve postural muscle strength.

The art and science of successful exercise prescription involves understanding all the following points:

- Goals and objectives of training (needs analysis)
- Fitness level of the individual (exercise testing)
- Variables involved with prescription and stimulus-effect relationships of the exercise stimuli
- Training adaptations associated with different exercise stimuli
- Psychological ability to perform the exercise (interaction and training observations)

SUMMARY

Proper exercise prescription can result in the successful design of exercise programs that address the specific component(s) of physical fitness needed by the individual for health, fitness, and performance. The program emphasis will shift according to the specific needs of the individual. It is important to understand, however, that no one form of training (e.g., resistance training) can produce all the required training effects for every sport or individual. This chapter addressed how to develop a total conditioning program. How to individualize the resistance training program is discussed in the next chapter.

SELECTED READINGS

American College of Sports Medicine. 1990. The recommended quantity and quality of exercise for developing and maintaining cardiorespiratory muscular fitness in healthy adults. *Medicine and Science in Sports and Exercise* 22:265-74.

Chromiak, J.A., and Mulvaney, D.R. 1990. A review: The effects of combined strength and endurance training on strength development. *Journal of Applied Sport Science Research* 4:55-60.

Dudley, G.A., and Fleck, S.J. 1987. Strength and endurance training: Are they mutually exclusive? *Sports Medicine* 4:79-85.

Hennessy, L.C., and Watson, A.W.S. 1994. The interference effects of training for strength and endurance simultaneously. *Journal of Strength and Conditioning Research* 8:12-19.

Hutton, R.S. 1992. Neuromuscular basis of stretching exercises. In *Strength and power in sport,* ed. P.V. Komi, 29-38. Oxford: Blackwell Scientific.

Osternig, L.R.; Robertson, R.N.; Troxel, R.K.; and Hansen, P. 1990. Differential responses to proprioceptive neuromuscular facilitation (PNF) stretch techniques. *Medicine and Science in Sports and Exercise* 22:106-11.

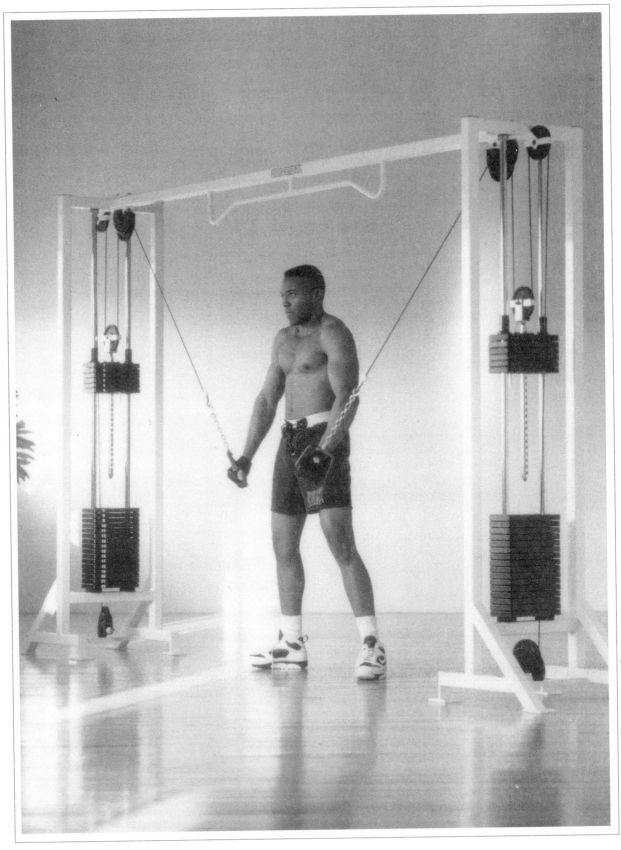

PART II

RESISTANCE TRAINING AND EXERCISE PRESCRIPTION

any factors need to be considered in designing a resistance training program to successfully meet the needs and goals of the trainee. If the trainee is preparing for a sport or particular activity, a general program for that sport is developed. The general program for the sport must then be individualized, however, to address the strengths and weaknesses of each trainee. Chapter 5 examines factors that must be considered when individualizing a resistance training program. Chapter 6 discusses various types of resistance training that can be used to meet the needs of a team or trainee. In chapter 7 adaptations to resistance training are discussed. Knowledge of the body's adaptations to training is useful in understanding how to best design programs to meet an individual's needs and goals. Chapter 8 discusses detraining, or the changes that take place when training is reduced or stopped. Knowledge of detraining is useful in developing programs that will maintain training adaptations for as long as possible. The information contained in part II will help you to design individualized resistance training programs.

CHAPTER 5

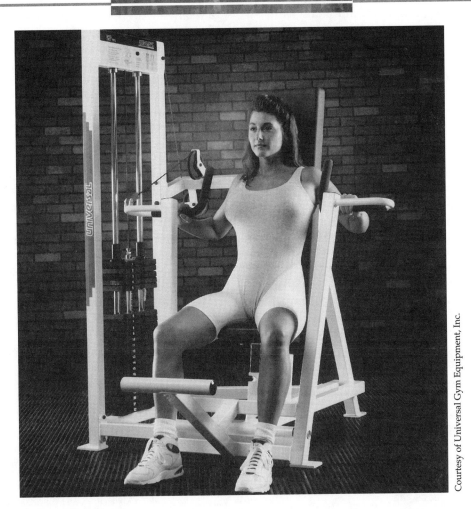

Courtesy of Universal Gym Equipment, Inc.

Individualizing Exercise Prescriptions

P rograms of the future will be completely individualized. This will promote optimal training adaptations. Furthermore, research attempting to identify program differences will need to be conducted over longer periods of time (> 6 mo) to allow for individual responses and to differentiate program characteristics. Individual differences in the magnitude of an adaptational response to a given exercise stimulus support the need for individualized programs. For example, if a group of 30 people perform three sets of 10 RM of the bench press exercise for 3 mo, the percentage gains in 1-RM strength will differ among individuals in the group. Their progression of resistances over the training period will vary. Such results can be empirically observed by monitoring the training progress of lifters or by examining data from scientific investigations. People respond differently to the same training program. Thus, general programs written for fitness, sports, or other activities should be viewed only as a starting point for an individual program.

The key to improved program design is the identification of specific variables that need to be controlled in order to better predict the training outcomes. The most challenging aspect of resistance training exercise prescription is making decisions related to the development and changes of an individual's training goals and program design. One is faced with making appropriate changes in the resistance training program over time. This means that sound clinical or coaching decisions must be made based on factual understanding of resistance training, the needs of the sport or activity, individual training responses, and testing data. Therefore, planning and changing the exercise prescription is vital for the success of any resistance training program (figure 5.1).

Understanding resistance training exercise prescription allows for better quantification of the exercise stimulus. Planning ranges from the development of a single training session to the variation of the program over time. The ability to better quantify the workout and evaluate the progress made toward a specific training goal are the basic hallmarks of solid program design, which leads to optimal physical development.

Resistance training programs have for many years been shrouded in mystery and intrigue. Expected gains are often unrealistic. Teachers and coaches of resistance training are often asked, "What is the best resistance training program?" This is a tough question because the best program is really related to the training goals of the individual. Training goals are related to the specific types of adaptations desired. Thus, the "best" program does not really exist, unless it is designed to meet the needs and goals of a specific individual.

The gains made in any variable related to muscular performance are linked to an individual's genetic potential. If an individual starts to train in a relatively deconditioned state (at the bottom of the curve in figure 5.2), the initial gains are great because of a large adaptational potential that exists. It is apparent that almost any program might work for an untrained individual in the early phases of training. As training proceeds, gains decrease as the trainee approaches his or her genetic potential (at the top of the curve). Understanding this concept is important to understanding the adaptations and changes that occur over time.

This concept can be called the *window of adaptation,* meaning that at the start of training the opportunity for change in a specific variable (e.g., 1 RM in the bench press) can be great. The window of adaptation may be small at the end of a training program or at the start of a training program if the individual already has a high level of adaptation or fitness in a particular variable because of prior training. Thus, training expectations must be kept in perspective. Gains will be related to an individual's potential for adaptation and fitness level. It is also important to note that all adaptations, such as strength and muscle hypertrophy, are not on the same time line of development (see chapter 7).

In highly trained athletes the gains made may be quite small or difficult to measure over short training periods (e.g., 8-12 wk). In a study by J.R. Hoffman and colleagues (1990), college football players chose among different frequencies of train-

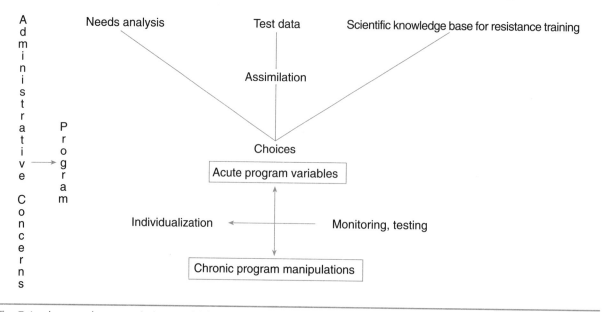

Fig. 5.1   An exercise-prescription model for resistance training.

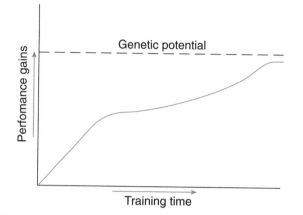

Fig. 5.2 A theoretical training curve. Notice that at the start of a training program large gains in fitness are made quickly. After this period of rapid initial fitness gains, further improvement occurs at a slower rate.

ing per week over a 10-wk off-season conditioning program. The groups that chose 3, 4, and 6 d/wk made no gains in 1-RM bench press (table 5.1). It can be speculated that the 3-d/wk program was not a sufficient stimulus to elicit significant strength increases in already conditioned football players who had already participated in an intensive heavy resistance training program. The lack of changes in 1-RM bench press strength for players using a 6-d/wk program may have been caused by the development of an overtraining syndrome. Squat 1 RM improved for all groups but the 3-d/wk group. These data indicate that the length of the training program, the fitness level of the athlete in a particular lift or performance task, and the frequency of training can all influence the training adaptations. The expectation of large continual strength gains in the same exercise (e.g., bench press) by some athletes is unrealistic.

SETTING AND EVALUATING GOALS

Common program goals in resistance training are improvements in function, such as increased

TABLE 5.1
Results of Performance and Anthropometric Testing in College Football Players Using a Selected Frequency of Training

Variable	Test	3 d	4 d	5 d	6 d
BW (kg)	Pre	80.3±5.1	94.2±12.7	99.2±14.4	112.3±12.4
	Post	79.6±6.4	93.1±12.0*	98.7±13.7	111.0±12.1
BP (kg)	Pre	107.2±11.6	127.7±13.9	131.1±20.1	143.9±12.0
	Post	109.1±28.7	132.2±14.5	135.3±9.0*	149.7±17.3
SQ (kg)	Pre	140.1±18.6	173.6±36.2	170.6±19.4	191.6±34.9
	Post	147.4±38.9	186.3±31.9*	183.4±22.1*	204.1±39.5*
40 (s)	Pre	4.83±0.14	5.01±0.22	4.97±0.23	5.23±0.20
	Post	4.82±0.19	4.97±0.18	4.93±0.24	5.18±0.20
VJ (cm)	Pre	70.2±7.7	65.9±8.4	64.5±8.6	59.9±6.7
	Post	71.1±7.6	66.0±8.8	66.0±7.9	62.5±7.1
2 MI (s)	Pre	933.1±49.7	945.0±61.3	960.8±99.3	982.2±65.0
	Post	811.1±77.1*	830.7±55.5*	834.2±84.8*	879.8±68.7*
SF (mm)	Pre	54.7±12.2	79.7±15.3	83.6±20.0	100.3±13.0
	Post	50.9±10.5*	72.9±12.7*	79.0±19.7*	92.4±15.2*
TH (cm)	Pre	56.0±2.5	59.5±4.6	59.8±4.6	63.9±3.4
	Post	56.7±1.6	61.4±3.5*	61.5±4.2*	65.0±3.2
CH (cm)	Pre	92.8±3.9	103.3±7.2	105.9±8.4	111.9±7.1
	Post	94.8±3.1*	105.5±6.9*	107.1±8.2*	112.3±6.1

$* = p < 0.05$

BW = body weight, BP = bench press, SQ = squat, 40 = 40-yd sprint, VJ = vertical jump, 2 MI = 2-mi run, SF = sum of skinfolds, TH = thigh circumference, CH = chest circumference

Adapted, by permission, from Hoffman, J.R. *Journal of Applied Sport Science Research* (1990) 4 (3):80 Table 6.

muscular strength, power, and local muscular endurance (Kraemer and Koziris 1992). Other functional gains, such as an increase in coordination, agility, balance, and speed, are also common goals of a program. It is becoming clear that such factors as balance may also have implications for injury prevention by limiting falls in older individuals. Physiological changes related to increased body mass through muscle hypertrophy and improvement of other physiological functions such as decreased blood pressure, decreased body fat, and increased metabolic rate to help burn calories may be goals of athletes as well as fitness enthusiasts. Resistance training affects almost every physiological function and has the ability to enhance physical development and performance at all ages (Kraemer et al. 1990).

For the most part, training goals or objectives should be testable variables (e.g., 1-RM strength, vertical jump height) so their achievement can be objectively judged. A workout log is invaluable in evaluating the effects of various resistance training programs. Formal strength tests to determine functional changes in strength can be done on a variety of equipment, including isokinetic dynamometers, free weights, and machines (Knuttgen and Kraemer 1987). The results of these objective tests can help in determining how to modify the exercise program to reach training goals or develop new goals.

It should be noted here that improved athletic performance and health are distinct goals. Many elite athletes do things in their training programs for performance gains that far exceed what is needed for good health (e.g., lifting 7 d/wk, running 150 mi in a week, or training 4-6 hr/d). Therefore, goals in resistance training have to be put into the context of the needed outcome for the individual. Factors such as age, physical maturity, training history, and psychological and physical tolerance need to be considered in any goal development process or individual program design. Better decisions about the use of training time must be made to achieve goals that directly influence performance in the sport or activity. This is what makes an optimal program design.

MAINTENANCE OF TRAINING GOALS

A concept called *capping* may need to be applied to various training situations where small gains will require very large amounts of time to achieve and

in the long run are not necessary. Capping is deciding not to spend large amounts of training time to bring about a physiological change that is not needed for fitness or performance. These gains may be related to performance (e.g., bench press 1-RM strength) or some form of physical development (e.g., calf size). At some point, a value judgment about how to best spend training time must be made. This is a tough decision that comes only after an adequate period of training and determination of the realistic potential for further change for a particular variable. A maintenance training program is begun when the decision is made not to add any further training time to develop a particular characteristic (e.g., strength, size, power). Thus, more training time is available to address other training goals. Ultimately this decision may result in greater total development of the individual.

In sports many examples of training overkill can be found. For example, while the continued development of whole-body power is important in football, an exercise such as the bench press may not be a good measure of playing ability (Fry and Kraemer 1991). The physical attributes needed to bench press a great amount of weight are a large, muscular torso—including a large chest and large back musculature—and short arms. Large upper-body musculature is a positive attribute for football players because of the sport's dependence on body mass. However, because of the need for taller players—especially linemen—in today's game, few elite football players have the short arms needed for great success in the bench press.

Should the bench press lift be used as a part of the exercise prescription for football players? It should, but the expectations for and performance of that lift for each individual football player must be kept in perspective. Furthermore, its safe performance without injuring the shoulder is a concern. Thus, each player's individual physical dimensions must be considered when developing short-term (e.g., bench press strength after a 10-wk summer conditioning program) and especially long-term (e.g., bench press strength increase from freshman to senior year) goal development. Furthermore, the importance of the bench press to sport performance should also be evaluated. Spending extra time on the bench press to gain an extra 10 or 20 lb (4.5 or 9.1 kg) in the lift at the cost of not training, for example, hang-cleans, which help develop structural power vital for performance in football, would be an unwise use of training time (Barker et al. 1993; Fry and Kraemer 1991). For example, a player has been training for over a year and his bench press 1 RM is 355 lb (161 kg). The extra training time needed to achieve a 400-lb (181.4-kg) bench press may be best used instead to train another lift (e.g., hang-cleans) or sprint speed. Furthermore, the player may not have the physical dimensions (e.g., short arms) needed for a 400-lb bench press. Maintenance training of the bench press may be called for in this case.

Such a training decision is one of the many clinical or coaching decisions that must be made when monitoring the progress of resistance training programs. Are the training goals realistic in relationship to the sport or health enhancement being trained for? Is the attainment of a particular training goal vital to the program's success? These are difficult questions that need to be continually asked in the goal-development phase of each training cycle for any program.

UNREALISTIC GOALS

Careful attention must be paid to the magnitude of the performance goal and the amount of training time needed to achieve it. While scientific studies may last up to 6 mo, most real life training programs are developed as a part of an individual's sports career or whole life. Goals change, and resistance training programs must change to reflect these changing goals.

Too often goals are open ended and unrealistic. For many men the 23-in. (58.4-cm) upper arm, 36-in. (91.4-cm) thighs, 20-in.(50.8-cm) neck, 50-in.(127-cm) chest, or 400-lb (181.4-kg) bench press are unrealistic goals because of most men's genetic limitations to such extreme performance and muscle size. Women too can develop unrealistic goals, frequently in their desire for drastic decreases in limb size and body shape. Again, such changes may not be possible for many women because of a genetically determined larger anatomical structure. Many women mistakenly believe large gains in strength, muscle definition, and body fat loss can be achieved through the use of very light resistance training programs (e.g., 2- to 5-lb [0.9- to 2.3-kg] hand-held weights), in an attempt to "spot build" a particular body part or muscle. Although "spot hypertrophy" of a particular body part is possible, it is not accomplished with resistances this light. Ultimately, for both men and women setting realistic goals is a question of whether the resistance training program utilized can result in the desired body changes. The desired changes must be carefully and honestly examined.

Unrealistic expectations can also develop when equipment and programs are not evaluated using sound scientific principles. In today's "high-tech" and "big hype" marketing of products, programs, and equipment, training expectations can develop that are unrealistic for the average person. Movie actors, models, and elite athletes can project desirable body images and performance levels, but for most people such high levels of physical development and performance are unrealistic. Proper goal development is accomplished by starting out small, making progress, and then evaluating where the individual is and what is now possible. Most people make mistakes in goal development by wanting too much too soon with too little effort expended. Making progress in a resistance training program depends on a long-term commitment to a total training program. In addition, proper nutrition and lifestyle behaviors can help support training objectives and physical development. Careful evaluation of training goals and objectives and the equipment needed to achieve them can eliminate wasted time, money, and effort.

INDIVIDUALIZATION

Each program must be designed to meet the individual's needs and training goals. It is especially important that the individual's fitness level be evaluated and understood by the individual, teacher, personal trainer, and coach. It is important to remember that evaluation of a fitness level (e.g., 1-RM strength test) is typically not done until it is known that the individual can tolerate the test demands and that the data generated is meaningful (Kraemer and Fry 1995). One of the most serious mistakes made in designing a workout is placing too much stress on the individual before it can be tolerated. A coach or personal trainer must be sensitive to an individual's starting fitness level and ability to tolerate the exercise stress, including any exercise testing. Progress in a resistance training program should follow the staircase principle (figure 5.3). An individual begins a training session at a particular strength level. During the training session strength decreases because of fatigue; at the conclusion of the session strength is at its lowest point. After recovering from the first session the individual should begin the next training session at a slightly higher strength level. This staircase process should be repeated for each training session. Designing training programs that allow this staircase effect is the biggest challenge in the field of resistance training.

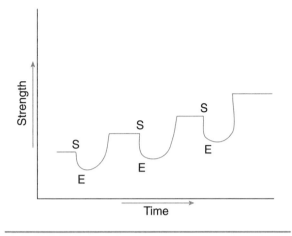

Fig. 5.3 A resistance training program should allow for a staircase effect. *S* and *E* designate the start and end of a workout, respectively.

When designing training programs for an athletic team, it is common to design one program for all team members to perform. Again, generalized programs will not produce the same results in all individuals. Thus, a general program written for a particular sport should be viewed as a starting point for each individual. Program changes and progression should be based on the needs of each athlete. Additions or deletions to a general program are often needed to address individual athletes' developmental goals that are not addressed in the general program. With the greater use of computers, improved monitoring and program feedback for achieving truly individualized resistance training programs is becoming more prevalent and easier.

EXERCISE PRESCRIPTION

Resistance training exercise prescription for a long time has been more of an art than a science, yet the science is a vital part of the whole process. The teacher, personal trainer, or coach must make program decisions based on a sound rationale. Therefore, the prescription of any exercise requires a solid understanding of the underlying scientific principles involved. Such knowledge will assist in the development of better resistance training programs and a logical development of successive training sessions. The developmental process of program design is presented in this chapter. The basic questions involved in the manipulation of training variables must be addressed. The specific combination of choices made for each training variable will determine the type of exercise stimulus presented to the body.

The major resistance training program design components are

- needs analysis,
- acute program variables,
- chronic program manipulations, and
- administrative concerns.

Each of these components is discussed in the following sections in the context of designing resistance training programs.

NEEDS ANALYSIS

A needs analysis consists of answering some initial questions that affect the other three program design components (Kraemer 1983a; figure 5.4). It is important that time be taken to examine these questions.

These are the major questions in a needs analysis:

1. What muscle groups need to be trained?
2. What are the basic energy sources (e.g., anaerobic, aerobic) that need to be trained?
3. What type of muscle action (e.g., isometric, eccentric) should be used?
4. What are the primary sites of injury for the particular sport or prior injury history of the individual?

What Muscles Need to Be Trained?

The first question requires an examination of the muscles and the specific joint angles to be trained. For any activity, including a sport, this involves a basic analysis of the movements performed and the most common sites of injury. With the proper equipment and a background in basic biomechanics a more definitive approach to this question is possible. With the use of a slow-motion videotape, the coach can better evaluate specific aspects of movements and can conduct a qualitative analysis of the muscles, angles, velocities, and forces involved. The decisions made at this stage help define one of the acute program variables: choice of exercise.

Specificity is a major tenet in resistance training and is based on the concept that the exercises and resistances used result in training adaptations that transfer to better performance in sport or daily activity. Resistance training is used, as it is often dif-

Needs analysis

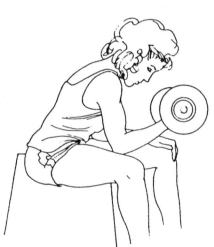

Exercise movements
• Specific muscles
• Joint angles
• Contraction mode
• Loading needs

Metabolism used estimated % contribution from:
• ATP-PC source
• Lactic acid source
• Oxygen source

Injury prevention
• Most common sites of possible injury
• Sites of previous injury

Acute program variables

1. Choice of exercise
   • Structural
   • Body part
   • Contraction mode

2. Order of exercise
   • Large muscle group first
   • Small muscle group first (pre-exhaust)
   • Arm to leg or arm-arm, leg-leg

3. Number of sets

4. Rest periods
   • Short < 1 minute
   • Moderate 1 to 3 minutes
   • Long > 3 minutes

5. Load (intensity)

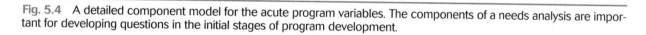

Fig. 5.4 A detailed component model for the acute program variables. The components of a needs analysis are important for developing questions in the initial stages of program development.

ficult if not impossible to overload sport movements without risk of injury or dramatically altering sport skill technique. Specificity assumes that muscles must be trained similarly to the sport or activity in terms of

• the joint around which movement occurs,

• the joint's range of motion,

• the pattern of resistance throughout the range of motion,

• the pattern of limb velocity throughout the range of motion, and

• the types of limb movement (concentric, eccentric, or isometric).

Resistance training for any sport or activity should include a full range of motion exercises around all the major joints of the body. However, training designed for specific sport or activity movements should also be included in the workout to maximize the contribution of strength training to performance. The best way to select such exercises is to quantitatively analyze the biomechanics of the sport or physical activity and to match it to exercises according to the aforementioned variables. Few such analyses of sports or activities have been done to date. Yet biomechanical principles can be used in a qualitative manner by an interested athlete or coach to intelligently select exercises. Through the use of slow-motion videotapes, the following steps allow a physical activity to be roughly analyzed in terms of the variables listed previously. Dr. Everett Harman, a biomechanist for the U.S. Army Research Institute of Environmental Medicine, has developed the following steps to be used for this purpose.

1. View a videotape of an athletic performance or activity.

2. Select a movement that appears to involve high-intensity physical exertion critical to the performance (e.g., the impact of two football linemen, the drive portion of a sprint stride, the push-off in a high jump).

3. Identify the body joints around which the most intense muscular actions occur. Running and jumping, for example, involve intense muscle actions at the knee, hip, and ankle. Intense exertion does not necessarily involve movement. Considerable isometric force may have to be applied to keep a body joint from flexing or extending under external stress.

4. Determine whether the movement is concentric, isometric, or eccentric. While force is being produced or applied externally, the muscle shortens during a concentric muscle action, is held at a constant length during an isometric muscle action, and is lengthened during an eccentric muscle action.

5. For each joint identified in step 3, determine the range of angular motion. Measure the angle between the two body segments adjacent to the joint with a protractor. See how the joint angle changes through the movement. Record the range of motion.

6. Try to determine where the most intense effort occurs in the range of motion around each particular body joint. Sometimes facial grimaces or tense muscles seen on videotape can help identify points of peak intensity. Record the joint angle of peak intensity.

7. Estimate the velocity of movement in the early, middle, and late phases in the range of motion. For videotape the time between frames in seconds is 1 divided by the frame rate. For example, if the rate is 30 frames per second, the interval time is 1/30 or 0.033 s. The angular velocity of a motion equals degrees traveled divided by total time. For example, if the limb moves 5° in 3 frames, the movement speed is 5/(3 × 0.033) = 50°/s.

8. Select exercises to match the limb ranges of motion and angular velocities, making sure that the exercises are appropriately concentric, isometric, or eccentric. As an example, in a jump takeoff the supporting leg usually bends, allowing elastic energy to be stored. Training for this part of the movement could be accomplished by a form of eccentric training. In the jump, after the knee reaches its smallest angle and the jumper begins to extend the leg for takeoff, high-intensity concentric contraction occurs at slow speed. To train for that part of the movement, the athlete can perform concentric actions through the specific range of joint motion using heavy weights at slow speed. To train for a faster part of the movement, use lighter weights at higher speeds for the specific range of motion. Stretch-shortening cycle training, with or without weight, could also be used to simulate the complete stretch-shortening cycle of a jump.

9. It is best for the exercise to be most difficult at the point in the range of motion where intensity during the target activity is greatest. This can be accomplished by trial and error or by using the principle that during a lifting movement involving little acceleration, the greatest resistance to movement around a joint occurs when the limb is horizontal and the weight is furthest from the joint's center of rotation (for example, around the midpoint of an arm curl movement). The most commonly performed weight exercises can be modified to locate peak tension at a desired joint angle. A basic exercise like the arm curl can be done standing or bending over or on a preacher bench to modify the angle of peak tension. To apply additional force to a muscle at a particular point in the range of angular motion, the athlete can attempt to accelerate the weight as the limb travels through the target range of motion.

Ideally, this analysis is followed up in the weight room with appropriate resistance exercises that train the specific muscles and joint angles involved. For general fitness and muscular development, all the major muscle groups of the body are usually trained.

Each exercise and resistance used in a program will transfer to another activity or sport to different degrees. The transfer specificity of a training program for improved health and well being is more related to its effects on medical variables (e.g., cholesterol levels) than to physical performance. The concept of transfer specificity is unclear to many coaches and health and fitness professionals. Every training activity has a percentage of carry-over to other activities. Except for practicing the specific task or sport itself, no conditioning activity has 100% carry-over. Some activities have a higher percentage of carry-over than others because of similarities in neuromuscular recruitment patterns, energy sources, and biomechanical characteristics. Yet most of the time the sport or activity cannot be overloaded to provide the needed effect on the neuromuscular system, which is why resistance training is used in the training process. The optimal training program maximizes carry-over to the sport or activity for which an individual is training.

What Energy Sources Need to Be Trained?

Performance of every sport or activity uses all three energy sources (Fox 1979). The energy sources to be trained have a major impact on the program design. Resistance training is usually more appropriate for enhancing anaerobic energy sources (ATP-PC and lactic acid sources) than for aerobic energy sources.

What Type of Muscle Action Should Be Used?

Decisions regarding the use of isometric, dynamic concentric, dynamic eccentric, and isokinetic exercise modalities are important in the preliminary stages of planning a resistance training program for sport, fitness, or rehabilitation. The basic biomechanical analysis previously described is used to decide what muscles to train and to identify the types of muscle action involved in the activity. Most resistance training programs use several types of muscle action. One factor that separates elite power lifters from less competitive power lifters is the rate at which the load is lowered in the squat and bench press. Elite power lifters lower the weight more slowly than less competitive lifters, even though the former use greater resistances. In this case some eccentric training may be advantageous for competitive power lifters. As another example, many holds in wrestling involve isometric muscle actions of various muscle groups. Therefore some isomet-

ric training may help in the conditioning of wrestlers.

What Are the Primary Sites of Injury?

It is important to determine the primary sites of injury in a sport and to understand the prior injury profile of the individual. The prescription of resistance training exercises is intended to enhance the strength and function of tissue so that it better resists injury and recovers faster when injured and to reduce the extent of damage related to an injury. The term *prehabilitation* has become popular to refer to the prevention of injury by training the joints and muscles that are most susceptible to injury in an activity, unlike *rehabilitation*, which deals with injuries after they occur. The prevention of reinjury is also an important goal of a resistance training program. Thus, understanding the sport's or activity's typical injury profile (e.g., knees in American football) and the individual's prior injury history can help in properly designing a resistance training program.

ACUTE PROGRAM VARIABLES

After the needs analysis has been completed, a specific training program is designed that addresses the exact needs of the individual. Acute program variables concern the design of one specific training session. Chronic program manipulations concern the changes made in the acute program variables over time. Changes in the acute program variables make up the progression plan for an entire training period. Periods of training are now planned many months or several years in advance, which has made periodization of training a vital feature in the manipulation of acute program variables in chronic program design.

Kraemer (1983b) developed an approach to evaluating a specific set of variables for each workout. Using statistical analyses, five specific variables that contribute to making various workouts different were determined. The acute program variables describe all possible single training sessions. By examining each of the variables in figure 5.4 and making decisions about them, a training session is designed. An almost infinite number of workout protocols can be created by manipulating the acute program variables. The choices made regarding each variable determine the training session.

Choice of Exercise

The number of possible joint angles and exercises is as limitless as the body's functional movements. A change in angle affects which muscle tissue is activated. Using magnetic resonance imaging (MRI) technology, Dr. Gary Dudley at the University of Georgia and Dr. Tesch at the Karolinska Institute in Sweden (Tesch and Dudley 1994) have shown that changes in the type of resistance exercise used cause changes in the activation pattern of the muscle. Muscle tissue that is not activated (i.e., no tension develops in the fiber) will not benefit from the resistance exercise. Exercises should be selected that stress the muscles and joint angles designated by the needs analysis. Exercises can be designated as primary exercises and assistance exercises. Primary exercises train the prime movers in a particular movement. They are typically major muscle group exercises (e.g., squat, bench press, hang-pulls). Assistance exercises train smaller muscle groups and aid in the movement produced by the prime movers (e.g., triceps press, lat pull-down, biceps curl).

Exercises can also be classified as structural (i.e., multijoint) or body part–specific (i.e., involving an isolated joint). Structural exercises include whole-body lifts that require the coordinated action of many muscle groups. Power cleans, power snatches, deadlifts, and squats are good examples of structural whole-body exercises. Exercises can also be classified as multiple-joint exercises, or exercises where movement occurs at more than one joint. For example, the bench press, which involves movement of both the elbow and shoulder joints, is a multijoint exercise. Some examples of other multijoint exercises are lat pull-downs, military presses, and leg presses. Most primary exercises can also be called structural exercises.

Exercises that isolate a particular muscle group are considered body-part or single-joint exercises. Biceps curls, sit-ups, knee extensions, and knee curls are good examples of isolated body-part exercises. Most assistance exercises can be classified as body-part exercises.

Structural or multijoint exercises require neural communication between muscles and promote coordinated use of multijoint movements. It is especially important to include structural and multijoint exercises in a program when whole-body strength movements are required for a particular activity, such as football, basketball, wrestling, and track and field. In these sports whole-body strength or power movements are the basis of success in blocking, tackling, jumping, takedowns, and throwing. Often structural exercises involve advanced lifting techniques (e.g., power cleans, power snatches), which require additional coaching beyond simple movement patterns. Teachers and coaches should have experience teaching these lifts or locate someone who does (e.g., a United States Weightlifting Club coach) before including them in a training program. For the individual interested in basic fitness, structural exercises may be advantageous only when training time is limited and it is necessary to train more than one muscle group at a time. The time economy achieved with structural and multijoint exercises is an important consideration for an individual or team with a limited amount of time per training session.

Order of Exercise

For many years large–muscle group exercises have been performed prior to exercising the smaller muscle groups in resistance training programs. It has been theorized that by exercising the larger muscle groups first, the greatest possible training stimulus is presented to all of the muscles involved in an exercise. This is also the theory behind performing structural or multijoint exercises (e.g., power cleans) before single-joint exercises (e.g., biceps curls). The rationale behind this exercise order is that the exercises performed in the beginning of the workout are the ones that require the greatest amount of muscle mass to perform. Thus, this ordering scheme focuses on gaining a greater training effect for the large muscle groups.

If structural exercises are performed early in the workout, more resistance can be used because fatigue is limited. To examine this concept, the authors compared the workout logs of 50 football players when squats were placed in the beginning of the workout with those when squats were placed at the end of the workout. Significantly heavier resistances (195 ± 35 kg vs. 189 ± 31 kg) were used by the players on heavy days (3 to 5 RM) when the squats were performed first. These observations can be explained by many factors, such as not enough rest prior to the last exercise, rest periods that are too short between sets and exercises, a dramatically greater amount of exercise (in this case 22 to 30 sets) performed prior to the squat, psychological fatigue, or greater physiological fatigue before the exercise.

Contrary to the preceding exercise order, different types of preexhaustion methods have been used by body builders in the United States and by weight lifters in the former Soviet Bloc countries in their training. These methods reverse the order of the exercises so that the small muscle groups are exercised before the larger muscle groups. An example is performing knee-extension and -flexion exercises followed by squats. Another method of preexhaustion involves fatiguing synergistic or stabilizing muscles before performing the primary exercise movement. An example of this strategy is performing lat pull-downs or military presses prior to performing the bench press. It is theorized that the fatigued smaller muscles will contribute less to the movement of later exercises, thereby placing greater stress on the large muscle groups. Often the result is just less resistance in the large–muscle group exercise, as observed in the preceding example. The advantages and disadvantages of preexhaustion exercise orders in optimizing strength and power gains remain anecdotal and need further direct study. However, some data exist to indicate that fatigue may stimulate strength development. Rooney, Herbert, and Balnave (1994) showed that continuous repetitions resulted in greater strength gains than when rest was taken between repetitions. Thus, accumulation of fatigue may be a physiological signal for adaptations such as increased muscle mass. How this finding relates to preexhaustion techniques remains to be studied.

The priority system is another method that has been used extensively in resistance training. Using the priority system, exercises that are most important to meeting the goals of the program are performed early in the session. This system allows the trainee to concentrate effort on the priority exercises and so increase the chance of adaptation to these exercises. Each exercise in a training session can be listed in order. The priority system will help the athlete to focus on the specific goals for each training session and eliminate excessive fatigue during the performance of the priority exercises.

A corollary of the priority system is that power exercises (e.g., power cleans, plyometrics) should be performed early in a session. This allows the lifter to develop and train maximal power before becoming fatigued, which would limit development of maximal power. In some instances, however, power exercises may be performed later in the session. For example, in basketball it is important that athletes not only have a high vertical jump, but also be able to jump during the fourth quarter when fatigued. In this instance, power exercises may be performed later in the session to train the ability to develop maximal power (e.g., vertical jump ability) in a fatigued state.

Another consideration is placing exercises that are being taught or practiced (especially complex movements) in the beginning of the exercise order.

For example, if an athlete is learning how to perform power cleans, this exercise would be placed in the beginning of the workout so motor skill performance is not inhibited by fatigue.

The ordering of exercises is also an important consideration in various types of circuit weight training protocols. The question of whether one follows a leg exercise with another leg exercise or whether it is appropriate to proceed to another muscle group must be addressed. The concept of preexhaustion can come into play here. Arm-to-leg ordering allows for some recovery of the arm muscles while the leg muscles are exercised. This is the most common order used in designing circuit weight training programs. Beginning lifters are less tolerant of preexhaustion, arm-to-arm and leg-to-leg exercise ordering, or stacking exercises for a particular muscle group because of high blood lactate concentrations (10-14 mmol/L), especially when rest periods between exercises are short (10 s to 60 s) (Kraemer et al. 1990; Kraemer, Gordon, et al. 1991). Stacking exercises is a common practice among elite body builders as a way to attempt to bring about muscle hypertrophy.

One final consideration for exercise order is the fitness level of the individual. As discussed earlier, training sessions should never be designed to be too stressful for an individual, especially a beginning trainee, and therefore not allow the staircase effect. The exercise order can have a significant impact on the training stimulus stress level in a training session.

Number of Sets

The number of sets used in a workout is directly related to training results. Typically, three to six sets are used to achieve optimal gains in strength when using a total body program. It has been suggested that multiple-set systems work best for development of strength and local muscular endurance (Atha 1981) and that the gains will be made at a faster rate than gains achieved through single-set systems (McDonagh and Davies 1984). The importance of resistance exercise volume (sets × repetitions) for strength and especially for muscle size gains during the early phases of a program have been demonstrated over long-term training programs (Dudley et al. 1991).

The use of a single set of an exercise is effective for individuals who are untrained or just starting a resistance training program. One-set programs might also be used for maintenance programs. Strength changes are not different among one, two, or three sets of 10 to 12 RM during the first several months of training by untrained individuals when the programs are not periodized (Graves et al. 1988). When a single set is compared to a multiple-set periodized program, however, significantly superior results are observed with the multiple-set periodized program (figure 5.5). In more highly trained athletes, strength gains are not achieved with low-volume, single-set training programs (table 5.2; Kraemer in press; Stowers et al. 1983; Willoughby 1993). Therefore, the use of one or two sets of an exercise may be more appropriate for beginners in the initial stages of a base program (first 6 to 12 workouts), for circuit weight training protocols, or for short-term, in-season programs for athletes. It is important to note that low-volume (single-set) programs may increase strength in un-

trained individuals, but more complex physiological adaptations (e.g., hypertrophy beyond initial changes) and performance increases may require higher-volume training for optimal results.

Multiple sets of an exercise present a training stimulus to the muscle during each set. Once initial fitness has been achieved, multiple presentations of the stimulus (three to six sets) using the desired resistance with specific rest periods between sets are superior to a single presentation of the stimulus. That a muscle or muscle group can only perform maximal exercise for a single set has not been demonstrated. In fact, sets at the same 10-RM load can be repeated using the same resistance with as little as 1-min rest by highly trained body builders (Kraemer, Noble, Culver, and Clark 1987).

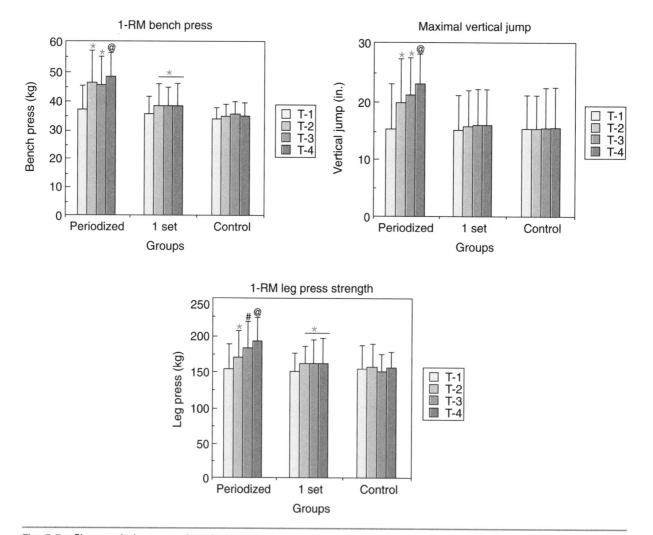

Fig. 5.5   Changes in leg press, bench press, and vertical jump performance in female tennis players using one-set or periodized multiple-set training programs. Courtesy of Dr. Kraemer's laboratory.

T-1 = pretraining, T-2 = 4 mo, T-3 = 6 mo, and T-4 = 9 mo

* = significantly (p ≤ 0.05) different from T-1
# = significantly different from T-1 and T-2
@ = significantly different from T-1, T-2, and T-3

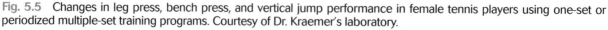

TABLE 5.2
Muscle Strength Changes in NCAA Division I College Football Players in the Leg Press (lbs)

	Pretest	Posttest
Multiple-set group	385±95	455±96*
Single-set group	389±87	399±78

All players participated in an in-season program up to the start of the 10-wk off-season study period.

* $p < .05$ from corresponding pretest

Adapted, by permission, from W.J. Kraemer, in press, "A series of studies: The physiological basis for strength training in American football: Fact over philosophy," *Journal of Strength and Conditioning Research.*

Exercise volume (sets × repetitions × intensity) is a vital concept in training progression. Exercise volume is especially important for individuals who have already achieved a basic level of training fitness or strength. The interaction of the number of sets with variation in training, or more specifically *periodized training,* may also help augment training adaptations. The time course of volume changes is important to the change in the exercise stimulus in periodized training. A constant-volume program may lead to staleness and lack of adherence to training.

Rest Periods Between Sets and Exercises

One frequently overlooked variable in exercise prescription is the length of the rest periods between sets and exercises. Recently the influence that rest periods have in dictating the stress of the workout and in influencing the amount of resistance that can be used has been shown. Rest periods between sets and exercises influence how much of the ATP-PC energy source is recovered and how high lactate concentrations are in the blood.

In studies by Kraemer, Noble, Culver, and Clark (1987), Kraemer et al. (1990, 1993), and Kraemer, Gordon, et al. (1991), the dramatic influence of rest periods on blood lactate, hormonal concentrations, and metabolic responses to resistance-exercise protocols was demonstrated in both men and women. In figure 5.6 the response of blood lactate to two different exercise protocols is shown for both men and women. Each workout consisted of eight exercises performed with either a 5- or 10-RM resistance. Sets and exercises were separated by rest periods of either 1 or 3 min.

The S workout consisted of using a 5-RM resistance for all exercises with 3 min of rest between sets and exercises. The H workout consisted of 10-RM exercise with a 1-min rest between sets and exercises. Comparisons of the S and H workouts

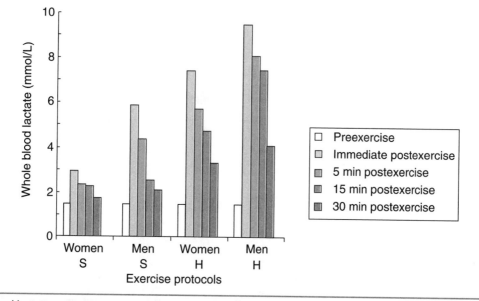

Fig. 5.6 Blood lactate responses to a strength protocol (S) (5 RM, eight exercises, 3-min rest between sets and exercise) and to a short-rest, body-building, hypertrophy protocol (H) (10 RM, eight exercises, 1-min rest between sets and exercise).

Adapted, by permission, from W.J. Kraemer, L. Marchitelli, D. McCurry, R. Mello, J.E. Dziados, E. Harman, P. Frykman, S.E. Gordon, and S.J. Fleck, 1990, "Hormonal and growth factor responses to heavy resistance exercise," *Journal of Applied Physiology* 69:1442-50; and from W.J. Kraemer, S.J. Fleck, J.E. Dziados, E.A. Harman, L.J. Marchitelli, S.E. Gordon, R. Mello, P.N. Frykman, L.P. Koziris, and N.T. Triplett, 1993, "Changes in hormonal concentrations following different heavy resistance exercise protocols in women," *Journal of Applied Physiology* 75:594-604.

demonstrate the dramatic effect rest periods have on blood lactate concentrations. Short rest periods significantly elevate blood lactate concentrations compared with longer rest periods. The effects of rest periods between sets and exercises and of total work performed on blood lactate concentrations are the same for both genders.

These studies indicate that heavier resistance does not result in higher blood lactate concentrations. It is the amount of work performed and the duration of the force demands placed on the muscle that determine the blood lactate concentrations. The 10-RM resistance allows a higher number of repetitions and longer sets, and exercise still takes place at a relatively high percentage of the 1 RM (75% to 85% of 1 RM), which results in higher blood lactate concentrations.

From a practical standpoint it has been demonstrated that short-rest programs can cause greater psychological anxiety and fatigue (Tharion et al. 1991). This might be caused by greater effort, more discomfort, and metabolic demands (e.g., high lactate production). The psychological ramifications of using short-rest workouts must be carefully considered when designing a training session. The increased anxiety appears to be caused by the dramatic metabolic demands characteristic of short-rest workouts (i.e., 1-min or less rest). While the psychological demands are higher, the changes in mood states do not constitute abnormal psychological changes and may be a part of the arousal process before a demanding workout.

The frequent use of workouts with short rest periods and heavy resistances should be slowly introduced into a training program as the acid-base buffer mechanisms in the body adapt to increased muscle and blood acid levels (decreased pH) (S.E. Gordon, Kraemer, and Pedro 1991). If such adaptations are vital to a sport (e.g., wrestling or 400- to 800-m track events), however, the training protocol must progress from long to short rest periods for better performance in these sports. Usually such a program is performed within the context of a more classic strength/power training program for a sport (e.g., two high-lactate workouts and two strength/power workouts in a week cycle) or as a preseason program for 8 to 12 wk prior to the start of the season.

Short rest periods are characteristic of circuit weight training, but the resistances used are typically lighter (i.e., 40% to 60% of 1 RM) (Gettman and Pollock 1981). This type of training session does not result in blood lactate concentrations as high as those of short-rest-period 10-RM sessions (figure 5.7).

Lactic acid may not be the "bad guy" we have

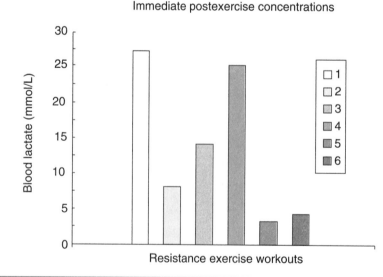

Immediate postexercise concentrations

Fig. 5.7 Postexercise blood lactate responses to different workouts: (1) body-building workout, (2) low-intensity circuit weight training, (3) high-intensity circuit weight training, (4) short-rest, high-intensity workout, (5) power lifting, (6) Olympic weight lifting.

Data from W.J. Kraemer, B.J. Noble, B.W. Culver, and M.J. Clark, 1987, "Physiologic responses to heavy-resistance exercise with very short rest periods," *International Journal of Sports Medicine* 8:247-52; from W.J. Kraemer, L. Marchitelli, D. McCurry, R. Mello, J.E. Dziados, E. Harman, P. Frykman, S.E. Gordon, and S.J. Fleck, 1990, "Hormonal and growth factor responses to heavy resistance exercise," *Journal of Applied Physiology* 69:1442-50; from L.R. Gettman and M.L. Pollock, 1981, "Circuit weight training: A critical review of its physiological benefits," *Physician and Sportsmedicine* 9:44-60; and from J. Keul, G. Haralambei, M. Bruder, and H.J. Gottstein, 1978, "The effect of weight lifting exercise on heart rate and metabolism in experienced lifters," *Medicine and Science in Sports and Exercise* 10:13-15.

always thought it to be (Brooks and Fahey 1984). Although it may contribute to fatigue, it can be utilized as a source of energy. Furthermore, it provides a relative comparison of stress and accumulative utilization of the lactic acid energy source. The type of training session, including rest periods, will determine to a great extent the amount of lactic acid that is produced and removed from the body.

If a needs analysis identifies lactic acid as the primary energy source, the rest periods may be gradually shortened to allow the buildup of blood lactate, thus encouraging an increased tolerance for and buffering of more acidic conditions. This type of training design (particularly for preseason training) may allow better tolerance for such anaerobic athletes as wrestlers, sprinters (400 to 800 m), and basketball players. Other anaerobic athletes, such as baseball players, rely primarily on the ATP-PC energy source to perform their skills. Performing resistance training programs that elevate lactic acid concentrations may not be necessary to improve performance in such sports. Careful manipulation of rest periods is essential to avoid placing inappropriate and needless stress on the individual during training. Furthermore, because of fatigue created by a high-volume, short-rest workout, it may be inappropriate to place such a workout immediately prior to a training session designed to develop skill in the sport or activity. Exceptions to this rule of thumb may be in sports such as wrestling where skills have to be performed under conditions of high lactate concentrations.

Rest Periods Between Workouts

The amount of rest required between training sessions depends on the recovery ability of the individual. Traditionally, three workouts per week with 1 d of rest between sessions were found to allow adequate recovery, especially for the novice (Atha 1981). If the resistance training is not excessive, only moderate amounts of delayed muscular soreness should be experienced 1 d after the session. The greatest amount of delayed muscular soreness results from heavy eccentric muscle actions rather than from concentric isokinetic, dynamic concentric, or isometric muscle actions (Clarkson and Tremblay 1988; Fleck and Schutt 1985; Talag 1973). As the lifter advances and is better able to tolerate resistance exercise sessions, the frequency of training can be increased. One report indicates that four days in succession per week may be superior to three alternate days in effecting increases in strength (Hunter 1985). The onset of perceived discomfort may be masked during consecutive

training sessions, and the 3-d recovery period may allow for a more complete recovery. This indicates that the interaction of stress and recovery may be more complex than previously thought.

Elite athletes may be capable of and need training frequencies of 5 d in a row to improve significantly over short periods of training (J.R. Hoffman et al. 1990). Empirically it has been observed that competitive lifters train five to seven days per week in order to achieve muscle size and strength gains (Kraemer, Noble, Culver, and Clark 1987). Training frequency per week is a function of the individual's need for exercise stimulus to cause fitness gains. It is important that the individual is able to tolerate the physical stress so that an overtraining phenomenon does not develop (Fry, Kraemer, et al. 1994). Periodized training cycles use variations in training frequency to alter and enhance the exercise stimulus and to provide for recovery. The individual's experience and physical condition as well as the amount of work performed in one training session will dictate the individual's tolerance to higher weekly training frequencies.

When consecutive-training-day sequences are used, it may be beneficial to use different exercises for the same muscle groups (e.g., bench press and incline bench press) and different resistances (e.g., 5 RM and 10 RM). Competitive lifters who train 6 or 7 d/wk have developed a greater exercise tolerance compared with beginners, who may tolerate training only 3 d/wk. When training is performed on consecutive days, it often involves the use of a split routine (different body parts exercised each day) or a split program (different exercises for the same body part performed each day). Consecutive training days should employ some type of variation. A 3 d/wk training program for all situations and sports is far from the optimal training frequency. The individual's needs and goals determine the amount of exercise required to increase a particular physiological or performance variable. Progression in frequency is also a key component of resistance training. Frequency of training will vary depending on the phase of the training cycle, the athlete's fitness level and training history, and the goals of the program. Careful choices need to be made regarding the rest between training days. These choices are based on the planned progress toward specific training goals and the tolerance of the individual to the program changes made. Excessive soreness the next morning may indicate that the exercise stress is too demanding. If this is the case, the workout resistances, sets, rest periods between

Resistance Used

The amount of resistance used for a specific exercise is probably the most important variable in resistance training (McDonagh and Davies 1984). It is the major stimulus related to changes observed in measures of strength and local muscular endurance. When designing a resistance training program, a resistance for each exercise must be chosen. The use of repetition maximums (RM) or the exact resistance that allows only a specific number of repetitions to be performed is probably the easiest method for determining a resistance. Research supports an RM continuum (figure 5.8; Anderson and Kearney 1982; Atha 1981; Clarke 1973; McDonagh and Davies 1984), which simply relates RM resistances to the broad training effects derived from their use. It appears that RM resistances of 6 or less have the greatest effect on strength measures and maximal power outputs. RM resistances of 20 and above show the greatest effect on muscular endurance measures. This continuum makes it possible to develop a particular feature of muscular performance to varying degrees over a range of RM resistances. Typically, one uses a training RM target (a single RM target, e.g., 10 RM) or an RM target zone (a range such as 3 RM to 5 RM). As the strength level of the lifter changes over time, the resistance is adjusted so a true RM target or target zone resistance is used.

Moving away from the 6-RM-or-fewer-repetitions strength stimulus zone, the gains in strength diminish until they are negligible. The strength gains achieved above 25-RM resistances are small

or nonexistent (Atha 1981) and perhaps are related to enhanced motor performance or learning effects when they occur. A variety of individual responses caused by genetic predisposition and pretraining status affect the training increases observed. But after initial gains have been made because of learning effects, heavier resistances will be needed to optimize muscle strength and size gains.

Another method of determining resistances for an exercise involves using a percentage of the 1 RM (e.g., 70% or 85% of the 1 RM). If the trainee's 1 RM for an exercise is 100 lb (45.4 kg), an 80% resistance would be 80 lb (36.3 kg). This method requires that the maximal strength in various lifts used in the training program be evaluated regularly. If 1-RM testing is not done regularly (e.g., each week), the percentage of 1 RM used in training decreases and therefore the training intensity is reduced. From a practical perspective, determination of the percentage of 1 RM for many lifts may not be administratively effective because of the amount of testing time required. Use of an RM target or RM target zone allows the individual to change resistances to stay at the RM target or within the RM target zone and thus to develop the characteristics associated with that portion of the RM continuum.

The use of percentage of 1-RM resistances is warranted for the clean and jerk, the snatch, and related competitive Olympic lifts. Since these lifts require coordinated movements and optimal power development from many muscles to result in correct lifting technique, the movements cannot be performed at a true RM or to momentary failure. The reductions in velocity and in power output experienced in the last repetition of an RM set are not conducive conditions for such structural

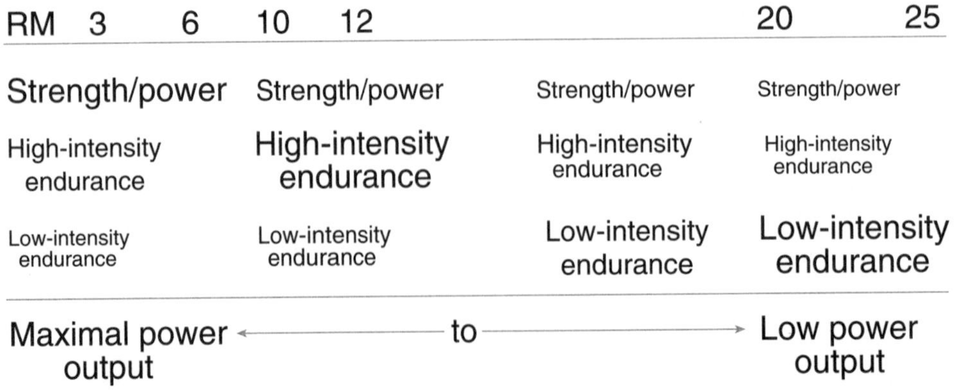

Fig. 5.8 Theoretical repetition maximum (RM) continuum.

Adapted, by permission, from S.J. Fleck and W.J. Kraemer, 1987, *Designing resistance training programs*, 1st ed. (Champaign, IL: Human Kinetics Publishers), 61.

lifts (e.g., power cleans, snatches, power snatches, hang-cleans). Therefore, percentage of the 1 RM is warranted to correctly calculate resistances for such lifts.

In two studies by Hoeger and colleagues (1987, 1990; table 5.3), the relationship between the percentage of 1 RM and the number of repetitions that can be performed was studied in both trained and untrained men and women. It was demonstrated that this relationship varies with amount of muscle mass needed to perform the exercise (i.e., leg press requires more muscle mass than knee extensions). When using machine resistances with 80% of 1 RM, previously thought to be primarily a strength-related prescription, the number of repetitions that could be performed was typically greater than 10, especially for large–muscle group exercises such as the leg press. The larger muscle group exercises appear to need much higher percentages of 1 RM to keep them in the strength RM zone of the repetition continuum.

The following example illustrates how using the percentage of 1 RM can result in a less than optimal resistance for increasing strength. A strength coach puts a sign on a leg press machine that states, "Use 80% of 1 RM for all sets." An athlete uses 80% of 1 RM and easily performs 22 repetitions. Will performing 22 repetitions per set result in optimal strength increases? Based on the RM continuum, a 22 RM is related primarily to development of local muscular endurance, not optimal development for strength and power.

The authors collected data on the number of repetitions possible in a leg press exercise in trained power lifters and untrained controls. The results showed that the power lifters could lift 80% of their 1 RM in the leg press for 22 repetitions, or a 22 RM, and the untrained controls could lift 80% of their 1 RM in the leg press for 12 repetitions, or a 12 RM. These data along with the data presented in the two important studies by Hoeger et al. (1987, 1990) clearly indicate that the method used to determine

TABLE 5.3
The Number of Repetitions That Can Be Performed With a Set Percentage of RM

	40%		60%		80%		1 RM[b]	
	$\bar{x}$	SD	$\bar{x}$	SD	$\bar{x}$	SD	$\bar{x}$	SD
Untrained males $n = 38$								
LP	80.1±7.9A[a]		33.9± 14.2A		15.2±6.5A		137.9±27.2	
LD	41.5±16.1B		19.7±6.1B		9.8±3.9B		59.9± 11.6	
BP	34.9±8.8B		19.7±4.9B		9.8±3.6B		63.9± 15.4	
KE	23.4±5.1C		15.4±4.4C		9.3±3.4BC		54.9± 13.3	
SU	21.1±7.5C		15.0±5.6C		8.3±4.1BCD		40.9± 12.6	
AC	24.3±7.0C		15.3±4.9C		7.6±3.5CD		33.2±5.9	
LC	18.6±5.7C		11.2±2.9D		6.3±2.7D		33.0±8.5	
Trained males $n = 25$								
LP	77.6±34.2A		45.5±23.5A		19.4±9.0A		167.2±43.2	
LD	42.9±16.0B		23.5±5.5B		12.2±3.72B		77.8± 15.7	
BP	38.8±8.2B		22.6±4.4B		12.2±2.87B		95.5±24.8	
KE	32.9±8.8BCD		18.3±5.6BC		11.6±4.47B		72.5± 19.8	
SU	27.1±8.76CD		18.9±6.8BC		12.2±6.42B		59.9± 15.0	
AC	35.3±11.6BC		21.3±6.2BC		11.4±4.15B		41.2±9.6	
LC	24.3±7.9D		15.4±5.9C		7.2±3.08C		38.8±7.1	

(continued)

	40%		60%		80%		1 RM[b]	
	$\bar{x}$	SD	$\bar{x}$	SD	$\bar{x}$	SD	$\bar{x}$	SD
Untrained females $n = 40$								
LP	83.6±38.6A[a]		38.0±19.2A		11.9±7.0A		85.3±16.6	
LD	45.9±19.9B		23.7±10.0B		10.0±5.6AB		29.2±5.6	
BP	—[c]		20.3±8.2B		10.3±4.2AB		27.7±23.7	
KE	19.2±5.3C		13.4±3.9C		7.9±2.9BC		26.7±7.8	
SU	20.2±11.6C		13.3±8.2C		7.1±5.2C		19.3±8.3	
AC	24.8±11.0C		13.8±5.3C		5.9±3.6C		13.8±2.7	
LC	16.4±4.4C		10.5±3.4C		5.9±2.6C		15.8±3.7	
Trained females $n = 26$								
LP	146.1±66.9A		57.3±27.9A		22.4±10.7A		107.5±16.0	
LD	81.3±41.8B		25.2±7.9CB		10.2±3.9C		34.8±6.0	
BP	—[c]		27.9±7.9B		14.3±4.4B		35.6±4.9	
KE	28.5±10.9C		16.5±5.3ED		9.4±4.3CD		40.3±10.2	
SU	34.5±16.8C		20.3±8.1CD		12.0±6.5CB		23.8±6.4	
AC	33.4±10.4C		16.3±5.0ED		6.9±3.1ED		17.3±3.8	
LC	23.2±7.7C		12.4±5.1E		5.3±2.6E		21.7±5.0	

LP = leg press (knees bent at a 100° angle for the starting position), BP = bench press, LD = lateral pull-down (resistance pulled behind the head to the base of the neck), KE = knee extension, SU = sit-up (horizontal board, feet held in place, knees at a 100° angle, and resistance held on chest), AC = arm curl (low pulley), LC = leg curl (to 90° of flexion).

[a] Letters indicate significantly different groupings, alpha level = 0.05; same letter = no difference.

[b] 1 RM expressed in kg.

[c] Data unobtainable due to resistance limitations on the Universal Gym equipment.

Adapted, by permission, from Hoeger et al. *Journal of Applied Sport Science Research* (1990) 4 (3):47-54 Tables 3 &4.

the resistance to be used for specific exercises in a training program must be carefully considered for each muscle group, for each specific type of lift, and for the exercise mode used (e.g., free-weight squat vs. leg press machine). In general, a certain percentage of the 1 RM with free-weight exercises will allow fewer repetitions than the same percentage of 1 RM on a similar exercise performed on a machine. This is most likely caused by the need for greater balance and control in space with free weights.

Often charts are used to predict the 1 RM from the number of repetitions performed with a submaximal load or to help determine an RM (e.g., from 1 to 10) from the 1-RM resistance that can be lifted. Unfortunately, most of these charts assume a linear relationship between these variables, and this is not the case. Thus, such charts and the resulting values should be used only as rough estimates of a particular RM resistance or to predict an individual's 1 RM. A variety of prediction equations are available to predict 1 RM, but these equations have the same inherent weaknesses as the prediction charts.

The configuration of the acute program variables results in the exercise stimulus for a particular workout. Workouts must be altered to meet changing training goals and to provide training variation. With this paradigm for the description of resistance exercise workouts, careful control of various components can be gained in manipulating variables to create new and optimal workout programs (Kraemer 1983a). Because so many different combinations of these variables are possible, an almost unlimited number of workouts can be developed. Understanding the influence and importance of each of the acute program variables in achieving a specific training goal is vital to creating the optimal exercise stimulus.

Table 5.4 reviews the program characteristics for some of the major resistance training goals and matches them with combinations of the acute program variables. Using the acute program variables to develop workouts that enhance certain

---

TABLE 5.4
Program Characteristics for Basic Goals in Resistance Training

1-RM strength

- Choice of exercise, the specific movement patterns, and types of muscle action needed are emphasized.
- Exercises to be emphasized are performed early in the training session.
- Heavy resistances (typically < 6 RM)
- Moderate to long rest periods (> 2 min) depending on the weight being lifted.
- Moderate to high number of sets (4-10) for the primary specific exercises (e.g., the squat), low to moderate number of sets (1-3) for assistance exercises.

Power

- Choice of exercise and the specific movement patterns for power development are typically related to multijoint structural movements (Olympic-type exercises such as power clean, hang-pulls, snatches, hang-cleans, etc.). Eccentric actions are not emphasized in these types of lifts.
- Exercises to be emphasized are performed early in training session.
- High-intensity (typically < 10 RM) resistances that are varied over time (periodized), for example: 1-5 RM, 6-10 RM, > 10 RM, yet rarely are more than 5 repetitions performed in a set, whether using a heavy, moderate, or light resistance. Power development lags behind strength. Therefore, in a specific set the number of repetitions performed will be slightly lower than the number the RM resistance allows.
- Moderate to long rest periods between sets and exercises (> 2 min).
- Moderate to high number of sets for power oriented exercises (4-10), low to moderate number of sets for assistance exercises (1-3).

Hypertrophy

- Large variety of exercise choice or movement patterns. Includes a considerable amount of isolation exercises. Concentric and eccentric actions are important. Multiple exercise angles for a joint are used.
- Large variety of exercise order. Muscles to be emphasized are exercised early in the training session.
- Moderate to high intensity (6-12 RM); higher numbers of repetitions are sometimes used, especially with super setting (back-to-back sets for the same muscle group).
- Short rest periods between sets and exercises (< 1.5 min).
- High total number of sets per muscle or muscle group (> 3).

Local muscular endurance

- Choice of exercise, the specific movement patterns, and types of muscle action needed for the sport or activity are emphasized.
- Muscles to be emphasized are exercised early in the training session.
- Low intensity (12-20 RM).
- Moderate rest periods between sets and exercises (2-3 min) for long-repetition sets (20 or greater), and short rest periods (30 to 60 s) between sets and exercises for lower-repetition sets (12-19).
- Moderate number of sets (2-3).

Adapted from W.J. Kraemer and L.P. Koziris, 1992, "Muscle strength training: Techniques and considerations," *Physical Therapy Practice*, 2:54-68.

characteristics is vital to physical development. It is also possible to train different muscles or muscle groups in different ways, resulting in workout programs that are a combination of the factors presented in table 5.4. For example, it is possible to train the chest musculature for 1-RM strength while training the leg musculature for power and the abdominal muscles for local muscular endurance. Proper manipulation of the acute program goals in developing a single workout or changing the workout over time (chronic program manipulations) are the basis of successful program design.

CHRONIC PROGRAM MANIPULATIONS: PERIODIZATION

Over the past 10 years the need for variation in a resistance training program has started to become obvious to both the scientist and the practitioner. Much of the early American research in this area centered around the concept that there is an optimal combination of sets and repetitions to bring about increases in strength (Atha 1981; Clarke 1966; O'Shea 1966). As discussed previously, this line of research assumes, among other things, that an optimal combination actually exists. However, by varying the resistance, the number of sets, and the number of repetitions, greater gains can be made. The most popular term for changing program variables is *periodization*. Periodization is a planned variation of the acute program variables.

Periodization was developed among Eastern European weight lifters as a way of changing their workouts over time to allow for better recovery and therefore greater gains in strength and power. (Matveyev 1981; Vorobyev 1978). Eastern European coaches and sport scientists noted that the training volume and intensity of successful athletes followed a certain pattern during the training year. At the start of the training year volume was high and intensity low. As the year progressed training volume decreased and intensity increased. Prior to a major competition volume was at its lowest for the year and intensity at its highest. Because of the need for recovery prior to a major competition, intensity was also decreased slightly immediately prior to the competition.

All traditional periodized programs follow this pattern for volume and intensity. The underlying concept promoting periodization is Selye's general adaptation syndrome. This theory proposes that the body's adaptation passes through three phases when it is confronted with a stress (in this case, resistance training). The first phase is shock: When the body is confronted with a new training stimulus, soreness develops and performance actually decreases. The second phase is adaptation to the stimulus: The body adapts to the new training stimulus and performance increases. The third phase is staleness: The body has already adapted to the new stimulus, and adaptations no longer take place. In this third phase it is possible for performance to plateau or, in the case of many highly motivated athletes, performance may decrease from overtraining.

Many programs that do not provide variation in exercise and rest result in a classic sawtooth pattern of strength changes. For example, the athlete increases his or her strength in response to a resistance training program but, because of a lack of variation and needed rest in the training program, either gets sick, loses motivation, overtrains, or quits training, resulting in a decrease in strength. The athlete with time recovers and starts to train again, making increases up to previously achieved levels, but again, because of a lack of training variation, the cycle of a decrease in strength repeats itself. These up and down changes over time may result in fitness and performance gains, but the gains are not maximized, nor are they maintained. Elimination of a sawtooth profile in favor of a staircase profile is preferable for physical development and is one of the goals of periodized training. Periodization is used to avoid staleness and overtraining, in addition to allowing for adequate rest, which ultimately keeps the exercise stimulus-response effective. Thus, a key factor to continuous gains is variation in the exercise stimulus.

The classic form of periodization breaks the training program into specific periods of time. The longest period of time is called the macrocycle (about 1 yr). The macrocycle is broken down into three or four periods of time called mesocycles (3 to 4 mo), and the mesocycle is broken down further into a microcycle (typically about 1 to 4 wk). Each training phase has a particular goal and is a part of the total training plan.

This type of periodized training was originally designed for use in the sports of track and field and weight lifting, in which athletes attempt to peak for a particular competition within the training year. Only the large–muscle group exercises were normally periodized. Other athletes and fitness enthusiasts have learned the benefits of such training variations and have adapted periodization for use in other sports and activities (O'Bryant, Byrd, and Stone 1988; Willoughby 1993).

Classic Periodization Program

In 1981 Stone, O'Bryant, and Garhammer in the United States developed a hypothetical model for strength/power sports of the classic periodization program that had been used by Eastern European weight lifters. Their model breaks a training program down into five mesocycles. The resulting periodization program is characterized by initiating the training with a high volume of exercise (i.e., more sets and repetitions) of low intensity (i.e., low resistance) as depicted in table 5.5. During each of the following mesocycles the volume of exercise is decreased and the intensity or resistance is increased.

In this model the initial phase of training is termed the *hypertrophy phase*, which is characterized by high-volume and low-resistance exercise. The major goals of this phase are to increase tolerance to resistance exercise and to increase muscle mass.

The major goals of the strength and power phases are to bring about increases in maximal strength and power, respectively. The goal of the peaking phase is to increase peak strength and power for a particular competition. The decrease in volume helps to compensate for the increasingly heavier resistances (increased intensity), which must be used to promote maximal strength and power increases.

The active rest phase consists of either low-volume, low-intensity resistance training or some other light physical activity. The goal of this phase is to allow recovery from the previous training, both physically and psychologically. In fact, this aspect

of periodized training may be the most important, as highly motivated athletes will often not want to take the rest their bodies require for optimal adaptations. If periods of rest and recovery within a training program are not planned, the possibility of staleness or overtraining is increased.

The goal of the entire training cycle is to achieve the highest strength/power level possible in the time allowed for the whole training cycle and peak strength/power for a major competition. Time for the active-rest mesocycle is then allowed, and the entire macrocycle is repeated.

Periodization was originally used to peak for one major competition a year, such as the world championships. Therefore each of the mesocycles was 2 to 3 mo long. Practitioners then discovered that even greater gains in strength/power could be achieved if two to three complete training cycles a year were performed. Consequently, each of the training phases (hypertrophy, strength, etc.) is now only 1 to 2 mo in length. The greater gains in strength/power are probably related to the basic concept of periodization that variation in training is needed to achieve optimal gains. More than one complete training cycle in a year provides more variation in training.

Table 5.5 presents a periodized program for strength/power sports such as weight lifting, power lifting, or shot-putting. Periodization can be used for other sports as well. This requires an alteration in the basic periodization plan to fit the individual sport or activity. The basic concepts of periodization can be maintained but must be translated into training cycles that result in the fitness gains needed for success in the particular sport or activity.

It would not be appropriate to design a resistance program for a 10-km runner or road cyclist to maximize 1-RM strength/power. The strength/

TABLE 5.5
Periodization of Training for a Strength/Power Sport

Mesocycle	1 Hypertrophy	2 Strength	3 Power	4 Peaking	5 Active rest
Sets	3-5	3-5	3-5	1-3	Light physical activity
Reps	8-20	2-6	2-3	1-3	
Intensity	Low	High	High	Very high	

Adapted, by permission, from M.H. Stone, H. O'Bryant, and J. Garhammer, 1981, "A hypothetical model for strength training," *Journal of Sports Medicine* 21:344.

power program outlined in table 5.5 is designed to maximize 1-RM strength/power and is inappropriate for an endurance athlete. However, the concepts of periodization can still be applied to resistance training for an endurance athlete or to any other activity. The set-and-repetition scheme for an endurance athlete's resistance program might consist of three mesocycles. The first mesocycle would have a training frequency of three sessions per week and would consist of two to three sets of each exercise at 15 to 20 RM, with 1.5 to 2.0 min of rest between sets and exercises. The second mesocycle would have a training frequency of three times per week and would consist of three sets of each exercise for the lower body at 12 to 15 RM, two to three sets of each exercise for the upper body at 12 to 15 RM, and 1.0 to 1.5 min of rest between sets and exercises. The peaking mesocycle would have a training frequency of one to three training sessions per week and would consist of two to three sets of each exercise at 8 to 12 RM, with 0.5 to 1.0 min of rest between sets and exercises. The training intensity is increased by increasing the resistance used and decreasing the rest between sets and exercises. Training volume is decreased by decreasing the number of sets, the number of repetitions per set, and the training days per week during the peaking mesocycle. Such a training plan will better meet the goals of endurance athletes. The training variables can be manipulated in any fashion imaginable as long as the training plan meets the needs of the trainee.

The intensity and the volume of exercise are the two most notable variables manipulated in many periodization models. For beginners, higher-volume protocols using lower intensities are followed by a gradual increase in the exercise intensity over the macrocycle with a drop in the volume of exercise. Conversely, more highly trained strength athletes do not decrease the volume of exercise as much over the training cycle because of their ability to tolerate and recover from higher-volume and high-intensity resistance exercise stress. In fact, longer periods of training (i.e., > 3 mo) may be needed for highly trained athletes to realize gains from periodization, as the potential to increase strength and power potential is small (Baker, Wilson, and Carlyon 1994). The general relationship between volume and intensity in a classic periodized model for beginning and advanced resistance-trained athletes is depicted in figure 5.9.

Nonlinear Models of Periodization

What have come to be called nonlinear or undulating models for resistance training periodization are becoming popular. Furthermore, they are proving to be as effective as classic periodization methods in short-term studies (Baker, Wilson, and Carlyon 1994; Poliquin 1988) and are superior to nonperiodized training protocols over longer training periods. This type of periodization is called nonlinear because of the dramatic change in the resistances used. For example, an athlete trains with moderate 8- to 10-RM resistances on Monday,

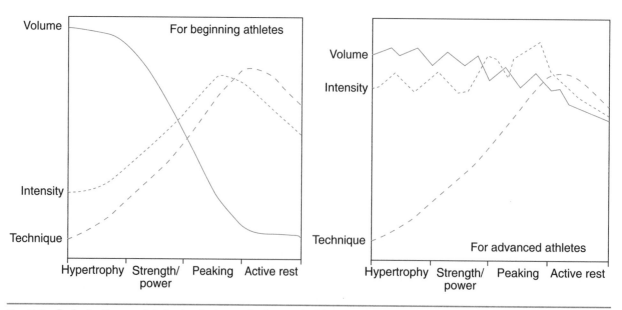

Fig. 5.9   Periodization models for beginning and advanced athletes.

heavy 3- to 5-RM resistances on Wednesday, and light 12- to 15-RM resistances on Friday for 12 wk. The 12-wk period is followed by a short active-rest phase, and the training cycle is then repeated. This type of periodization model may be most appropriate for team and individual sports in which peaking for one competition is not of prime importance because many competitions take place in a season.

With nonlinear models a higher volume of training is performed when light and moderate resistances are used. Therefore, not only does the training intensity vary dramatically on a daily basis, but also the training volume. The basic nonlinear model consists of varying the workout within 1- or 2-wk periods among light, moderate, heavy, and even very heavy resistances for appropriate exercises (e.g., core exercises). Nonlinear periodized plans are appropriate for team sports such as basketball, baseball, and volleyball and for individual sports such as tennis, wrestling, and racquetball. This type of periodized plan better meets the needs of athletes who must compete successfully weekly or biweekly. Intensive or high-volume training can be planned to occur during short breaks in competition, before competitions of little importance, or even before competitions against opponents who should be easily defeated.

Table 5.6 gives an example of a nonlinear periodization model used in the study of female tennis players in Dr. Kraemer's laboratory by Kraemer et al. (in press). A key element in linear periodization is the buildup to higher intensities over time, whereas in nonlinear models the intensity varies drastically within the week. Intensity also varies in linear plans on a daily and weekly basis, but the change in intensity is normally not as dramatic on a daily basis as in nonlinear periodization. Further studies are needed to determine optimal nonlinear models.

ADMINISTRATIVE CONCERNS

Administrative concerns are factors involved in the implementation of resistance training programs for large groups, such as classes or athletic teams. Addressing the administrative concerns is paramount in the realization of the desired exercise stimulus. The optimal program should be designed first, however, and the administrative concerns addressed after the program is designed. This allows for the optimal exercise stimulus to be created for a workout before it is compromised by limitations in equipment, time, or space. Administrative considerations that severely limit the optimal program should be remedied as soon as possible. This usually involves acquiring more equipment or space. Creativity and safely improvising with the equipment and space available make a program work. The major administrative concerns are

- availability of equipment,
- number of individuals,
- availability of space, and
- availability of time.

Availability of Equipment

A major problem in developing a resistance training program is equipment availability. Although sophisticated equipment is not needed to develop a resistance training program, the proper outfitting of a weight room allows more flexibility and diversity when designing a resistance training program (Rieger 1985). Weight training equipment represents the tools used in conditioning different muscles.

For people who are training alone with an interest simply in basic strength, power, or endurance

---

TABLE 5.6
An Example of Nonlinear Workout Variables for a Week of Training Using Various Primary Exercises

	Monday	Wednesday	Friday
Intensity (RM zone)	8-10 RM	3-5 RM	12-15 RM
Number of sets	3-4	4-5	3-4
Rest between sets and exercises	2 min	3-4 min	1 min

fitness, a host of different types of equipment have been developed for home use over the past 10 years. The safety aspects of such equipment should be evaluated prior to purchase. The ability of the equipment to supply proper resistance through the ranges of motion of various exercises should also be evaluated. When evaluating a piece of home-use equipment for purchase, various questions should be answered (table 5.7). In addition, many facilities exist for training outside the home (e.g., health clubs, recreation centers, and school facilities). Formal exercise programs should be evaluated prior to joining, using the basic consumer guidelines presented in table 5.8. The consumer can be overwhelmed by the process of choosing a club at which to work out because of the variety of certifications, exercise programs, and equipment offered. Making the selection is based on the individual's training goals, economy of purchase, and the expertise of the facility's instructors and staff.

Equipment availability is often a problem for coaches who must train large groups of athletes and for fitness directors who must establish programs for large numbers of people. The development of a resistance training facility is related to

---

TABLE 5.7
Basic Questions About Equipment for Home Use

- Can the resistance used be determined?
- Does it provide resistance through the full range of motion of the exercise?
- Is it well constructed, safe, and sturdy when using its intended range of resistances?
- Can it provide a range of resistances that will allow progress during a training program?
- Can it provide a variety of exercises for all the major muscle groups and joints in the body?
- What type of resistance training modality does it provide (e.g., isokinetic, constant external resistance, isometric)?
- Can resistance be increased or decreased in small increments?
- Does it fit all the people (children, large men, small women, etc.) who will use it?
- Is there a warranty, and how long is it?

TABLE 5.8
Basic Consumer Guidelines

- Is the instructor certified by a professional nonprofit organization in strength and basic first aid training?
- Is the instructor certified to perform cardiopulmonary resuscitation (CPR)?
- Does the instructor have an educational background and at least an undergraduate degree in an exercise-related discipline (e.g., exercise and sport science, physical education, or exercise physiology)?
- Are members screened for possible disease prior to exercise?
- Are members pretested to determine initial levels of physical fitness?
- Are individual goals determined for members from testing, evaluation of needs, and medical history?
- Is the exercise program individually prescribed?
- Is the progress of your program individually monitored?
- Is there a medical or scientific advisory board?
- Is there an emergency medical plan in case of injury?

the variety of exercise programs to be implemented and the equipment needed to perform the exercises. Obtaining needed equipment is a primary goal for the strength coach or fitness director who wants to provide a safe and effective training environment.

Exercises are performed with machines or free weights. Most machines are built to fit the average adult male. Thus children, some women, and other people of smaller or larger than average structure may find it difficult to properly position themselves on many machines and equipment. Improper positioning may not allow proper exercise technique or full range of exercise motion and may result in injury. If alterations—such as a seat pad or back pad—are made to a machine to allow proper fit, make sure the pad will not slide during performance of the exercise. Any materials used to alter a piece of equipment must not slide during exercise and must be sturdy enough to withstand the stress encountered during the exercise. Any alteration to equipment must be done carefully and must not compromise the safety of the lifter.

Many free-weight exercises require more time to learn proper technique than exercises performed on machines. However, if an individual can grasp and hold a dumbbell or barbell, it fits them, and they can perform the exercise with proper technique. Thus, the proper fit of free weights is not a major administrative concern.

Proper fit is a serious consideration when examining equipment needs for a program and choosing equipment for optimal use by a wide range of individuals. As discussed earlier in this chapter, the biomechanical requirements of the muscle actions to be trained with an exercise must be carefully matched to the equipment. Of importance is the type of strength curve (see chapter 2) needed for each exercise. For example, rubber cords, which fit all body sizes, can produce only an ascending strength curve. Movements with other than ascending strength curves will not be optimally trained with the use of rubber cords. The characteristics of the specific exercise movements to be trained must be matched with those of the equipment available. Comparing the present equipment inventory with the program's equipment requirements will quickly result in a list of needed equipment. This list provides the basis for future equipment purchases and indicates which exercise programs will suffer from administrative limitations related to equipment availability.

If the equipment available is minimal, viable substitutions must be found. It is possible to make some equipment. However, safety must never be compromised when developing homemade equipment. It is possible to substitute other forms of exercise such as plyometrics, paired-partner exercises, or dynamic drills (e.g., stair running) in situations where no resistance training equipment is available. Nevertheless, these are only temporary solutions until the optimal training equipment can be obtained.

A specific planning list should be created for the needed equipment. Basic questions should be asked when buying a piece of equipment (table 5.9). Goals should be established for when to purchase specific pieces of equipment for the weight room. This is an exciting phase of program development.

TABLE 5.9
Factors to Consider When Buying Equipment

- Does the equipment fit the people that will be using it (e.g., children), or can it be safely altered to do so?

- What is its cost per exercise?

- How much will it cost to purchase sufficient equipment to exercise all major muscle groups of the body?

- How easy is it to adjust the resistance?

- How long is its warranty?

- What does its warranty cover?

- Is the equipment made from heavy-gauge steel?

- Is the equipment sturdily constructed (e.g., are the welds solid)?

- Does the resistance increase in increments suitable for all users?

Prioritize each piece of needed equipment. High priority is usually given to equipment that exercises large muscle groups and offers a wide variety of exercise movements. Low priority is given to specialized pieces of equipment that exercise small muscle groups and can be used for only one exercise.

To obtain new equipment, all budget resources should be explored. Future equipment needs and what can be accomplished with the present equipment must be kept in perspective. Organization and planning are the key to obtaining needed equipment.

The Number of People Training

The existing facility frequently has the proper equipment but is inadequate for the large number of people using it. The first step in such situations is to better organize the flow of people using the facility. This task can be hampered by individual schedules, individual training time preferences, and the use of the facility by large groups, classes, or athletic teams.

To overcome these obstacles, first document facility usage to determine the number of individuals training at various times of the day and the days of the week on which they train. The heaviest volume usually occurs at noon and late afternoon, when individuals have free time and athletic teams are most likely to train. When working with large groups, classes, or athletic teams, obtain a list of preferred and alternate times from each group. Have coaches and instructors indicate their preferences for their groups. Awareness of usage fluctuation throughout the day aids in allocating training schedules that satisfy most parties using the facility. Accurate information regarding the facility's use also provides strong support for budget requests.

Organization of user flow in the training facility also involves the usage patterns of the equipment. First, determine how many people use particular exercises in their training programs. This information is used to adjust the exercise order of the various training programs in order to eliminate lines of people waiting to use one or several pieces of equipment. This is especially important when timed exercise workouts (e.g., 1-min rest periods) are critical to the effectiveness of the exercise stimulus.

Efficient patterns of movement are accomplished by training charts that specify the sequence of exercises and rest periods. Innovative techniques include tape-recorded exercise sequences for use either on a facility-wide audio system or on personal cassette recorders, color-coded taped floor movement patterns, and workout sheets with a flow chart. Whichever method is chosen, it must be appropriate for the facility. Although these specific organizational methods are mandatory when there are a large number of people using the facility, they might also be used simply to stress the proper exercise sequence and adherence to rest periods. Efficient, patterned trainee movement in the facility can be accomplished by four basic tips:

- Use predetermined exercise progressions.
- Make sure individuals who are involved in a particular exercise flow pattern need the same rest periods.
- Group individuals with identical training regimens together when possible.
- Carefully plan training programs and exercise flow patterns during time periods when more than one group or team is training.

Acquiring Appropriate Space

The availability of training space refers to the room available for exercise equipment. In the past university and high school weight rooms were given low-priority areas in the basement, the boiler room, the men's locker room, or a storage shed. This led to problems of access (e.g., women being unable to train because the weight room was in the men's locker room), temperature control, ventilation problems, and inadequate space to place equipment properly and safely in the room. If the facility is carefully designed and planned, these problems can be eliminated. Remodeling or relocation of the facility can also solve many of these problems. In either case, it is important to plan for the facility's future use and needs, not just today's needs. This will help ensure that the facility is functional long after it is built or remodeled.

No equipment purchases should be made without first measuring the space available within the facility, and the basic floor plan should be drawn prior to developing a new facility or area. Placement of equipment in the facility that best allows for population flow is vital, as is the provision of space to house new equipment. Sufficient room must be allowed between pieces of equipment to allow easy access to the equipment. Buffer areas with no equipment must be allowed around free weight areas, especially lifting platforms, in case a lifter loses a lift and must drop the barbell or dumbbell. Furthermore, the facility should be clean and have good ventilation and a comfortable temperature. Future equipment purchases are directly related to additional space if the facility is to be a safe and desirable place in which to train.

Scheduling Training

The amount of training time available can cause problems if the designed training programs do not match the projected training time. The length of a training session, including rest periods, should be calculated immediately after the session is planned. The session must consider the individual's as well as the facility's schedule. Though individuals should use the best training program possible, for some people, such as multisport athletes and individuals with demanding personal schedules, time is so limited that the training session has to be modified. Any modifications caused by time limitations should be made carefully. Large–muscle group exercises and short rest periods are acute variable choices that can provide time economy but should only be prescribed in appropriate situations. If it is necessary to limit small–muscle group exercises, the fewest number possible should be eliminated to allow the training session to fit into the available time. In addition, the exercises eliminated should be those least important to achieving the program's goals. Also, short rest periods (less than 1 min) should be used only when higher blood lactate levels are desired and the trainee has the fitness level to tolerate high blood lactate levels.

SAFETY ISSUES

Although there is a great deal of organization involved in the management of a resistance training facility, remember that the first responsibility is to provide, in a safe manner, the best exercise stimulus possible.

Proper Spotting Technique

Good spotting technique is vital for a safe resistance training program. Here is a checklist that spotters should use at all times:

1. Know proper exercise technique.
2. Know proper spotting technique.
3. Be sure you and any additional spotters are strong enough to assist the lifter with the resistance being used.
4. Know how many repetitions the lifter intends to do.
5. Be attentive to the lifter at all times.
6. Stop the lifter if exercise technique is incorrect.
7. Know the plan of action if a serious injury occurs.

The goal of correct spotting is to prevent injury. A lifter should always have access to a spotter. If the trainees cannot spot each other safely, as may be the case in some special education classes, young children's classes, classes of people with handicaps, or classes in which training pairs are unequal in strength, enlist the help of other individuals or reduce the number of trainees.

Spotting and Exercise Technique Practice

When teaching a new exercise, demonstrate proper exercise and spotting techniques, and discuss the major points of the techniques. Then allow each trainee to try the exercise with a light resistance, such as a barbell or dumbbell with no weight plates on it or even a broomstick. For an exercise performed with a machine, using a light resistance may mean removing all weight from the machine or taking the pin out of the weight stack. After the trainee attempts the exercise, point out any flaws in technique. Then continue further technique practice with light resistances; this will minimize the effects of fatigue while learning the exercise. In addition to practicing the exercise, all trainees should demonstrate and practice proper spotting techniques for each of the exercises used in a program.

Usually free-weight exercises will require more time to teach proper exercise and spotting techniques than do machine exercises. This is because free weights require the lifter to balance the resistance in all directions (left, right, forward, backward, up, down). Most machines restrain the exercises into one plane of movement and require little, if any, balancing. Additional time may also be needed to teach proper exercise techniques for multijoint exercises, such as squats, because coordination of movement at several joints is needed for proper technique.

Attempting to teach techniques for too many exercises at once, especially multijoint exercises, will slow down the learning process. How many exercise techniques someone can learn at one time will vary. A general guideline is seven to eight exercises, of which one to three may be multijoint exercises.

Emergency Plan

Safety and proper supervision are concerns for all conditioning programs. Injuries in a properly supervised resistance training program are rare, with the most common type of injury being muscle strains. The following are some possible causes of injury during resistance training:

- Attempting to lift too much weight
- Attempting too many repetitions with a certain weight
- Using improper lifting technique
- Improperly placing feet or hands on a resistance training machine so they slide off the pedals or handles
- Placing hands on the pulley system of a resistance training machine
- Placing hands between the weight stack of a resistance training machine
- Inattentive spotters
- Improper behavior in the facility
- A bench or piece of equipment sliding during the exercise

- Worn-out equipment (e.g., machine cables or pulleys) that breaks during lifting
- Not using collars on free weights
- Accidentally dropping free-weight plates while loading or unloading a bar

Even though injuries are rare (Hamill 1994; Zemper 1990), a resistance training facility should have an emergency plan to deal with serious injuries that require medical attention. The plan should be posted in the weight room, and all supervisors should be familiar with it. An emergency plan should include the phone number and location of the nearest ambulance service and/or hospital. Make sure to give the local emergency personnel the address and any pertinent information needed to locate the training facility. It is also a good idea to have an alphabetized card catalog of trainees' home and business phone numbers and addresses.

A phone should be located in the weight room. If not, all supervisors should know the location of the nearest phone. In addition, all supervisors should have basic first aid and cardiopulmonary resuscitation (CPR) skills.

EXERCISE PRESCRIPTION CASE STUDIES

The prescription of resistance training is both a science and an art. Ultimately, individualized programs provide for optimal changes in the exercise prescription process and result in the best overall training response for the individual. A paradigm for exercise prescription has been developed and presented in this chapter that provides the framework for optimal design of resistance training programs. Although guidelines can be given, the art of designing effective resistance training programs requires logical exercise prescription followed by evaluation, testing, and interaction with the trainee. Resistance training prescription is a dynamic process that requires the strength and conditioning professional to respond to the trainee's changing adaptation levels and functional capacities with altered program designs to meet the changing training goals.

The following case studies demonstrate manipulations of acute and chronic program variables. The case studies offer one possible solution to the needs and goals of the person in question.

CASE STUDY ONE

John just took a job at a senior high school as the head wrestling coach and physical education teacher. He was an avid weight trainer in college and felt this played a large role in his athletic career. John's undergraduate courses in exercise science stimulated an interest in strength training. On the basis of his interest and previous experi-

Continued

ence he was appointed head of the high school's strength and conditioning program. John decided to develop a workout program for his wrestling team.

John started with a needs analysis for the sport and determined that the movements and angles involved with wrestling vary but primarily involve the large muscles of the hip, leg, and back. Dynamic muscle actions are the most common, although some isometric actions take place during various wrestling moves. The energy is derived primarily from the lactic acid energy source and aerobic metabolism, because wrestling entails intense activity extended over 6 min with a limited amount of rest. A discussion of his needs analysis for the wrestling team follows.

Muscle Groups to Be Trained. Wrestling requires overall physical training, but the large muscle groups of the back, hip, and legs are especially important for the performance of most moves. Wrestling requires a great deal of dynamic strength and power but also requires local muscular endurance.

Injury Sites. The main injury sites are the neck, shoulder, ankle, and knee.

Muscle Action. Dynamic concentric and eccentric muscle actions are the primary movement types. Isometric muscle actions are used to a lesser extent.

Energy Sources. The lactic acid source is the major contributor of energy during a match, with significant support from the aerobic source and the remainder derived from the ATP-PC source.

Off-Season Training

John designed the workout shown in table 5.10 for his wrestlers. The M-F program is designed to strengthen the various body parts of the wrestler using primarily body-part exercises and one structural exercise (squat). Exercises are ordered within a group to exercise the same body part at different angles. This exercise order and short rest periods (1.0 to 1.5 min) stress the lactic acid energy source, which results in an accumulation of lactic acid similar to that observed during wrestling (12 to 20 mmol/L). Longer rest periods (2 to 5 min) are allowed between squat sets. This allows heavy weights to be used for the prescribed 5 repetitions per set and so stresses maximal strength development. This workout is primarily used in the off-season and pre-season before the wrestler is able to put in much time on the mat. During the season such a high-lactic-acid workout program is less important and may be performed only once a week, because the wrestling provides the specific metabolic conditioning needs. Progression from 1.5-min to 1-min rest periods is used at the start of the program to allow exercise tolerance to develop. This type of program will reduce the symp-

TABLE 5.10
M-F Body-Part Workout
(Stresses Lactic Acid Energy Source)

Exercise	Sets/Reps
Bench press	10 ↓ 10 ↓ 10 ↓
Upright row	10 ↓ 10 ↓ 10 ↓
	* * *
Lat pull-down	10 ↓ 10 ↓ 10 ↓
Seated row	10 ↓ 10 ↓ 10 ↓
	* * *
Knee extensions	10 ↓ 10 ↓ 10 ↓
Knee flexions	10 ↓ 10 ↓ 10 ↓
	* * *
Squats	10 / 5 / 5 / 5 / 5
	→ → → →
Sit-ups	50 ↓ 50 ↓
Knee-ups	25 ↓ 25 ↓
	* *
Arm curls	10 * 10 * 10 *
	→ → →
Calf raises	10 * 10 * 10 *
	→ → →
Four-way neck isometrics	15 reps, 3-5s each

/ = 2- to 5-min rest

* = 1-min rest

↓ = alternating exercise order

→ = do all sets of an exercise before moving to next exercise

Note. All sets listed are at RM resistances.

Continued ☞

toms of nausea, dizziness, and vomiting associated with intolerance of high levels of

TABLE 5.11
Tu-Th Structural Workout

Deadlifts	8 / 8 / 8 / 8 / 8 /
Hang-cleans	5 / 5 / 5 / 5 / 5 /
Sit-ups	4 × 25
Split squats	10 / 10 / 10 / 10 /
High-pulls	8 / 8 / 8 / 8 /

/ = 2- to 5-min rest between sets and exercises
Note. All sets listed are at RM resistances.

acidity, helping the wrestler to adapt to the high concentrations of lactic acid encountered during a wrestling match.

In order to address the structural strength needs of the wrestler, a Tu-Th training session was also developed, which is used at the onset of the program and is subject to chronic program manipulations (table 5.11). This workout is designed to develop explosive power in the legs, hips, and back. Structural exercises are chosen to accomplish this goal. Adequate rest is given between sets and exercises to allow the use of heavy resistance primarily to promote strength/power gains.

Chronic Manipulations (Periodization)

Several possibilities exist concerning chronic manipulation. As the season approaches, the number of repetitions can be decreased to five or six or even to two or three for the junior and senior wrestlers in the structural exercises on M-F and Tu-Th workouts. The rest periods between sets and exercises can be gradually decreased to 20 s for the body-part workouts (M-F). These two manipulations help strength levels to peak while maintaining a high amount of stress on the lactic acid energy source. In addition, one or two additional sets or one or two fewer sets at a higher intensity could be performed to create variation in training. These increases and/or decreases in the volume and intensity of the daily workouts help to prevent the staleness of the general adaptation syndrome. Two- or three-week cycles where the intensity (RM) is changed on the Tu-Th workouts (e.g., 10, 5, 3 RM) and the rest is altered on the M-F workouts (e.g., 60 s, 45 s, 20 s) could also be used to add variation to the program. As previously mentioned, the structural training program might also be put on M-F, and the high-lactic-acid program on Tu-Th once wrestling practice starts. As the season approaches, it becomes necessary to focus training on the practice of actual wrestling skills. One way to decrease the time spent in the weight room is to decrease the number of sets and repetitions along with decreasing the rest periods. This may be a key consideration for the in-season program. Another way to decrease time in the weight room is to increase the number of structural workouts at the expense of the body-part workouts, with the goal of eventually eliminating the body-part workouts altogether and having only three structural workouts per week. Structural exercises stress several muscle groups at once, whereby all major muscle groups are stressed in a shorter period of time than in body-part workouts. Structural workouts become vital during the in-season program, as do injury-prevention exercises for the neck, knees, shoulders, and ankles. Therefore, the structural and injury-prevention exercises should constitute the majority of in-season exercises.

Individual Considerations

John realized that all of his wrestlers did not have the same level of experience with resistance training and physical conditioning. He therefore made individual modifications in the beginning resistances and rest periods until each of his wrestlers could tolerate the basic body-part and structural sessions. He also developed individual workout cards and later a computer program to individualize the workouts of each

Continued ☞

wrestler so that each could make progress. He also ran teaching sessions in the weight room to instruct his athletes on the basic techniques of the lifts. One of his wrestlers had a chronic shoulder problem from the previous season. In this case, John added a few more exercises for the shoulder area to improve the athlete's overall shoulder strength. Some of the heavier wrestlers had very low aerobic fitness. For these individuals John developed some basic aerobic fitness programs for use in the off-season program. All of the wrestlers were on aerobic fitness programs to facilitate better recovery between rounds and between matches (especially during tournaments). In addition, in the preseason he utilized an interval sprint program to enhance anaerobic capacities. Finally, John stressed off-season weight control after appropriate body-composition analysis and consultation with the team physician. This helped his wrestlers find their optimal weight.

CASE STUDY TWO

Maelu was primarily interested in a personal fitness program. She was actively involved in an aerobic running program and was ready to include a resistance training program to balance her conditioning activities, improve her upper-body strength, and prevent lower-limb injury during aerobic exercise. Her basic needs analysis indicated additional upper-body strength along with quadriceps, hamstring, and calf exercises to aid in her injury-prevention program. Based on this needs analysis the following beginning workout was developed (table 5.12).

This program is designed to achieve moderate strength gains in the upper-body musculature. Two minutes of rest were allowed between both sets and exercises. Initially, light resistances are used to aid in developing proper exercise technique. The resistances are then increased until RM resistances are used for the desired number of repetitions. Because long rest periods are allowed, the training session can be performed in multiple-set fashion (complete all sets of an exercise before performing the next exercise) or in a circuit format. Maelu initially performs only one exercise per body part and one or two sets of each exercise until her tolerance to the workouts improves.

TABLE 5.12
Training for Case Study 2

Chest exercise:	
Bench press	12, 10, 10
Back exercise:	
Lat pull-down	10, 10, 10
Abdomen exercises:	
Bent-leg sit-ups	15, 15
Knee-ups	15, 15
Arm/shoulder exercises:	
Military press	12, 10, 10
Arm curls	12, 10, 10
Leg exercises:	
Knee extensions	15, 15, 15
Knee flexions	15, 15, 15
Toe raisers	15, 15

Chronic Changes

Maelu is not a competitive athlete and therefore is not attempting to prepare for a particular competition or season. She is interested in general fitness, and the purpose of her resistance training is to increase upper-body and lower-body strength to prevent injury. The major goals of chronic manipulations (periodization) are to prepare the athlete for a particular season or competition and to ensure continued gains in fitness and strength. Because these are not the goals of Maelu's program, a great deal

Continued ☞

of chronic manipulation is unnecessary. Because new data indicate that increased strength and power enhance aerobic performance, however, heavy days using 3- to 5-RM and 6- to 8-RM resistances would provide a change and enhance strength development.

Maelu may consider two chronic manipulations of her program. One is to periodically substitute different exercises that stress the same muscle group for exercises already in her program. Examples of this are substituting squats or leg presses for knee extensions and knee flexions, the incline press for the military press, and bent-over rowing for lat pull-downs. This will help to keep the program from becoming tedious. Maelu should also continually try to shorten her rest periods to decrease the time necessary to complete a workout and to improve her local muscular endurance.

CASE STUDY THREE

Joan is a women's collegiate volleyball coach. Because of a rather poor season last year, she decided to initiate an off-season resistance training program to improve the team's performance. Joan has ideas about what the goals of a resistance training program for women's volleyball should be. But to make these goals more specific, she conducted a literature search concerning women's volleyball and discovered that several training factors have been found to improve performance, including vertical jumping ability (Fleck et al. 1985; Gladden and Colacino 1978; Spence et al. 1980), upper-body and arm strength (Morrow et al. 1979), and low percentage of body fat (Morrow et al. 1979; Fleck et al. 1985). The goals of Joan's program were to increase vertical jumping ability and upper-body strength and to decrease percentage of body fat. The exercises chosen to fulfill these needs are outlined in table 5.13.

Because of the arrangement of the weight room and available time, Joan decided to run the program as a timed circuit, allowing 30 s to perform the exercise and 1-min rest between exercises. She placed the athletes in groups of three, which provided spotters for each exercise and assistance in changing the resistance needed for each exercise. The athletes would begin training using a 10 RM; when they could complete all three circuits of an individual exercise with the 10 RM, the resistance would be increased. Resistance training was performed on Monday, Wednesday, and Friday. Joan also had team meetings in which proper diet and caloric balance were discussed. The aim of these meetings was to educate her players about the role these factors play in weight control and athletic performance.

TABLE 5.13
Training for Case Study 3

	Sets	Repetitions
Hang-cleans	3	5
Incline presses	3	10
Squats	3	10
Lat pull-downs	3	10
Sit-ups	3	20
Toe raisers	3	10
Wrist curls	3	10
Back extensions	3	10
Leg extensions	3	10
Leg curls	3	10

Chronic Manipulations

Joan decided to start the resistance training program 9 wk prior to the onset of the volleyball season. She decided to incorporate the concept of periodization: For the first 4 wk the original workout was performed; weeks 5, 6, and 7 called for exercises

Continued ☞

at 8 RM; and for the last 2 wk the exercises were performed with 5 RM. The rest periods diminished from 60 s to 50 s to 40 s and finally to 30 s during the last 2 wk of the program for the single-joint exercises. In addition, for the last 5 wk of the program plyometric jumping exercises were performed on Tuesday, Thursday, and Saturday. Joan found that an alternative workout using only structural exercises or integration and substitution of various structural exercises into her 3-d/wk program could benefit the development of total-body power and single-leg strength. Such exercises are hang-cleans, hang-pulls, split squats, side squats, power snatches, lunges, and push presses.

SUMMARY

Using a needs analysis, acute program design, chronic program design, and consideration of administrative factors results in the optimal program for any situation. It is then necessary to be creative and search out ways to improve the design of the program and the resistance training facility. The next chapter discusses various resistance training systems (i.e., sets and repetitions) that can be used when designing a program.

SELECTED READINGS

Dudley, G.A.; Tesch, P.A.; Miller, B.J.; and Buchanan, P. 1991. Importance of eccentric actions in performance adaptations to resistance training. *Aviation, Space, and Environmental Medicine* 62:543-50.

Fleck, S.J., and Kraemer, W.J. 1996. *Periodization breakthrough*. New York: Advanced Research Press.

Kraemer, W.J. 1982. Weight training: What you don't know will hurt you. *Wyoming Journal of Health, Physical Education, Recreation and Dance* 5:8-11.

Kraemer, W.J. 1994. The physiological basis for strength training in mid-life. In *Sports and exercise in midlife*, ed. S.L. Gordon, 413-33. Park Ridge, IL: American Academy of Orthopaedic Surgeons.

Kraemer, W.J., and Baechle, T.R. 1989. Development of a strength training program. Chap. 2 in *Sports medicine*, 2d ed., eds. F.L. Allman and A.J. Ryan, 113-27. Orlando, FL: Academic Press.

Kraemer, W.J., and Koziris, L.P. 1992. Muscle strength training: Techniques and considerations. *Physical Therapy Practice* 2:54-68.

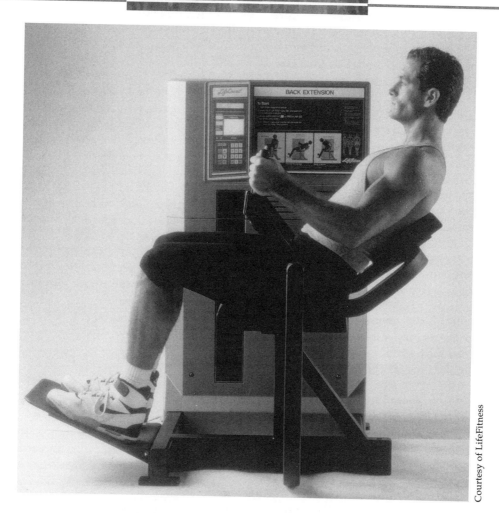

CHAPTER 6

Courtesy of LifeFitness

Resistance Training Systems

Most resistance training systems were originally designed by strength coaches, power lifters, Olympic weight lifters, or body builders. They are popular not because they have been scientifically shown to result in greater increases in strength, power, or hypertrophy than other training systems. Rather, they are popular because experienced practitioners believe they work better than other systems or because the system has been marketed by an individual or company. A great deal of speculation exists about why various systems are effective or how they physiologically cause a training adaptation. More research is needed concerning all the training systems described within this chapter. Still, knowledge of the various systems described in this chapter can be of value to a practitioner. The fact that a system has been used by enough people to have name recognition indicates that it has a good success rate in bringing about the desired changes. The system may therefore be worth examining to see how it might fit into the design of a program.

Knowledge of the various systems is also valuable because it demonstrates the many possibilities for manipulating acute training variables. Many resistance trainers adapt one system of training and then attempt to apply it to all individuals and muscle groups. This will inevitably lead to less than optimal gains in some muscle groups as well as in many individuals. The indefinite use of one program also leads to plateaus in progress and possibly overtraining. Manipulation of the acute and chronic training variables must be used to avoid these problems. Optimal gains in strength or muscular hypertrophy are achieved by mixing the various training programs and manipulating the training variables appropriately.

Several common mistakes are made by novice resistance trainers when examining programs. One mistake is to assume that the system used by a champion body builder, power lifter, or Olympic weight lifter is the best for the novice. Programs used by competitive weight lifters and body builders often are too intense for the novice resistance trainer. It has taken years of training for the competitive athlete to achieve the fitness level necessary to tolerate the program he or she is presently using. The champion weight lifter or body builder also has a genetic potential for superior strength and muscle size that allows him or her to tolerate very intense programs and to achieve the accompanying gains in strength and muscular size.

A training record or log is invaluable for determining which training system or variation of a system works best for each individual or team. Without a record of workouts, the progression of a program that was found to be successful in causing strength, power, or muscular hypertrophy will not be remembered in enough detail to repeat it. Furthermore, the sets, repetitions, and resistances used in a program need to be documented for use in planning the next workout. A training record answers many questions concerning an individual's response to a particular program—including which system works best and how long until a plateau develops with a particular system. Training logs are also a motivational tool because athletes can see their own progress over the course of a specific training period.

MULTIPLE-SET SYSTEM

The multiple-set system originally consisted of two to three warm-up sets of increasing resistance fol-

lowed by several sets at the same resistance. This training system became popular in the 1940s (Darden 1973) and was the forerunner of the multiple-set and repetition systems of today. The optimal resistance and number of repetitions for strength development using a multiple-set system has undergone considerable research (see chapter 2, "Dynamic Constant External Resistance Training"). For some multijoint exercises a 5 to 6 RM performed for a minimum of three sets appears to be the optimal resistance and number of repetitions to cause optimal increases in strength.

A multiple-set system can be performed at any desired resistance, for any number of repetitions and sets to meet the desired goals of a training program. Performance of a multiple-set system with no change in training variables for a long period of time, however, normally results in the plateauing of strength and power gains. The majority of training systems are variations of the multiple-set system. If strength and power are the objectives of training, multiple-set systems can be optimized by periodizing the training (Willoughby 1993).

SINGLE-SET SYSTEM

The single-set system, the performance of each exercise for one set, is one of the oldest resistance training systems. First published in 1925 (Liederman 1925), the original single-set system consisted of using heavy resistances and few repetitions per set with a 5-min rest between exercises. Single-set systems are still quite popular, and a single set of 8 to 12 repetitions was recommended by one of the leading resistance training equipment manufacturers in the 1970s. Significant gains in strength using a single-set system have been demonstrated (Hurley, Seals, Ehasani et al. 1984; Peterson 1975; Stowers et al. 1983). However, it has also been demonstrated that a single-set system (one set of 10 repetitions) resulted in a significantly smaller strength gain than either a multiple-set system of three sets of 10 repetitions or a periodized program progressing from sets of 10 to sets of 5 to sets of 3 repetitions, all performed with a heavy resistance for that number of repetitions (Stowers et al. 1983). Vertical jump ability was increased only in the periodized group. This study clearly demonstrates the superiority of multiple-set programs over a single-set program in producing increases in strength and vertical jump ability. In addition, periodized training using multiple sets appears superior to using the same multiple-set system for the entire training period for the development of strength and power (Willoughby 1993). However, comparisons of increases in strength caused by different training regimens may vary dramatically from one muscle group to another.

Recent information indicates that the volume of resistance training performed has a major effect on the cellular adaptations to resistance training and on the rate at which strength is lost after cessation of training (Dudley et al. 1991; Hather et al. 1992). This information indicates that a single-set system may not promote the cellular adaptations needed to support long-term gains in strength and power. The faster loss of strength gains with a smaller volume of resistance training indicates that the single-set system is not the best choice for a competitive athlete. When the athlete quits resistance training, the strength gained will be lost quickly (within 4 wk). Even though a single-set system may not be the best overall program, it may be a viable program for an individual who has very little time to dedicate to resistance training or as a specific 3- to 4-wk phase of an in-season program.

BULK SYSTEM

The bulk system refers specifically to a multiple-set system of three sets of five to six repetitions per exercise. A comparative study of 10 resistance training systems resulted in some very interesting conclusions (Leighton et al. 1967). The major weakness of this study was that groups trained dynamically (except for the isometric group) and were tested isometrically. Nevertheless, some insights can be gained from this particular investigation. This study trained college students two times per week for 8 wk. Each group was composed of 20 to 29 subjects. All groups performed two-armed arm curls, two-armed arm presses, lat pull-downs, half squats, sit-ups, side bends, leg presses, knee curls, toe raises, and bench presses. Static or isometric strength was determined both before and after the 8-wk training period for all groups. The bulk system turned out to be one of the most effective systems in causing increases in static strength over the short-term training period for the back and legs (see table 6.1). Therefore, this system may be valuable for increasing general leg and back strength during short-term training programs (e.g., preseason).

CHEAT SYSTEM

The cheat system is quite popular among body builders. As the name implies, it involves cheating or breaking strict form of an exercise (Weider 1954).

As an example, rather than maintaining an erect upper body when performing standing barbell arm curls, the trainee uses a slight body swing to start the barbell moving. The body swing is not grossly exaggerated but is sufficient to allow the trainee to lift 10 to 20 lb (4.5 to 9.1 kg) more resistance than is possible with strict form. In the barbell curl the weakest position is when the arms are fully extended. The strongest position is when the elbow joint is at an approximately 90° angle. When barbell curls are performed with strict form, the maximal amount of resistance that can be lifted depends on the resistance that can be moved from the weakest, or fully extended, position. The muscles involved in flexing the elbow therefore are not maximally active during the stronger portions of the movement. The object of cheating is to allow the use of heavier weights, which will force the muscle(s) to develop a force closer to maximal through a greater range of the movement and thus enhance strength gains.

Care must be taken when using the cheat system. The heavier resistances and the cheating movement increase the chance of injury. As an example, the swinging movement of the hips and lower back when performing arm curls places additional stress on the lower back.

Comparisons of strength gains caused by the cheat system versus those from various other training systems indicate that this system is quite effective (see table 6.1). The cheat system appears to be one of the most effective systems in increasing two-arm and back-and-leg static strength. The cheat system can be used in conjunction with virtually any other training system (e.g., cheating during multisets).

EXHAUSTION-SET SYSTEM

Exhaustion sets can be incorporated into virtually any training system. Body builders use sets to exhaustion in their training programs. A set to exhaustion means performing as many repetitions as possible with good technique until momentary concentric failure occurs (i.e., the resistance cannot be lifted). Advocates of this system believe that with sets to exhaustion more motor units will be recruited and therefore receive a training stimulus than when sets are not performed to exhaustion. It has been reported that one set to exhaustion of 10 repetitions causes significant gains in squat ability, but that three sets of 10 repetitions, two sets of which were to exhaustion, cause significantly greater increases in squat ability (Stowers et al. 1983). Training in this study was conducted twice

TABLE 6.1
Comparison of Isometric Strength Gains Caused by 10 Resistance Training Systems

	Bulk	Cheat	DeLorme[a]	Descending half triangle	Double progressive	Heavy-light training days[b]	Isometric[c]	Oxford[d]	Super setting	Triset
Elbow flexion	8*	23*	9*	11*	7	3	0	7*	12*	25*
Elbow extension	9	66**	16	9**	25*	34**	35*	28**	9	30**
Back and leg	24**	27*	0	24*	13	19*	-5	11	21*	17*

Note. Strength values given are percentage change pre- to posttraining.

[a] DeLorme is a light-to-heavy system.

[b] Heavy-light refers to maximal resistance being used during only one training session per week, 2/3 maximal used during the second session.

[c] Isometric training consisted of one maximal action.

[d] Oxford is a heavy-to-light system.

* Significant increase pre- to posttraining at .05 level of significance

** Significant increase pre- to posttraining at .01 level of significance

Note. From "A study of the effectiveness of ten different methods of progressive resistance exercise on the development of strength, flexibility, girth and body weight," by J.R. Leighton et al., 1967, *Journal of the Association for Physical and Mental Rehabilitation, 21,* p. 79. Copyright 1967 by The American Kinesiotherapy Association. Adapted with permission.

weekly for 7 wk. This same study also demonstrated that a group trained with periodization had significantly greater increases in squat and vertical jump ability than either of the exhaustion-set groups. However, no significant differences among the three groups in bench press ability were demonstrated. Thus, sets to momentary concentric failure result in increased strength, but a periodized training program may result in greater increases in strength and power, especially of the legs.

FORCED REPETITION SYSTEM

Forced repetitions are an extension of the exhaustion-set system and the cheat system used by some power lifters. After a set to exhaustion has been performed, training partners assist the trainee by lifting the resistance just enough to allow the trainee to complete three to four additional repetitions. Forced repetitions can be performed with many exercises after a set to exhaustion has been performed. This system forces the muscle to continue to produce force when it is partially fatigued and therefore may be valuable when attempting to increase local muscular endurance.

This system must be used carefully because it can easily cause muscular soreness. Because the forced repetitions are performed under conditions of fatigue, the lifter must concentrate on the forced repetitions and never give up during a movement, and the spotter or spotters need to be extremely attentive and capable of lifting the weight if the lifter loses proper exercise technique. The efficacy of forced repetitions to increase strength remains unclear.

BURN SYSTEM

The burn system is an extension of the exhaustion-set system. The burn system can be incorporated into any other training system. After a set has been performed to momentary concentric failure (the weight can no longer be lifted for a complete repetition), half or partial repetitions are performed. Normally five to six partial repetitions are performed, which cause an aching or burning sensation, giving this system its name (Richford 1966). Advocates of this system claim it is especially effective when training the calves and arms.

CIRCUIT PROGRAM

Circuit programs consist of a series of resistance training exercises performed one after the other with minimal rest (15 s to 30 s) between exercises. Approximately 10 to 15 repetitions of each exercise are performed per circuit at a resistance of 40% to 60% of 1 RM. The exercises can be chosen to train any muscle group. This type of program is very time efficient when large numbers of people are trained, because each piece of equipment is in virtually constant use. It is also very time effective for an individual with a limited amount of training time.

One proposed benefit of a circuit weight training program is improved cardiovascular fitness. Circuit programs of short-term duration (8 wk to 20 wk) increase maximal oxygen consumption approximately 4% and 8% in men and women, respectively (Gettman and Pollock 1981). This is substantially less, however, than the 15% to 20% increase in maximal oxygen consumption caused by traditional running or cycling cardiovascular conditioning programs over the same time period. In fact, if subjects are already physically active or aerobically fit, even less improvement in maximal oxygen consumption can be expected from circuit weight training programs.

If one goal of a training program is to increase cardiovascular endurance, circuit training is the resistance program of choice. However, if a major goal of the conditioning program is to dramatically improve cardiovascular fitness, then an endurance training program (e.g., running, cycling, swimming) needs to be included in the total program.

PERIPHERAL HEART ACTION SYSTEM

The peripheral heart action system is a variation of circuit training. In this system a training session is divided into several sequences (Gajda 1965). A sequence is a group of four to six different exercises, each for a different body part. The number of repetitions per set of each exercise in a sequence varies with the goals of the program, but normally 8 to 12 repetitions per set are performed. One training session consists of performing all the exercises in the first sequence three times in a circuit fashion. The remaining sequences are then performed one after the other in the same fashion as the first sequence. An example of the exercises in a peripheral heart action training session is given in table 6.2.

This system is extremely tiring. The heart rate should be kept at 140 beats per minute or higher. The short rest periods and maintenance of a relatively high heart rate make this program very similar to normal circuit training. The peripheral heart

	TABLE 6.2			
	Example of a Four-Sequence Peripheral Heart Action Training Session			
	Sequence			
Body part	**1**	**2**	**3**	**4**
Chest	Bench press	Incline press	Decline press	Fly
Back	Lat pull-down	Seated row	Bent-over rows	T-bar row
Shoulders	Military press	Upright row	Lateral raise	Front raise
Leg	Squat	Knee extension	Back squat	Split squat
Abdomen	Sit-up	Crunch	Roman-chair sit-up	V-up

action system is therefore a good resistance training system to increase cardiovascular endurance as well as local muscular endurance.

TRISET SYSTEM

The triset system is similar to the peripheral heart action system in that it incorporates groups or sequences of exercises. As the name implies, it consists of groups of three exercises for the same body part. The exercises can train different muscle groups and are performed with little or no rest between exercises and sets. Normally three sets of each exercise are performed. Three exercises constituting a triset are, for example, arm curls, triceps extensions, and military presses. Trisetting is one of the most effective systems for increasing static strength (see table 6.1). The short rest periods and the use of three exercises in series for a particular body part make this a good system to increase local muscular endurance.

COMPOUND-SET SYSTEM

The compound-set system is used by some body builders to develop hypertrophy (Hatfield 1981). It may also be used to develop local muscular endurance. The compound-set system involves performing an exercise for one muscle group and then, after little or no rest, performing another exercise for a muscle group in a different part of the body. This alternating of muscle groups continues until the desired number of sets is completed. Alternating of muscle groups allows the first muscle group to partially recover while the second is being exercised, and vice versa. As an example, triceps extensions and knee extensions may be alternated in the compound-set system.

DOUBLE PROGRESSIVE SYSTEM

The training stimulus in the double progressive system is varied by changing both the number of repetitions and the resistance used. Initially the resistance is held constant while the number of repetitions per set is increased until a specified number of repetitions is reached. The resistance is then increased and the number of repetitions is decreased until the number of repetitions performed is back to the initial number. This process is then repeated. An example of this system is given in table 6.3. Of the systems compared in table 6.1 the double progressive system appears to be one of the least effective. Although the research is sparse, it indicates that use of the double progressive system is unwarranted.

TABLE 6.3		
Example of the Double Progressive System		
Sets	**Repetitions**	**Resistance (lb)**
1	4	120
2	6	120
3	8	120
4	10	120
5	12	120
6	10	140
7	8	160
8	6	175
9	4	185

FLUSHING

This system was developed by body builders to produce hypertrophy, definition, and vascularity. The number of exercises, sets, repetitions, and rest periods is not clearly defined. Flushing involves performing two or more exercises for the same muscle or for two muscle groups in close proximity. The idea behind flushing is to keep blood in the muscle group or groups for a long period of time. It is believed that this will help develop muscle hypertrophy. Many body builders train a muscle group with several exercises in succession during the same training session, so empirically this practice appears to result in hypertrophy. It is unknown how blood flow mediates changes in hypertrophy. The physiological mechanisms that mediate such training adaptations remain speculative. It could be hypothesized that higher blood flow allows more of the body's natural anabolic factors (e.g., growth hormone or testosterone) found in the blood to bind to receptors in muscle and connective tissue, but such speculation lacks supporting scientific evidence.

FUNCTIONAL ISOMETRICS

The functional isometrics system attempts to take advantage of the joint-angle specificity of strength gains caused by isometric training. Functional isometrics entail performing a dynamic concen- tric action for 4 to 6 in. (10.2 to 15.2 cm) of a movement, until the resistance hits the pins at the top of the power rack (figure 6.1). The trainee continues to attempt to lift the resistance with maximal effort for 5 to 7 s. The pins in the power rack are often placed at the sticking point of the exercise being performed.

The objective of this system is to use joint-angle specificity to cause increases in strength at the weakest point within the range of motion. The maximal amount of resistance that can be lifted in any exercise is determined by the amount of resistance that can be moved through the sticking point (the weakest point in that movement). Functional isometrics used in conjunction with normal DCER training has been shown to cause significantly greater increases in 1-RM bench press strength than DCER training alone (Jackson et al. 1985).

Many power lifters use this system without a power rack during the last repetition of a heavy set (e.g., 1-6 RM). They attempt to perform as much of a repetition as possible, and when the weight cannot be moved they continue to produce force isometrically at the exact angle where the sticking point occurs. This type of training requires very attentive spotters. In this system it is important to know where the sticking point is in the range of motion to allow optimization of the training, particularly because sticking points can change with training. This system is appropriate when the major goal of the program is to increase the 1-RM capability of a particular exercise.

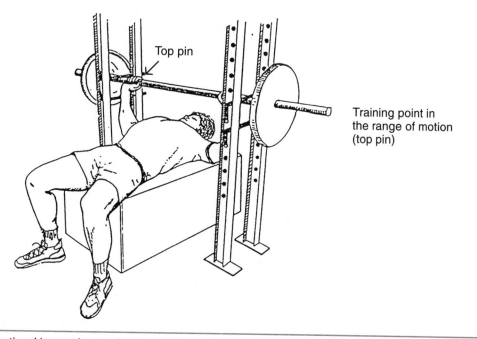

Top pin

Training point in the range of motion (top pin)

Fig. 6.1   Functional isometrics used at the sticking point in a bench press. The top pin is placed at the exact point in the range of motion desired to be trained.

TRIANGLE PROGRAM

Triangle or pyramid programs are used by many power lifters. A complete triangle or pyramid program starts with a set of 10 to 12 repetitions with a light resistance. The resistance is then increased over several sets so that fewer and fewer repetitions can be performed, until only a 1 RM is performed. Then the same sets and resistances are repeated in reverse order, with the last set consisting of 10 to 12 repetitions (see figure 6.2).

LIGHT-TO-HEAVY SYSTEM

As the name implies, a light-to-heavy system involves progressing from light to heavy resistances. This system became popular in the 1930s and 1940s among Olympic lifters (Hatfield and Krotee 1978). It consists of performing a set of three to five repetitions with a relatively light resistance. Five pounds (2.3 kg) are then added to the resistance, and another set of three to five repetitions is performed. This is continued until only one repetition can be performed.

The DeLorme regimen of three sets of 10 repetitions with the resistance progressing from 50% to 66% to 100% of 10 RM is a light-to-heavy system. The DeLorme system causes significant increases in strength over short-term training periods (DeLorme, Ferris, and Gallagher 1952; DeLorme and Watkins 1948; Leighton et al. 1967). The DeLorme training group in the study depicted in table 6.1 demonstrated a significant increase in static elbow-flexion strength but no significant increases in static elbow-extension or back-and-leg strength. A second light-to-heavy system (descending half triangle or descending half pyramid, see figure 6.2) demonstrated significant increases in all three static strength tests. This appears to be one of the more effective systems of the study depicted in table 6.1 for increasing static back-and-leg strength.

HEAVY-TO-LIGHT SYSTEM

In a heavy-to-light system, after a brief warm-up, the heaviest set is performed, then the resistance is lowered for each succeeding set (figure 6.2). The Oxford technique is a heavy-to-light system consisting of three sets of 10 repetitions progressing from 100% to 66% to 50% of 10 RM. Significant gains in strength have been achieved with the Oxford system (Leighton et al. 1967; McMorris and Elkins 1954; Zinovieff 1951).

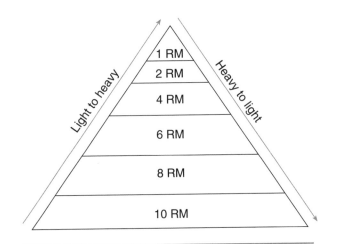

Fig. 6.2   Performing sets that progress from light to heavy resistances is a light-to-heavy system (an ascending pyramid). Performing sets that progress from heavy to light resistances is a heavy-to-light system (a descending pyramid). A full pyramid, or triangle, consists of both the ascending and descending portions of the pyramid.

Comparisons of the heavy-to-light (descending half triangle) and light-to-heavy (ascending half triangle) systems are equivocal but tend to favor the heavy-to-light system. One study found the heavy-to-light system to be superior to the light-to-heavy system in strength gains but indicated that further research is necessary (McMorris and Elkins 1954). A second study (Leighton et al. 1967; see table 6.1) found little difference between the two in increasing elbow flexion but found that the heavy-to-light system (Oxford) is clearly superior compared to a light-to-heavy system (DeLorme) in increasing elbow-extension and back-and-leg strength.

MULTIPOUNDAGE SYSTEM

The multipoundage system with free weights requires one or two spotters to assist during a training session. If machines are used, spotters may not be needed. The trainee performs four or five repetitions at a 4- or 5-RM resistance. Then 20 to 40 lb (9.1 to 18.1 kg) are removed from the resistance, and the trainee performs another four or five repetitions. This procedure is continued for several sets (Poole 1964). The number of sets possible depends on the original resistance used and the goals of the program. Some body builders believe that this system results in increased vascularity and that the large volume of training that can be done in a short period of time contributes to the development of muscular hypertrophy. The performance of several sets of an exercise in rapid succession makes this a good system for increasing local muscular endurance.

NEGATIVE SYSTEM

During most resistance exercises the *negative*, or eccentric, portion of the repetition is lowering the weight. During this phase the muscles involved are actively lengthening so that the resistance can be lowered in a controlled manner. Conversely, the lifting of the resistance during the repetition of an exercise is termed the *positive*, or concentric, portion.

It is possible to lower more weight in the negative portion of a repetition than is lifted in the positive portion. Negative resistance training involves lowering more weight than can be lifted in the concentric phase of the repetition. Negative training can be done by having spotters help the lifter raise the weight, which the lifter then lowers unassisted. It can also be performed on some resistance training machines by lifting the weight with both arms or legs and then lowering the resistance with only one arm or leg. On some machines it is possible to lift the weight with both the arms and legs and then to lower the weight using just the arms or just the legs. Proper exercise technique and safe spotting techniques must be used for all exercises performed during heavy negative training. There are also electronic weight machines with which negative training can be performed.

Advocates of negative training believe that the use of more resistance during the negative portion of the exercise results in greater increases in strength. However, studies using 120% of the concentric (positive) 1 RM for negative training have not resulted in greater gains in strength than normal DCER training. Only limited data are available concerning the optimal eccentric resistances for particular muscle groups. Ranges of 105% to 140% of the concentric 1 RM have been proposed, but the resistance depends on whether a machine or free weights are used. Machines reduce the need for balance and involvement of assistance muscles, thus heavier eccentric (negative) resistances may be possible. It has been shown that a repetition that uses a heavier eccentric resistance (105% of the concentric 1 RM) immediately prior to the concentric phase of the repetition results in a heavier concentric 1 RM (Kraemer et al. in press). Eccentric training may enhance the neural facilitation of the concentric movement. Further study is needed to determine whether such training affects training-related gains in strength. For free weights, resis-

tance of 105% to 110% of the concentric 1 RM probably represents the upper limit of effective eccentric resistances for most exercise movements.

SUPER OVERLOAD SYSTEM

The super overload system is a type of negative weight training. Partial repetitions are performed using 125% of the 1 RM weight. For example, if an individual's 1-RM bench press is 200 lb (90.7 kg), 250 lb (113.4 kg) is used (200 lb [90.7 kg] $\times$ 1.25 = 250 lb [113.4 kg]). Spotters help the lifter get the weight in the straight-arm position of the bench press. The lifter lowers the weight as far as possible before lifting the weight back to the straight-arm position without assistance from the spotters. The lifter performs 7 to 10 such partial repetitions per set. The lifter then slowly lowers the weight to the chest-touch position, and the spotters help lift the weight back to the straight-arm position. Three such sets per exercise are performed in a training session.

The super overload system has been shown to be as effective as conventional weight training in developing 1-RM strength (Powers, Browning, and Groves 1978). Over 8 wk of training, 3 d/wk, with at least 1 d of rest between training sessions, the super overload system resulted in 1-RM bench and leg press increases equal to conventional weight training. Because resistances greater than 1 RM are used in this type of training, spotters are mandatory when using free weights. It is also possible to use some machines with this system. As in the negative system, the resistance may be lifted with both arms or legs and the partial repetitions performed with only one arm or leg.

PRIORITY SYSTEM

The priority system can be applied to virtually all resistance training systems. The priority system involves performing the exercises that apply to the training program's major goal(s) first, so that the trainee can perform the major training or exercises with maximal intensity. If the major exercises are performed late in the training session, fatigue may prevent the trainee from using maximal resistances, which may limit the adaptation to the training.

A body builder's weakest muscle group in terms of definition and hypertrophy may be the quadriceps group, for example. Using the priority concept, exercises for the quadriceps group would be performed at the beginning of a training session. A basketball coach may decide that a power forward's biggest weakness is lack of upper-body strength, which causes the player to be pushed around under the boards. Major upper-body exercises are placed at the beginning of the training session for this player. A football player may want to promote strength and power development of the thighs, hips, and lower back and therefore would perform heavy hang-cleans and squats in the beginning of the workout.

REST-PAUSE SYSTEM

This system involves using near-maximal resistances (1 RM) for multiple repetitions. This is made possible by taking a 10- to 15-s rest between repetitions. As an example, a lifter performs one repetition of an exercise with 250 lb (113.4 kg), which is near the 1 RM for the exercise. The lifter puts the weight down, rests 10 to 15 s, and then performs another repetition with 250 lb (113.4 kg). This is repeated for four to five repetitions. If the lifter cannot perform a complete repetition, spotters lend just enough assistance to allow completion of the four to five repetitions. Only one set of an exercise is performed, but two to three exercises per muscle group may be performed in the same training session. The goal of this system is to use the maximal resistance possible. Proponents of this system believe that by using a resistance as close as possible to maximal the greatest possible gains in strength will occur.

SPLIT ROUTINE SYSTEM

Many body builders use a split routine system. Body builders perform many exercises for the same body part to encourage hypertrophy. Because this is a time-consuming process, not all parts of the body can be exercised in a single training session. Solving this predicament has led to training various body parts on alternate days, or a split routine. A typical split routine system entails the training of arms, legs, and abdomen on Monday, Wednesday, and Friday and chest, shoulders, and back on Tuesday, Thursday, and Saturday. This system solves the predicament of limited time per session, but it means that training is performed 6 d/wk.

Variations of a split routine system can be developed so that training sessions take place 4 or 5 d/wk. Even though training sessions are quite frequent, sufficient recovery of muscle groups between training sessions is possible because body parts are not trained on successive days. The split

routine system allows the training intensity for a particular body part or group of exercises to be maintained at a higher level than would be possible if the four to six training sessions were combined into two or three long sessions. The maintenance of a higher intensity (heavier resistances) should result in greater gains in strength. In highly strength trained athletes (i.e., college football players) short-term (10-wk) strength gains in bench press and squat exercises depend on increased use of assistance exercises (J.R. Hoffman et al. 1991). Split routines allow more attention to the assistance exercises needed to enhance strength development. Thus, split routines offer the advantages of a higher intensity and volume of training and allowing the performance of more assistance exercises that may enhance strength development.

BLITZ PROGRAM

The blitz program is a variation of the split routine system. Rather than training several body parts during each training session, only one body part is trained per session. The duration of the training session is not reduced. Thus, more sets or exercises for a particular body part are performed. An example of a blitz program is to perform all arm, chest, leg, trunk, back, and shoulder exercises on Monday, Tuesday, Wednesday, Thursday, Friday, and Saturday, respectively. This type of program is performed by some body builders in preparation for a contest. A short-duration blitz program may also be appropriate if an athlete's performance is limited by the strength of a particular muscle group or groups. A long jumper might perform a blitz program for the legs prior to the start of a season, which might involve training only the legs 2 d/wk.

ISOLATED EXERCISE SYSTEM

The isolated exercise system devotes an entire training session to a single exercise (Horvath 1959). For example, on Monday only the bench press is performed; Tuesday, the squat; Thursday, arm curls; and Friday, upright rows. Other exercises can be added to achieve as many training days per week or sessions per week as desired. A resistance is selected that allows 8 to 10 repetitions to be performed. The trainee then performs set after set of that day's exercise for as many repetitions as possible for 1-1/2 hr. A 1-min rest is allowed between sets.

This system places a great deal of stress on the muscles and joints involved in each exercise; this system is not recommended for more than six consecutive weeks (Horvath 1959). Variations of this system similar to the blitz program may be appropriate for a short duration if an athlete's performance is limited by one particular muscle group. Some body builders use this system to stimulate hypertrophy of a particular muscle or muscle group. Long-term use of this system may result in an overuse injury or overtraining syndrome of the muscle group(s) involved. Therefore, careful monitoring and a strong rationale for using this system are needed.

SUPER PUMP SYSTEM

Proponents of the super pump system believe that advanced body builders need to perform 15 to 18 sets for each body part per training session in order to achieve the muscular development desired (Page 1966). To achieve this high number of sets, anywhere from one to three exercises per muscle group are performed per training session. This system uses 15-s rest periods between sets of five to six repetitions (Page 1966). The repetitions must all be performed with strict adherence to correct form, and each muscle group must be trained two to three times per week. The super pump system appears to be effective for advanced lifters who desire greater muscular hypertrophy of the arms, chest, and shoulders. This system may be too fatiguing to use in training the large muscles of the legs and back (Darden 1973).

SUPER SETTING SYSTEMS

Super setting has evolved into two distinct systems. One program uses several sets of two exercises for the agonist and antagonist muscles of one body part. Examples of this type of super setting are arm curls immediately followed by triceps extensions or knee extensions immediately followed by knee curls. Significant increases in strength from this type of super setting have been reported (see table 6.1). The super setting system is one of the most effective for increasing back-and-leg static strength of the 10 systems compared in table 6.1.

The second type of super setting uses one set of several exercises in rapid succession for the same muscle group or body part. An example of this is one set each of lat pull-downs, seated rowing, and bent-over rowing. Both types of super setting in-

volve sets of 8 to 10 repetitions with little or no rest between sets and exercises. Super setting is popular among body builders, suggesting that it results in muscular hypertrophy. If the goal of a training program is to produce increases in muscular hypertrophy, super setting warrants consideration. In addition, super setting appears to enhance local muscular endurance, because body builders have demonstrated the ability to maintain a higher percentage of their 1-RM strength when performing a consecutive series of exercises with very little rest (10 s to 60 s) between sets (Kraemer, Noble, Culver, and Clark 1987).

SUPER SLOW SYSTEM

The super slow system involves performing very slow repetitions ranging from 20 to 60 s per repetition. Proponents say that the increased amount of time that the muscle is under tension enhances its strength development. To date, few data are available to support this theory.

This system is typically used for isolated joint exercises or machine exercises where the movement can be controlled throughout the range of motion. Usually only one or two sets of one to five repetitions of an exercise are performed in a workout. The resistance varies, depending on the trainee's muscular endurance fitness level, and is not related to a normal-speed repetition using a given RM resistance. As the duration of the repetition increases, the amount of resistance that can be utilized decreases because the amount of force that a muscle can produce dramatically decreases with time due to fatigue. Thus, each point in the range of motion receives less than an optimal strength stimulus. Super slow systems appear to have some potential efficacy in developing slow-velocity muscular endurance and decreases in percentage of body fat.

COMPARISON OF SYSTEMS

The potential for creating a new resistance training system appears almost infinite. All the systems discussed in this chapter were designed to address specific training goals. They evolved from a variety of sources, including the sports of body building, power lifting, and weight lifting. Systems continue to be used if desired adaptations are realized by the groups using them. Commercial magazines and equipment companies have attempted to promote resistance training systems that suit their

TABLE 6.4
Acute Program Variables of Various Training Systems

Training system	Acute program variables						
	Repetitions/set	Resistance	Choice of exercise	Order of exercise	Rest between sets or exercises	Sets per exercise
Blitz	8-10	8-10 RM	One muscle group/d	NS	NS	NS
Bulk	5-6	NS	NS	NS	NS	3-5
Burn	After a set to failure 5 or 6 more partial reps are performed	NS	NS	NS	NS	NS
Cheat system	NS	>1 RM	NS	NS	NS	NS
Circuit	10-15	40%-60% of 1 RM	NS	NS	15-30s	1-3
Compound set	NS	NS	NS	Alternating 2 muscle groups in different parts of body	A few seconds	NS
Double progressive	NS	Constant resistance with increasing reps, then increasing resistance with decreasing reps	NS	NS	NS	NS
Exhaustion sets	NS	RM for desired number of reps	NS	NS	NS	NS
Flushing	NS	NS	2 or more exercises for same muscle group in sequence	NS	NS	NS
Forced repetitions	After a set to failure 3-4 more assisted reps are done	NS	Exercise where resistance movement can be assisted	NS	NS	NS
Functional isometrics	NS	NS	After some movement a 5- to 7-s isometric action is performed	NS	NS	NS
Heavy-to-light	NS	Progresses from heavy to light	NS	NS	NS	NS
Isolated exercise	8-10	8-10 RM	One exercise/d	NS	1 min	As many as possible in 1-1.5 hr

System						
Light-to-heavy	NS	Progresses from light to heavy	NS	NS	NS	NS
Multiple set	NS	NS	NS	NS	NS	3 or more
Multipoundage	4-5	4-5 RM initially, reduced 20-40 lb (9.1-18.1 kg) per set to allow 4-5 more reps		NS	NS	Several
Negative	NS	>1 RM	NS	NS	NS	NS
Peripheral heart action	NS	NS	Sequence of 5-6 exercises each for different body parts	NS	None or little	4-6
Priority	NS	NS	NS	Perform most important exercises first in session	NS	NS
Rest-pause	1	Near 1 RM	NS	NS	10-15 s	4-5
Single set	4-10	4-10 RM	NS	NS	NS	1
Split routine	NS	NS	Different muscle groups each training session	NS	NS	NS
Super overload	7-10 partial	>1 RM	NS	NS	NS	3
Super pump	5-6	5-6 RM	1-3 per muscle group	NS	15 s	15-18 per body part
Super setting 1	NS	NS	Agonist and antagonist	Agonist to antagonist	None	Several
Super setting 2	NS	NS	Several for same muscle group	NS	None-little	1-several
Super slow	1-5	NS	NS	NS	NS	1-2
Triangle	NS	Light to heavy, back to light	NS	NS	NS	Several
Triset	NS	NS	3 for a body part	NS	None-little	3

NS = not specified

equipment's characteristics or that fit into their marketing strategies. Nevertheless, it should be possible to describe each system in terms of its acute program variables (table 6.4). However, for most systems the acute program variables were never completely defined. This may explain why training responses to a system vary considerably.

SUMMARY

With manipulation of acute program variables it is easy to design many distinctly different systems. The resistance system should be designed to address the needs of the individual or the event for which the individual is training. Popular or fad training systems should be described and evaluated in terms of their acute program variables and their ability to address the needs of an individual or sport. The choice of training system depends on the goals of the program, time constraints, and how the goals of the resistance training program relate to the goals of the entire fitness program. A major goal of any program is to bring about physiological adaptations, which are the subject of the next chapter.

SELECTED READINGS

American College of Sports Medicine. 1990. The recommended quantity and quality of exercise for developing and maintaining cardiovascular and muscular fitness in healthy adults. *Medicine and Science in Sports and Exercise* 22:265-74.

Dudley, G.A.; Tesch, P.A.; Miller, B.J.; and Buchanan, P. 1991. Importance of eccentric actions in performance adaptations to resistance training. *Aviation, Space, and Environmental Medicine* 62:543-50.

Hoffman, J.R.; Fry, A.C.; Howard, R.; Maresh, C.M.; and Kraemer, W.J. 1991. Strength, speed, and endurance changes during the course of a Division I basketball season. *Journal of Applied Sport Science Research* 5:144-49.

Leighton, J.R.; Holmes, D.; Benson, J.; Wooten, B.; and Schmerer, R. 1967. A study of the effectiveness of ten different methods of progressive resistance exercise on the development of strength, flexibility, girth, and body weight. *Journal of the Association of Physical and Mental Rehabilitation* 21:78-81.

Willoughby, D.S. 1993. The effects of mesocycle-length weight training programs involving periodization and partially equated volumes on upper and lower body strength. *Journal of Strength and Conditioning Research* 7:2-8.

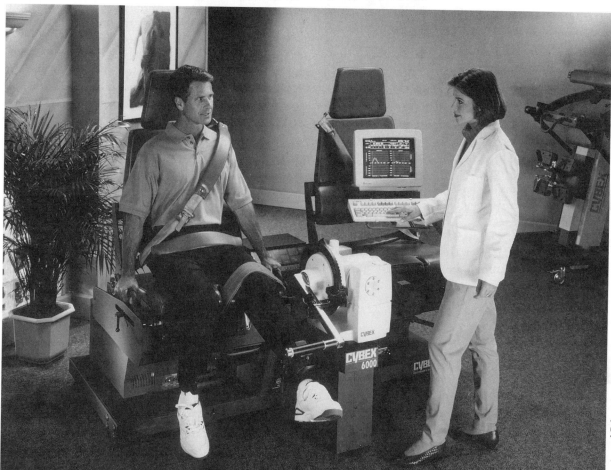

CHAPTER 7

Courtesy of Cybex

Adaptations to Resistance Training

Both acute and chronic physiological changes occur with exercise. An acute response to exercise usually results in an immediate change in the examined variable. For example, an increase in heart rate in response to a jog at 4.5 mph (7.2 km/hr) on a treadmill is called an acute exercise response. Chronic change has to do with the body's response to a repeated exercise stimulus over the course of a training program. The physiological process by which the body adapts to the exercise is called *adaptation* to training. For example, the heart rate response to that same 4.5-mph treadmill jog of submaximal exercise intensity decreases by the end of a 12-wk training program. Though the body responds acutely to a given exercise stress (in this case, by increasing heart rate), repeated exposure to the exercise stimulus by means of training reduces the acute response (lower heart rate). It is important to be familiar with both the acute and the chronic changes that occur with exercise; this knowledge facilitates exercise prescription as well as program design. The adaptation to training ultimately determines whether a resistance training program is effective and whether an athlete is capable of a higher level of physiological function or performance. A great deal of information on the adaptations to resistance training has accumulated over the past decade. The purpose of this chapter is to review some of the findings important to the understanding of resistance training program design.

All adaptations follow a specific time course. An acute exercise stimulus will initiate an adaptation in the body, but only through repeated exposure to the exercise stimulus (a training program) will a change take place in a specific cell, tissue, or system. A resistance training program's effectiveness in causing a change varies, depending on the amount of adaptation that has already taken place. For example, if an athlete has never trained using the bench press exercise, the initial changes in strength will be dramatic. But after he or she has progressively trained for a long period of time, the gains that are made will be small in comparison, because the potential for adaptation has been realized. In other words, the *window of adaptation* is now

much smaller because of prior training and improvement in physical performance, or physiological change (Newton and Kraemer 1994). Thus, from start to finish in a training program, gains or adaptations do not take place at a constant rate. Building and peaking programs and maintenance programs acknowledge the time course for adaptations of the body. This time course concept is shown in figure 7.1 for muscle fiber size and strength gains. The largest changes take place early in training and then slow down as training continues. A similar phenomenon exists for all training adaptations, but the time course and the point where the most dramatic adaptational response takes place vary from variable to variable.

MUSCLE FIBER ADAPTATIONS

One of the most prominent adaptations is the enlargement of muscles. Today, sport scientists, athletes, and coaches all agree that a properly designed and implemented strength training program leads to muscle growth. This growth in muscle size has

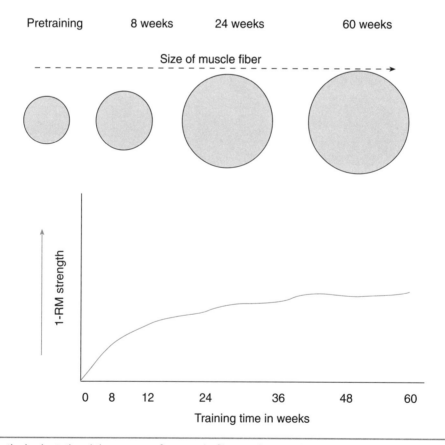

Fig. 7.1   Theoretical adaptational time course for muscle fiber and strength changes in response to a strength training program.

been thought to be caused primarily by muscle fiber hypertrophy, or an increase in the size of the individual muscle fibers (MacDougall 1992). It has also been suggested that the increase in muscle size may be caused by muscle fiber hyperplasia, or an increase in the number of muscle fibers, but this theory is controversial. Hyperplasia following resistance training in humans has not been directly proven because of methodological difficulties (e.g., one cannot take out the whole muscle for examination) but has been shown in response to various exercise protocols in birds and mammals (for reviews see Antonio and Gonyea 1994; MacDougall 1992).

Hyperplasia

Hyperplasia was first implicated as an adaptive strategy for muscle enlargement in laboratory animals (Gonyea 1980; Ho et al. 1980). Critics of these studies have claimed that methods of evaluation, damage to the muscle samples, and degenerating muscle fibers account for the observed hyperplasia. A few later studies attempted to correct such problems, however, and still demonstrated increases in muscle fiber number (Alway, Winchester, Davies, and Gonyea 1989; Gonyea et al. 1986).

Several studies comparing body builders and power lifters concluded that the cross-sectional area of the body builders' individual muscle fibers was not significantly larger than normal, yet these athletes possessed larger muscles than normal (MacDougall et al. 1982; Tesch and Larsson 1982). This indicates that these athletes had a greater total number of muscle fibers than normal, and hyperplasia may account for this increase. Yet another study using body builders concluded that they possessed the same number of muscle fibers as the control group but possessed much larger muscles (MacDougall et al. 1984). This study suggests that the large muscle size of body builders is caused by hypertrophy of existing muscle fibers rather than hyperplasia. A study of hyperplasia in cats indicated that for hyperplasia to occur, the exercise intensity must be sufficient to recruit fast-twitch (Type II) muscle fibers (Gonyea 1980). It is possible that only high-intensity resistance training can cause hyperplasia and that Type II muscle fibers may be targeted for this type of adaptation.

Though no concrete evidence supports the hyperplasia theory in humans, there are indications that hyperplasia occurs from resistance training. Because of these conflicting results, this topic continues to remain controversial, and further research on elite competitive lifters may help to resolve the controversy. Although hyperplasia in humans may not be the primary adaptational response of most muscle fibers, it might represent an adaptation to resistance training that is possible when certain muscle fibers reach a theoretical upper limit in cell size. In theory very intense, long-term training may make some Type II muscle fibers primary candidates for such an adaptational response. If hyperplasia does occur, it may account for only a small portion (e.g., 5%-10%) of the increase in muscle size.

Hypertrophy

An increase in muscle size in response to resistance training has been observed in both animal and human studies. In laboratory animals, muscle growth occurred from hypertrophy alone (Bass, Mackova, and Vitek 1973; Gollnick et al. 1981; Timson et al. 1985). Increased muscle size in strength-trained athletes has been attributed to hypertrophy of existing muscle fibers (Alway 1994; Alway, Grumbt, Gonyea, and Stray-Gundersen 1989; Haggmark, Jansson, and Svane 1978). This increase in the cross-sectional area of existing muscle fibers is attributed to the increased size and number of actin and myosin filaments and to addition of sarcomeres within existing muscle fibers (Goldspink 1992; MacDougall et al. 1979). However, not all muscle fibers undergo the same amount of enlargement. The amount of enlargement depends on the type of muscle fiber and the pattern of recruitment (Kraemer et al. 1995). The contractile proteins and fluid (sarcoplasm) in muscle fibers are constantly changing and turning over every 7 to 15 d (Goldspink 1992). Resistance training influences this process by affecting the quality and quantity of contractile proteins that are produced.

The increase in muscle fiber size can be seen by examining a group of muscle fibers under a microscope after they have been stained. In figure 7.2 a picture of a sample obtained from a woman's vastus lateralis (quadriceps muscle) is shown before (a) and after (b) an 8-wk heavy resistance training program. The fibers are cut in cross section; the dark fibers are the Type I, the intermediate dark fibers are Type IIB, and the white fibers are Type IIA. It is obvious that the size of all of this woman's muscle fibers, especially the Type II (fast-twitch) muscle fibers, increased with just 8 wk of heavy resistance training.

Adaptations in muscle fibers with heavy resistance training must be viewed in light of both quality and quantity of the contractile proteins (i.e., actin and myosin). The quality of protein refers to

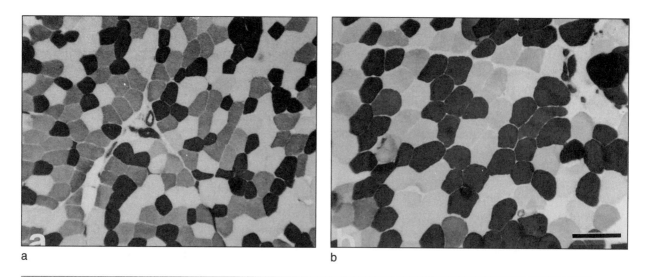

a   b

Fig. 7.2   Muscle sample obtained **A.** before and **B.** immediately after an 8-wk strength training program. Dark fibers are Type I, intermediate dark fibers are Type IIB, and white fibers are Type IIA. These data and micrograph set courtesy of Dr. Robert S. Staron, Ohio University, Athens, OH.

the type of proteins found in the contractile machinery. With the initiation of a heavy resistance training program, changes in the types of muscle proteins (e.g., myosin heavy chains) start to take place within a couple of workouts (Staron et al. 1994). As training continues, the quantity of contractile proteins starts to increase as muscle fiber cross-sectional areas increase. To demonstrate a significant amount of muscle fiber hypertrophy, it appears that a longer period of training time (more than eight workouts) is needed to increase the contractile protein content in all the muscle fibers. Thus, short-term programs (4-8 wk) may not result in very large changes in the size of muscles.

Muscle Fiber Transformation

A lot of resistance exercise research focuses on the myosin molecule and on examination of fiber types

using histochemical myosin adenosine triphosphatase (mATPase) staining activities at different pHs. Changes in muscle mATPase fiber types also give an indication of associated changes in the myosin heavy-chain (MHC) content (Fry, Allemeier, and Staron 1994). We now know that a continuum of muscle fiber types exists and that transformation within a particular muscle fiber subtype (e.g., from Type IIB to Type IIA) is a common adaptation to resistance training (G.R. Adams et al. 1993; Staron et al. 1991, 1994; Kraemer et al. 1995). It appears that as soon as Type IIB muscle fiber is stimulated, it starts a process of transformation toward the Type IIA profile by changing the quality of proteins and expressing different amounts and combinations of mATPase types. Figure 7.3 shows the transformation process that occurs with heavy resistance training in the muscle fiber subtypes. Using this classification scheme for

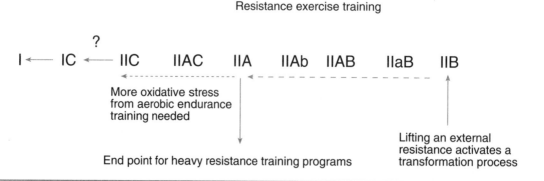

Fig. 7.3   The process of muscle fiber–type transformation. Changes in myosin ATPase and myosin heavy-chain proteins underlie this process.

evaluating muscle fiber–subtype changes, it is doubtful that under normal training conditions muscle fibers transform from Type II to Type I (Kraemer et al. 1995). Thus, the old concept of trying to change muscle fiber types appears to apply to changes only within a fiber type (for reviews see Kraemer et al. 1995; Staron and Johnson 1993).

In a study by Staron and colleagues (1994) a high-intensity resistance training protocol was performed by men and women two times per week for 8 wk. This protocol focused on the thigh musculature with heavy multiple sets of 6 to 8 RM on one day and 10 to 12 RM on the other day for several exercises (squats, leg presses, and knee extensions). Two-minute rest periods were used to induce hormonal changes with the exercise protocol (Kraemer et al. 1990). Maximal dynamic strength increased over the 8-wk training period without any significant changes in muscle fiber size or fat-free mass in the men or the women. This supports the theory that neural adaptations are the predominant mechanism in the early phase of training. It is interesting to note that a significant decrease in the Type IIB percentage was observed in women after just 2 wk of training (i.e., four workouts) and in the men after 4 wk of training (i.e., eight workouts). Over the 8-wk training program (16 workouts) the Type IIB muscle fiber types decreased from 21% to about 7% of the total muscle fibers in both men and women (Staron et al. 1994). The alteration in the muscle fiber types was supported by myosin heavy-chain (MHC) analyses. This was the first study to establish the time course of specific muscular adaptations in the early phase of a resistance training program for men and women.

It is not known to what extent muscle fiber remodeling contributes to muscle strength; however, gradual increases in the number and size of myofibrils and perhaps the fast fiber–type conversions of Type IIB to IIA might contribute to force production. In addition, changes in hormonal factors (testosterone and cortisol interactions) are correlated with such changes in the muscle fibers (e.g., percentage shift in Type IIA) and may help to mediate such adaptations. However, the nervous system alterations may still be the most dramatic adaptation mediating strength and power changes early in a training program. Many other changes take place during muscle fiber remodeling in the early phase of training that may influence when hypertrophy is initiated. Thus, the quality of the protein type being generated is an important aspect of muscular development, especially in the early phases of resistance training.

Longer studies of heavy resistance training have also examined changes in muscle fiber type and cross-sectional size with training. Staron and co-workers (1991) examined changes in skeletal muscle in women who trained for 20 wk, detrained for 30 to 32 wk, and then retrained for 6 wk. Increases in muscle fiber cross section were seen with training. The percentage of Type IIB fibers decreased from 16% to 0.9%. This study also demonstrated that during detraining muscle fiber cross-sectional areas return to pretraining values and a conversion from Type IIA to Type IIB fibers occurs. Thus, the percentage of muscle fiber types also return to pretraining values during detraining. In addition, it was demonstrated that retraining resulted in a quicker change in muscle size and conversion to Type IIA fibers than initial training from an untrained condition. Thus, the concept of "muscle memory" used by athletes and coaches has some validity in retraining after a period of detraining.

A series of studies using the same subject population examined the effect of resistance training on muscle strength, morphology, histochemical responses, and MHC responses (G.R. Adams et al. 1993; Dudley et al. 1991; Hather, Mason, and Dudley 1991). Three groups of men trained for 19 wk. One group (con/ecc) trained using both concentric and eccentric muscle actions, normal resistance training for 4 to 5 sets of 6 to 12 repetitions. A second group (con) trained with only concentric actions for 4 to 5 sets of 6 to 12 repetitions, and a third group (con/con) used only concentric actions for 8 to 10 sets of 6 to 12 repetitions. Thus, the third group performed twice the training volume as the second group. All groups showed significant gains in strength and an increase in the percentage of Type IIA fibers with an accompanying decrease in percentage of Type IIB fibers. Increases in Type I fiber area occurred only in the con/ecc group, whereas Type II fiber area increased in both the con/ecc and con/con groups. Capillaries per unit muscle fiber area increased only in the con/con and con groups. The changes in Type II fiber subtypes were paralleled by an increase in MHC IIA and a decrease in MHC IIB. The results indicate that hypertrophy, Type II fiber–type transformation, and capillaries per unit fiber area are all affected by muscle action type and training volume.

The remodeling of muscle tissue with heavy resistance exercise is a function of the program and the sequential changes in contractile proteins. All fibers appear to hypertrophy, but not to the same extent. It appears with Type II muscle fibers that the process involves an increase in the rate of protein synthesis and with Type I muscle fibers a decrease in the rate of degradation (Goldspink 1992). Conventional heavy resistance training programs in humans appear to hypertrophy both Type I and Type II muscle fibers (Kraemer, Patton, et al. 1995; Staron et al. 1991). Type II muscle fibers make larger relative gains when compared to the Type I muscle fibers in both humans and animals (Edgerton 1978; Gonyea and Sale 1982; Kraemer, Patton, et al. 1995).

The pattern of neural recruitment and the amount of muscle tissue recruited determine whether cellular and whole muscle changes occur. When enough muscle is affected, body composition will be altered in the resistance-trained individual. The amount of muscle mass gained and fiber transformation consequent to a resistance training program will also be affected by an individual's genetic potential.

Connective Tissue

Physical activity also increases the size and strength of ligaments, tendons, and bone (Fahey, Akka, and Rolph 1975; Stone 1992; Zernicke and Loitz 1992). As the skeletal muscles become stronger and can lift more weight, the ligaments, tendons, and bones must also adapt in order to support greater forces and weights. Bone has a tendency to adapt much more slowly (e.g., 6-12 mo for a change in bone density) than muscle (Conroy et al. 1992). Increased strength of the ligaments and tendons is a neces-

sary adaptation to help prevent possible damage to these structures caused by the muscles' ability to lift heavier weights and develop more tension. Although it is now acknowledged that the dense, fibrous tissues that make up tendons and ligaments respond to metabolic changes and are adaptable, no research has examined the effects of heavy resistance exercise on these structures (Stone 1992; Zernicke and Loitz 1992).

Conroy and colleagues (1992) reviewed the basic characteristics of resistance training that are needed to alter healthy bone. Bone is very sensitive to compression, strain, and strain rate. Such forces are common in resistance training and are related to the type of exercise utilized, the intensity of the resistance, and the number of sets. A study by Conroy and co-workers (1993) demonstrated that elite junior (14- to 17-yr-old) Olympic weight lifters had significantly higher bone density in the hip and femur regions than did age-matched control subjects. Even more amazing was that these young lifters who had been training for over a year had bone densities higher than adult men. In addition, bone density continued to increase over the next year of training (authors' unpublished data). These data indicate that the type of training characterized by high-power exercise movements (squats, power cleans, pulling exercises, overhead lifts) and by variations using heavy resistances and multiple sets produces dramatic changes in bone metabolism and most likely tendon and ligament growth as well (table 7.1).

TABLE 7.1
Bone Mineral Density Values for the Spine and Proximal Femur

Anatomical site	Bone mineral density ($g \cdot cm^{-2}$)		[Comparison with adult reference data] (Comparison with matched controls)
	Junior lifters	Controls	
Spine	1.41 ± 0.20*†	1.06 ± 0.21	[113%] (133%)
Femoral neck	1.30 ± 0.15*†	1.05 ± 0.12	[131%] (124%)
Trochanter	1.05 ± 0.13*	0.89 ± 0.12	ND (118%)
Ward's triangle	1.26 ± 0.20*	0.99 ± 0.16	ND (127%)

Values are means ± 1 *SD*. *$p \le .05$ from corresponding control data, † $p \le .05$ from corresponding adult reference data. ND = no reference data available.

Adapted, by permission, from B.P. Conroy et al., 1993, "Bone mineral density in elite junior weightlifters," *Medicine and Science in Sports and Exercise* 25(10):1105.

Connective tissue is abundantly distributed throughout the body. Physiological adaptations in ligaments and tendons occur as a result of physical training and may aid in injury prevention. Physical activity causes increased metabolism, thickness, weight, and strength of ligaments (Staff 1982; Tipton et al. 1975). Damaged ligaments regain their strength at a faster rate if physical activity is performed after the damage has occurred (Staff 1982; Tipton et al. 1975). Both the attachment site of a ligament or tendon to a bone and the muscle-tendinous junction are frequent sites of injury. Research involving laboratory animals demonstrates that with endurance-type training the amount of force necessary to cause separation at these areas increases (Tipton et al. 1975). There is reason to believe that resistance training would not produce similar results.

The connective tissue that surrounds the entire muscle (epimysium), groups of muscle fibers (perimysium), and individual muscle fibers (endomysium) may also adapt to resistance training. These sheaths are of major importance in the tensile strength and elastic properties of muscle; they form the framework that supports an overload on the muscle. Compensatory hypertrophy induced in the muscle of laboratory animals causes an increase in the collagen content of these connective tissue sheaths (Laurent et al. 1978; Turto, Lindy, and Halme 1974). It has been reported, however, that body builders do not differ from age-matched control subjects in the relative amount of connective tissue in the biceps brachii (MacDougall et al. 1985). Therefore, the connective tissue sheaths in muscle appear to increase at the same rate as muscle tissue.

Resistance training has been found to increase the thickness of hyaline cartilage on the articular surfaces of bone (Holmdahl and Ingelmark 1948; Ingelmark and Elsholm 1948). One major function of hyaline cartilage is to act as a shock absorber between the bony surfaces of a joint. Increasing the thickness of this cartilage could facilitate the performance of this shock-absorbing function.

NERVOUS SYSTEM ADAPTATIONS

Figure 7.4 presents a theoretical overview of the basic interactions and relationships among components of the neuromuscular system. A message

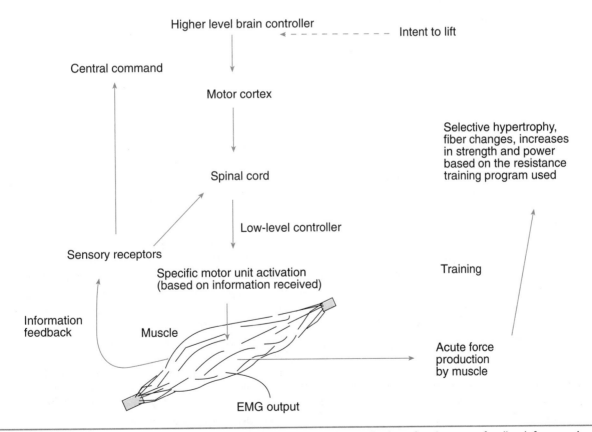

Fig. 7.4   A theoretical overview of the neural pathways involved in the activation of and sensory feedback for muscle.

is developed in the higher brain. This is transmitted to the motor cortex, where a stimulus for muscle activation is transmitted to a lower-level controller (spinal cord or brain stem). From there the message is passed to the motor neurons of the muscle and results in a specific pattern of motor unit activation.

The motor units activated meet the demands of force production by activating their associated muscle fibers. Various feedback loops send information back to the brain and can help modify force production as well as provide communication to other physiological systems (e.g., the endocrine system). The high- and low-level brain commands can be modified by feedback from both the peripheral sensory and the high-level central command controllers. Various adaptations from resistance training in the communications among the various parts of the neuromuscular system can be observed. Differences in the neural activation of different resistance training programs can produce different types of adaptations, such as increases in strength with little change in muscle size (Ploutz et al. 1994).

Size Principle

When the maximal possible force is desired from a muscle, all the available motor units typically are activated. The activation of motor units is influenced by a process called the size principle (see chapter 3). This principle is based on the observed relationship between motor-unit twitch force and recruitment threshold (Desmedt 1981): A motor unit with a low twitch force has a low recruitment threshold and so will be recruited first.

Typically Type II motor units have a high twitch force and so are not recruited unless high forces are needed. Motor units are recruited in order from low to high recruitment thresholds and so from low to high force output. An increase in motor unit firing rate also increases force. These two factors result in a continuum of voluntary force from the muscle (Henneman, Somjen, and Carpenter 1985). Most muscles contain motor units with a range in the number of fibers per motor unit and with Type I or Type II fibers. These factors allow force production ranges from very low levels to maximal force production (Noth 1992). Maximal force production requires not only the recruitment of all motor units—including the high-threshold motor units—but also the recruitment of these motor units at a high enough firing rate to produce maximal force (Sale 1992). It has been theorized that un-

trained individuals may not be able to voluntarily recruit the highest-threshold motor units or to maximally activate their muscles. Thus, part of the training adaptation is developing the ability to recruit all motor units when needed to perform a task.

Few exceptions to the size principle are thought to exist. However, some advanced lifters' or athletes' order of recruitment may not follow the order stipulated by the size principle. It may be possible to inhibit lower-threshold (i.e., Type I) motor units but still activate the higher-threshold motor units in an attempt to enhance the rate of force development and power production. This idea has been derived from the observations during very rapid stereotyped movements and during voluntary eccentric muscle action in humans (Dudley and Harris 1992; Sale 1992). Dudley and co-workers (1990) demonstrated that the activation of knee extensors by the central nervous system during maximal efforts depends on the speed and type of muscle action. The central nervous system is also capable of limiting force by engaging inhibitory mechanisms that may be protective in nature. Training may therefore result in changes in the order of fiber recruitment or in reduced inhibition, which may help in the performance of certain types of muscle actions.

Muscle Tissue Activation

Magnetic resonance imaging (MRI) allows for the visualization of whole muscle groups. Activated muscle can be observed via the color changes in the images before and after exercise. Lighter areas represent areas where muscle tissue has been activated by the exercise. This contrast shift has been shown to be directly related to force development from muscle actions evoked by both voluntary and surface electromyostimulation (K. Adams et al. 1992; Ploutz et al. 1994). A representative MRI image before and after multiple sets of 10-RM leg press exercise is shown in figure 7.5.

Ploutz and colleagues (1994) utilized MRI technology and a specific program that was designed to increase strength with little or no change in muscle size over a 9-wk training period. Training was performed 2 d/wk. Each session consisted of high-intensity single knee-extension exercise using the left quadriceps for three to six sets of 12 repetitions. Exercise-induced MRI contrast shifts were evoked by using five sets of 10 knee extensions for each resistance of 50%, 75%, and 100% of the maximum pretraining resistance that could be lifted for

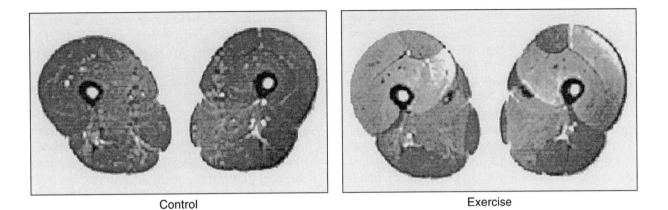

Control   Exercise

Fig. 7.5 A cross-sectional magnetic resonance image (MRI) of thigh musculature before and after a heavy-resistance workout. The white and lighter gray areas in the after-exercise scan represent muscle tissue that has been used to lift the weight. MRI allows one to examine the extent to which specific parts of intact muscle have been activated with acute exercise. This scan provided by Dr. Gary Dudley, University of Georgia, and Dr. Lori Ploutz, Ohio University.

five sets of 10 repetitions. One-repetition maximum (1-RM) strength increased by 14% over the training period in the trained left thigh musculature and by 7% in the untrained right thigh musculature. The left quadriceps femoris muscle cross-sectional area increased by 5%, while the right demonstrated no change. This indicated that neural factors mediated much of the improvement in 1-RM strength. Interestingly, the amount of muscle that needed to be activated in the posttraining test was less than that required to perform the same exercise protocol prior to training. This reduction in the amount of muscle needed to lift a given resistance in the posttraining state demonstrated that unless the resistance used is progressively increased over a training period, less muscle will be activated as muscular strength increases.

These data also give insights as to why a classic modification of the progressive overload concept, specifically periodized training, may in fact be effective in providing recovery for certain muscle fibers. While muscle strength increases over a training program, the use of heavy, moderate, and light resistances in training would allow specific muscle fibers not to be taxed by the lifting required on light and moderate training days. Yet the increased stress per cross-sectional unit area of activated muscle could potentially elicit a physiological stimulus for strength gains and tissue growth (Ploutz et al. 1994). The heavy training days would maximally activate the available musculature, but by alternating the intensities over time, overtraining or a lack of recovery could be minimized (Fry, Allemeier, and Staron 1994; Fry et al. 1994c; Kraemer and Koziris 1994). Such periodized training manipulations have

been found to be important, especially as the training level becomes more demanding.

Changes in the Neuromuscular Junction

Morphological changes in the nervous system of humans with heavy resistance training remain unclear. The adaptability of neuromuscular junctions (NMJs) with different intensities of exercise was demonstrated by Deschenes and colleagues (1993), who examined the effects of high- versus low-intensity treadmill exercise training on NMJ adaptations in the soleus muscle of rats. Both high- and low-intensity running produced an increase in the area of the NMJ. Although NMJ hypertrophic responses were observed in both groups, the high-intensity group showed more dispersed, irregularly shaped synapses, whereas the low-intensity training resulted in more compact, symmetrical synapses. The high-intensity training group also exhibited a greater total length of NMJ branching when compared with low-intensity and control groups. Thus, it might be hypothesized that heavy-resistance exercise training would produce morphological changes in the NMJ. These changes may be of much greater magnitude than adaptations from endurance training because of the differences in required quanta of neurotransmitter involved with the recruitment of high-threshold motor units.

Time Course of Neural Changes

The initial quick gains in strength from training appear to be mediated via neural factors (Moritani 1992; Sale 1992). Following a resistance training program there can be weak relationships between increases in strength and changes in muscle cross-sectional area (Ploutz et al. 1994), limb circumference (Moritani and DeVries 1979, 1980), and muscle fiber cross-sectional area (Costill et al. 1979; Ploutz et al. 1994; Staron et al. 1994), indicating that other factors are responsible for gains in strength. In one study isometric training produced a 92% increase in maximal static strength but only a 23% increase in muscle cross-sectional area (Ikai and Fukunaga 1970). On the basis of this kind of evidence scientists have concluded that neural factors have a profound influence on muscular force production. Such neural factors are related to the following processes: increased neural drive to the muscle, increased synchronization of the motor units, increased activation of the contractile apparatus, and inhibition of the protective mechanisms of the muscle (i.e., Golgi tendon organs).

Neural factors and quality of protein changes (e.g., alterations in the type of myosin heavy chains and type of myosin ATPase enzymes) may explain early (2-8 wk) strength gains. It is during this time that strength gains are much greater than can be explained by muscle hypertrophy. In addition, the ability to activate all the available motor units may also be a factor in the early phases of training, when trainees' muscles are "learning" how to exert force in various resistance exercises. The specific type of program utilized may be one of the most important factors in initial strength gains caused by neural factors, because programs that are of very high intensity (> 90% of 1 RM) but low in total exercise volume may not provide an adequate stimulus for muscle tissue growth (Sale 1992). Therefore, strength gains may depend more on neural factors with these types of programs. A program that does promote muscle tissue growth may diminish the contribution of the initial neural adaptations to strength and power gains. However, muscle fiber hypertrophy has been shown to require typically more than 16 workouts to show significant increases (Staron et al. 1994). Various types of training might therefore be able to more quickly enhance the hypertrophy of muscle in the early phases (1-8 wk) of training, thereby enhancing the hypertrophic contribution to strength and power gains. However, this has been observed only in a few studies (Cannon and Cafarelli 1987; Carolyn and Cafarelli 1992; Thorstensson et al. 1976). The large majority of studies have demonstrated that in the early phases of a heavy resistance training program increased voluntary activation of muscle is the largest contributor to strength increases (for reviews,

see Moritani 1992; Sale 1992). After this period muscle hypertrophy becomes the predominant factor in strength increases, especially for younger men.

Neural Drive

Scientists have investigated neural drive to a muscle using integrated electromyographic (EMG) techniques (Häkkinen and Komi 1983; Kamen, Kroll, and Zigon 1984; Moritani and DeVries 1980; Sale et al. 1983; Thorstensson et al. 1976). EMG techniques measure the electrical activity within the muscle and nerves and indicate the amount of neural drive (a measure of the number and amplitude of nervous impulses) to a muscle. In one of these studies 8 wk of DCER weight training shifted the EMG activity-to-muscular force ratio to a lower level (Moritani and DeVries 1980). Because the muscle produced more force with a lower amount of EMG activity, more force production occurred with less neural drive. Calculations predicted a 9% strength increase from training-induced hypertrophy; in actuality, however, strength increased 30%. It is believed that this increase in strength beyond that expected from hypertrophy resulted from the combination of the shift in the EMG-to-force ratio and the 12% increase in maximal EMG activity. This and other research supports the idea that an increase in maximal neural drive to a muscle increases strength. The studies reveal that less neural drive is required to produce any particular submaximal force after training; consequently, there is either an improved activation of the muscle or a more efficient recruitment pattern of the muscle fibers. Some studies have demonstrated that improved activation of the muscle does not occur after training (McDonagh, Hayward, and Davies 1983). Therefore, more efficient recruitment order is probably responsible for the increased force produced.

Sale and colleagues (1983) have investigated the possibility that additional motor units can be recruited after strength training. The theory of this process as a mechanism to increase force production assumes that an individual is not able to simultaneously activate all motor units in a muscle prior to training. Belanger and McComas (1981) found that this is true for some muscles but not for others, and so this mechanism could contribute to an increased force output in some, but not all, muscles.

Another neural factor that could cause increased force production is increased synchronization of motor unit firing. The greater the synchronization, the greater the number of motor units firing at any one time. Increased synchronization of motor units has been observed after strength training (Milner-Brown, Stein, and Yemin 1973). During submaximal force production, however, increased synchronization of motor units is actually less effective in producing force than asynchronous activation of motor units (Lind and Petrofsky 1978; Rack and Westbury 1969). It is thus unclear whether greater synchronization of motor units produces greater force or not.

Training has been shown to increase the period of time from several to 30 s that all motor units can be tonically active (L. Grimby, Hannerz, and Hedman 1981). An adaptation of this type may not cause an increase in maximal force but does aid in maintaining it for a longer period of time. It has also been observed that during maximal voluntary actions the high-threshold Type II motor units normally do not reach the stimulation rates required for complete tetanus to occur (DeLuca et al. 1982). If the stimulation rate to these high-threshold motor units were increased, actual force production would also increase.

Inhibitory Mechanisms

Inhibition of muscle action by reflex protective mechanisms, such as that provided by the Golgi tendon organs, has been hypothesized to limit muscular force production (Caiozzo, Perrine, and Edgerton 1981; Wickiewicz et al. 1984). These protective mechanisms appear to be especially active when large amounts of force are developed, such as maximal force development at slow speeds of movement. The effect of these inhibitory mechanisms can be partially removed by hypnosis. Ikai and Steinhaus (1961) found that force developed during forearm flexion by non-resistance-trained individuals increased 17% under hypnosis. In the same study the force developed by highly resistance trained individuals under hypnosis was not significantly different from force developed in the normal conscious state. The researchers concluded that resistance training may cause voluntary inhibition of protective mechanisms.

Information concerning protective mechanisms has several practical applications. Many resistance training exercises involve action by the same muscle groups of both limbs simultaneously, or bilateral actions. The force developed during bilateral actions is less than the sum of the force developed by each limb independently (Ohtsuki 1981;

Secher, Rorsgaard, and Secher 1978). The difference between the force developed during bilateral action and the sum of the force developed by each limb independently is called bilateral deficit. This bilateral deficit is associated with reduced motor unit stimulation (Vandervoot, Sale, and Moroz 1984). The reduced motor unit stimulation could be caused by inhibition by the protective mechanisms, resulting in less force production. Training with bilateral actions reduces bilateral deficit (Secher 1975), thus bringing bilateral force production closer to the sum of unilateral force production. Although bilateral exercise reduces the bilateral deficit, the performance of unilateral exercises may be important to maintain the deficit in sports, for example, where force production by one limb independently is required. Unilateral exercises can be performed using dumbbells and some types of weight training equipment.

Knowledge of the neural protective mechanisms is also useful in understanding the expression of maximal strength. Neural protective mechanisms appear to have their greatest effect in slow-velocity, high-resistance movements (Caiozzo, Perrine, and Edgerton 1981; Dudley et al. 1990; Wickiewicz et al. 1984). A resistance training program in which the antagonists are activated immediately prior to performance of the exercise is more effective in increasing strength at low velocities than a program in which preactivation of the antagonists is not performed (Caiozzo et al. 1983). The precontraction in some way partially inhibits the neural self-protective mechanisms, thus allowing a more forceful action. Preactivation of the antagonists can be used as a method both to enhance the training effect and to inhibit the neural protective mechanisms during a maximal lift. For example, immediately prior to a maximal bench press, forceful actions of the arm flexors and muscles that adduct the scapula (i.e., pull the scapula toward the spine) should make possible a heavier maximal bench press than when no preactivation of the antagonists is performed.

Neural Changes and Long-Term Training

The neural component may also play a major role in mediating strength gains in advanced lifters. In a study by Häkkinen and co-workers (1988b) minimal changes in muscle fiber size were observed in competitive Olympic weight lifters, but strength and power increased over 2 yr of training. EMG data demonstrated that voluntary activation of muscle was enhanced over the training period. Thus, even in advanced resistance-trained athletes, the mechanisms of strength and power improvement may be related to neural factors. It must be kept in mind that the subjects in this investigation were competitive weight lifters who compete in body-mass classification groups and that gains in muscle mass may not necessarily enhance their competitive advantage. Furthermore, the types of programs used by Olympic weight lifters are primarily related to strength and power development (Garhammer and Takano 1992; Kraemer and Koziris 1994). Programs for body builders or other athletes may have some similar characteristics related to power development but must also be designed to meet muscle mass or specific sport-performance needs. Training goals and specific protocols therefore play a key role in the neural adaptation to resistance training.

Sale (1992) has described the dynamic interplay of neural and muscular hypertrophy factors (figure 7.6). A dramatic increase in the adaptation of neural factors is observed over the time course (e.g., 6 wk to 10 wk) used for most resistance training studies in the literature. As the duration of training increases (> 10 wk), muscle hypertrophy eventually takes place and contributes more than neural adaptations to the strength and power gains observed. However, eventually muscle hypertrophy also reaches a maximum and levels off. It is interesting to note that increases in muscle fiber cross-sectional area range from about 20% to 40% in most training studies. Few studies have training periods long enough to increase muscle fiber size beyond this base level of change. Changes in muscle fiber cross-sectional area do not necessarily reflect the magnitude of changes in the whole muscle cross-sectional area determined by image systems (MRI, CAT scans). This lack of correlation may be because several different exercises or training angles are required to stimulate the entire cross-sectional area of a whole muscle, whereas changes in a specific fiber may be brought about by only one exercise (Ploutz et al. 1994). Eventually strength and power gains derived from the progressively and properly loaded and activated musculature appear to be bounded by a genetic upper limit of neuromuscular adaptation (Häkkinen 1989).

FORCE-VELOCITY CURVE

With strength training, the skeletal muscle force-velocity curve ideally moves up and to the left (figure 7.7). After training, the muscle is stronger at all velocities of movement, from an isometric action to an action performed at maximal speed. There is disagreement, however, regarding the optimal velocity of movement at which resistance training exercises should be performed. Some coaches and scientists feel that in order to be strong at a fast velocity of movement one must train at a fast velocity of movement. Others feel slow velocities of movement during resistance training are most beneficial (see chapter 2, "Isokinetics").

The information concerning the velocity at which training is performed points to four important conclusions. First, if the training program prescribes only one velocity of movement, it should

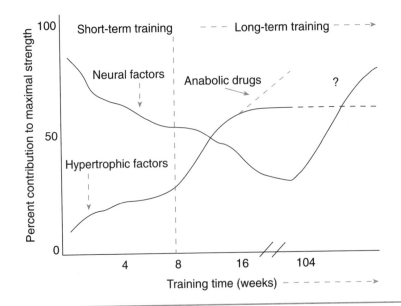

Fig. 7.6   Dynamic interplay of neural and hypertrophic factors for increased strength.

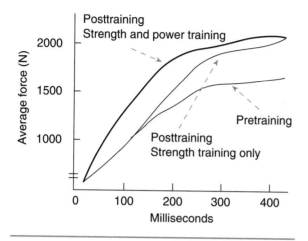

Fig. 7.7 Response of the force-velocity curve for the squat movement to different types of resistance training programs.

be an intermediate speed. Second, any training velocity increases strength within a range above and below the training velocity. Third, velocity-specific training may be needed for optimal performance in some sports. Fourth, further research is needed to distinguish between the effects of neural factors and muscle hypertrophy on the force-velocity curve.

POWER DEVELOPMENT

Explosive resistance training creates specific increases in muscle activation and rates of force development (Häkkinen, Alén, and Komi 1985). The increases in what is called *explosive strength* occur when stretch-shortening cycle exercises are used or when lighter loads (30% to 60% of 1 RM) are used in power-type exercises (e.g., pulls, cleans) where minimal inhibitory or antagonist facilitation is activated (Newton, Kraemer, Häkkinen, et al. 1996). Newton and co-workers (1996) demonstrated that in an acute "normal" bench press exercise power output was not maximal over about 50% of the range of motion when 45% of the 1 RM was lifted as explosively as possible. When the weight was allowed to be released from the hands at the end of the range of motion with the use of a special testing device, power output was enhanced throughout the range of motion. The reduction in power and rate of acceleration over the range of motion of a normal bench press was theorized to be due to activation of the antagonist muscles of the upper back, and lack of neural activation in the chest over much of the range of motion, which may protect the joints when the weight was not released. This was not observed when the weight could be

released at the end of the range of motion in the bench press. These data demonstrate why "speed reps" may be counterproductive to power development in some exercises (e.g., bench press, shoulder press) and support the use of resistance training tools (e.g., medicine balls) that allow the weight in such exercises to be released or the use of exercises in which momentum is not a problem with the apparatus (e.g., isokinetics, pneumatics, hydraulics).

The development of power may be one of the most important physiological adaptations. The ability to exert force earlier in a movement plays a vital role in many athletic and everyday activities. From an athletic perspective it may be more appropriate to think of strength as the force capability of the muscle for actions ranging from the fastest eccentric to the fastest concentric actions. The force-velocity relationship for muscle dictates that the faster the velocity of concentric muscle action, the lower the force that can be produced, yet maximal power is produced at intermediate velocities of movement (approximately 30% of maximum shortening velocity) (Knuttgen and Kraemer 1987). Pure 1-RM strength is required in the sport of power lifting, the name of which is inaccurate because there is no requirement for the weight to be moved quickly (so it has low power demands). If an athlete attempts to lift the maximum amount of weight, movement velocities are barely higher than zero. The lifter therefore exhibits maximal force but very low levels of power in 1-RM lifts.

Many strength and conditioning specialists believe that if the athlete's slow-velocity strength increases, then power output and dynamic performance will also improve. This is true to a certain extent because maximum strength, even at slow velocities, is a contributing factor to explosive power. All explosive movements start from zero or slow velocities, and it is at these phases of the movement that slow-velocity strength can contribute to power development. As the muscles begin to achieve higher velocities of shortening, however, slow-velocity strength capacity has a reduced impact on the ability to produce high force (Duchateau and Hainaut 1984; Kanehisa and Miyashita 1983a; Kaneko et al. 1983). This fact becomes increasingly important as the athlete attempts to train specifically for optimal power development.

Several studies have shown improved performance in power activities (e.g., vertical jump) following a strength training program (K. Adams et al. 1992; Bauer, Thayer, and Baras 1990; Clutch et al. 1983; Wilson et al. 1993). Research by Häkkinen and Komi (1985a) showed a 7% improvement in vertical jump ability following 24 wk of intense weight training. In a related study (Häkkinen and Komi 1985b) a group of subjects performed explosive jumps with a lighter resistance and produced significant (21%) improvement in vertical jump ability. The results indicate that there may be specific training adaptations to heavy resistance versus power-type training.

Heavy-resistance strength training using high resistance and slow velocities of concentric muscle action leads primarily to improvements in maximal strength (i.e., the high-force, low-velocity portion of the force-velocity curve), and the improvements are reduced at higher velocities. Power training, which utilizes lighter resistances and higher velocities of muscle action, results in increases in force output at higher velocities of movement and in the rate of force development (Häkkinen and Komi 1985b).

Although velocity-specific training adaptations are observed, changes in performance with training are not always velocity specific. The conflict results from the complex nature of explosive muscle actions and from the integration of slow and fast force production requirements within the context of a complete movement. Another factor confounding the observation of clear, specific training adaptations is that a wide variety of training interventions will produce increases in strength and power in untrained people. Komi and Häkkinen (1988) suggest that the response may not always follow the velocity-specific training principle, depending on the training status of the individual. For individuals with low levels of strength, improvements throughout the force-velocity spectrum may be produced regardless of the training resistance or style used. It appears that specialized types of training cause training adaptations of single factors (e.g., high force, high power) only after a base level of strength and power training has been established. This hypothesis is supported by the fact that if an athlete already has an adequate level of strength, increases in explosive power performance in response to traditional strength training will be poor, and training interventions that are more specific are required to further improve power output (Häkkinen 1989). Improvement of power performance in trained athletes therefore may require complex training strategies (Wilson et al. 1993).

Training for Power

Newton and Kraemer (1994) proposed a mixed model to develop all aspects of power (i.e., power,

coordination, strength, and muscle size). The fact that power is equal to force times the velocity of the muscle action is often given as the justification for low-velocity, heavy-resistance training for the development of explosive power. It has often been reasoned that an increase in an athlete's 1-RM strength is all that is required from a resistance training program.

If power performance is to be maximized, however, then both the force and velocity components must be trained. Because the movement distance is usually fixed by the athlete's ranges of joint motion, velocity is determined by the time taken to complete the movement. Therefore, training using methods that decrease the time over which the movement is produced increases the power output. Intimately linked to this concept is the rate of force development (RFD).

Rate of Force Development

Because time is limited during powerful muscle actions, the muscle must exert as much force as possible in a short period of time. One factor contributing to the muscle's ability to do this has been termed the *rate of force development* (RFD). RFD may explain to some extent why heavy resistance training has not always increased power performance. Squat training with heavy resistances (70% to 120% of 1 RM) has been shown to improve maximum isometric strength; however, it does not improve the maximum RFD (Häkkinen, Komi, and Tesch 1981) and may even reduce the muscle's ability to develop force rapidly (Häkkinen 1989). On the other hand, activities during which the lifter attempts to develop force rapidly (e.g., explosive jump training with light resistances) increase an athlete's ability to rapidly develop force (Behm and Sale 1993; Häkkinen, Komi, and Tesch 1981).

Specifically, explosive resistance training increases the slope of the early portion of the force time curve. Figure 7.7 compares the effects of heavy resistance (strength) training versus explosive (power) training on the RFD curve. Although heavy resistance training increases maximal strength and thus the highest point of the force-time curve, this type of training does not improve power performance appreciably, especially in athletes who have already developed a strength training base (i.e., more than 6 mo of training). This is because the movement time during explosive activities is typically less than 300 ms and most maximal force increases cannot be realized over such a short period of time. The athlete does not have the time to utilize his or her developed slow-velocity strength.

Deceleration Phase and Traditional Weight Training

The results of many studies (Berger 1963c; Wilson et al. 1993; W.B. Young and Bilby 1993) highlight a problem with traditional weight training and power development. It has been observed that when lifting a weight, the bar decelerates for a considerable proportion (24%) of the concentric movement (Elliott, Wilson, and Kerr 1989). The deceleration phase increases to 52% when performing the lift with a lighter resistance (e.g., 81% of 1 RM) (Elliott, Wilson, and Kerr 1989). In an effort to train at a faster velocity more specific to sport activity, athletes may attempt to move a light weight rapidly during the lift. This increases the duration of the deceleration phase (Newton and Wilson 1993b), as the athlete must slow the bar to a complete stop at the end of the range of motion and therefore does not optimally develop power.

Plyometric training and weighted jump squats avoid this problem by allowing the athlete to explode all the way through the movement to the point of load projection (i.e., takeoff in jumping, ball release in throwing, or impact in striking activities). It could be argued that traditional weight training promotes development of the deceleration action. The deceleration results from a decreased activation of the agonists during the later phase of the lift and may be accompanied by considerable activation of the antagonists, particularly when using lighter resistances and trying to lift the weight quickly (Newton et al. 1994). This deceleration obviously is very undesirable when attempting to maximize explosive performance. To offset this, a style of lifting must be incorporated that involves ballistic resistance training.

The problem of the deceleration phase can be overcome if the athlete actually throws or jumps with the weight. This has been termed *dynamic* or *explosive* resistance training but is probably best described as *ballistic* resistance training. The term *dynamic* is not really appropriate because all training that involves movement (i.e., not static or isometric) would be classed as dynamic. The term *explosive* is too general, as the athlete can move explosively from the bottom of a traditional squat but reduce effort near the top of the range of motion and never leave the ground. Ballistic infers acceleration to high velocity with actual projection into

free space, so this type of training is perhaps best described as ballistic resistance training (Newton and Wilson 1993a).

The resistance used for ballistic training has an impact on the ability to develop power. Kaneko and co-workers (1983) found velocity-specific effects for a task that involved lifting a weight as quickly as possible. Subjects trained with a resistance of either 0%, 30%, 60%, or 100% of maximal isometric strength. The results demonstrated a classic resistance-specific training effect. The groups training with the heavier resistances showed the greatest increases in isometric strength, and the group training with 0% resistance produced the greatest increase in unloaded movement velocity. Perhaps the most interesting finding was that the 30% resistance produced the greatest increase in force and power over the entire concentric velocity range and also resulted in the greatest increase in maximum mechanical power.

A study by Wilson and colleagues (1993) compared the effects of 10 wk of training using traditional back squats, loaded jump squats, or plyometric (stretch-shortening cycle) training (drop jumps) on vertical jump performance. The loaded jump squats were completed using a resistance of 30% of maximum. This allowed the subjects to produce the greatest mechanical power output. All the training groups showed increases in vertical jump performance; however, the loaded-jump-squats group showed significantly greater increases (18%) than the other two groups (heavy resistance training, 5%; stretch-shortening cycle training, 10%). These results were similar to that obtained by Berger (1963c) who also found that performance of jump squats with a resistance of 30% of maximum resulted in greater vertical jump ability increases than did traditional weight training, plyometric training, or isometric training.

Based on studies of muscle fiber contractile characteristics (Faulkner, Claflin, and McCully 1986; Green 1986) there appears to be a great range of adaptations within the muscle cell that alter its maximal velocity of shortening and force output at specific velocities. In particular, a considerable difference exists in the power capacity of fast-twitch (Type II) versus slow-twitch (Type I) muscle fibers (Faulkner, Claflin, and McCully 1986). One study by Duchateau and Hainaut (1984) removed the confounding variable of neural innervation and considered only contractile changes within the muscle. Subjects completed 12 wk of training using either dynamic actions with a resistance of 30%

of maximal voluntary muscle action (MVMA) or isometric training. The dynamically trained group showed increases in maximal shortening velocity, whereas the isometrically trained group did not. Whether the actual shortening velocity of the muscle fiber or the frequency of neural input is the reason for adaptations in force production at specific velocities remains speculative. Certainly, further research is required.

Behm and Sale (1993) presented evidence that it is the intention to move quickly that determines the velocity-specific response. Heavy-resistance weight training may be effective in increasing power if the athlete attempts to move the resistance as quickly as possible. This theory has been tested by W.B. Young and Bilby (1993), who compared the effects of slow and fast weight training on vertical jump ability and RFD. This study failed to find a velocity-specific effect on RFD, and the slow weight training was more effective for increasing vertical jump performance. The subjects had no prior weight training experience, and this may have influenced the results. More study is needed to determine if intention to move a weight is enough to alter the nervous system and its ability to produce force.

Whether performing traditional or ballistic resistance training, there is considerable controversy over the resistance to be used for the development of explosive power (Wilson et al. 1993; W.B. Young 1993). If an athlete is limited to traditional resistance training techniques, then heavy (> 80% maximal) resistances are preferable, because the muscle simply cannot be overloaded sufficiently using light resistances while stopping the weight at the top of the range of motion (Newton et al. 1994). For ballistic resistance training there is perhaps no optimal intensity or resistance. Both heavy (> 80% maximal) and light (< 60% maximal) resistances have application in the training of muscular power, with each affecting different components of explosive muscle action. If one had to choose a single resistance, the resistance that produces maximal power output (30% MVMA) has been shown to be optimal (Wilson et al. 1993).

The degree to which this increase in power output will transfer to athletic performance, however, may depend on whether the mass being moved represents a resistance similar to 30% of MVMA. Accelerating the leg to kick a football or throwing a baseball represents a much lighter resistance than 30%. Similarly, performing an Olympic lift involves a much heavier resistance. In reality there is a wide selection of resistances to use for power or ballistic

training. The greatest increase in power or performance may result when training with resistances that span the concentric force-velocity curve.

Although ballistic resistance training is effective for improving power performance, the high eccentric forces exerted on the athlete when landing from the jump or catching the falling weight are a problem (Newton and Wilson 1993b). However, weight training equipment can be adapted to reduce the eccentric resistance (Newton and Wilson 1993b). Ballistic weight training should progress gradually from the unloaded to loaded conditions, and the athlete should have completed a prior strength training program. Preparatory phases for the development of basic strength levels are vital in a progression to ballistic training techniques.

Neural Protective Mechanisms

Neural protective mechanisms can affect force output. Plyometric, or stretch-shortening cycle, training results in an increase in the overall neural stimulation of the muscle and thus in force output; however, qualitative changes are also apparent. In subjects unaccustomed to intense jump training, there is a reduction in EMG activity starting 50 to 100 ms before ground contact and lasting for 100 to 200 ms (Schmidtbleicher, Gollhofer, and Frick 1988). Gollhofer (1987) has attributed this to a protective mechanism caused by the Golgi tendon organ reflex acting during sudden, intense stretch loads to reduce the tension in the musculotendinous unit during the peak force of the stretch-shortening cycle. After a period of plyometric training the inhibitory effects are reduced—termed *disinhibition*—and force during stretch-shortening cycle increases as a result (Schmidtbleicher, Gollhofer, and Frick 1988).

Plyometric training places considerable force on the musculoskeletal system, and some researchers recommend that the athlete have a preliminary strength training base (e.g., squat ability 1.5 times body weight) before commencing a plyometric training program. The potential for injury is thought to be much higher for some types of plyometric training such as drop jumps, and these types should not be attempted by the beginner (Schmidtbleicher, Gollhofer, and Frick 1988).

CARDIOVASCULAR ADAPTATIONS

Cardiovascular adaptations to resistance training have received a significant amount of study during the last 10 years. As with all adaptations to resistance training, the response is affected by the training volume and intensity. It used to be thought that physical training resulted in a condition termed *athlete's heart*. Physical conditioning, including resistance training, does result in cardiovascular adaptations that resemble the adaptations to hypertension (i.e., increased ventricular wall thickness and chamber size). If the changes are examined closely, however, there are differences between the adaptations to hypertension and to resistance training. As an example, with hypertension the ventricular wall thickness increases beyond normal limits. With weight training this rarely occurs and is not evident if wall thickness is examined in relation to lean body mass, whereas with hypertension wall-thickness increases are evident even when examined in relation to lean body mass. This has led to the use of the terms *pathological hypertrophy* to mean the changes that occur with hypertension and *physiological hypertrophy* to mean the changes that occur from physical training.

Cardiovascular adaptations are caused by the training stimulus placed on the cardiovascular system during training. It has long been known that the cardiovascular adaptations to endurance training are different from those to resistance training (Morganroth et al. 1975). In general, these differences in adaptations are caused by the need to pump a large volume of blood at a relatively low pressure during endurance exercise, whereas during resistance training a relatively small volume of blood is pumped at a high pressure. This difference between endurance and resistance training results in different adaptations.

Training Adaptations at Rest

Cardiovascular adaptations at rest occur from performing resistance training (tables 7.2 and 7.3). Changes in cardiac morphology, pumping ability, heart rate, blood pressure, and the lipid profile indicate cardiovascular function. These factors are also indicators of cardiovascular risk.

TABLE 7.2 Chronic Resting Cardiovascular Adaptations From Resistance Exercise	
Heart rate	– or no change
Blood pressure	
Diastolic	– or no change
Systolic	– or no change
Double product	– or no change
Stroke volume	
Absolute	+ or no change
Relative to BSA	No change
Relative to LBW	No change
Cardiac function	
Diastolic	No change (+?)
Systolic	+ or no change
Lipid profile	
Total cholesterol	– or no change
HDL-C	+ or no change
LDL-C	– or no change

– = decreased, + = increased.

BSA = body surface area, LBW = lean body weight, HDL-C = high-density lipoprotein cholesterol, LDL-C = low-density lipoprotein cholesterol.

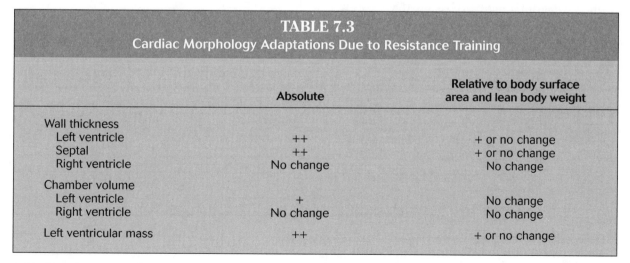

TABLE 7.3 Cardiac Morphology Adaptations Due to Resistance Training		
	Absolute	Relative to body surface area and lean body weight
Wall thickness		
Left ventricle	++	+ or no change
Septal	++	+ or no change
Right ventricle	No change	No change
Chamber volume		
Left ventricle	+	No change
Right ventricle	No change	No change
Left ventricular mass	++	+ or no change

+ = increased

Heart Rate. Strength-trained athletes have average (Fleck 1988) or lower than average (Stone et al. 1991) resting heart rates. Short-term resistance training studies result in significant decreases of 5% to 12% (Fleck 1988, 1992) and nonsignificant decreases (Fleck 1988, 1992; Goldberg, Elliot, and Kuehl 1994) in resting heart rate. Decreased resting heart rate from physical training is normally attributed to a combination of decreased sympathetic and increased parasympathetic stimulation to the heart (Blomqvist and Saltin 1983; Frick, Elovainio, and Somer 1967).

Blood Pressure. The majority of reports show strength-trained athletes to have average or slightly below average resting systolic and diastolic blood pressures (Fleck 1988, 1992). Short-term training studies on males also demonstrate no change or slight decreases in systolic and diastolic resting blood pressures (Fleck 1988, 1992; Goldberg, Elliot, and Kuehl 1994). Decreased resting blood pressures, when they do occur, are most likely related to decreased body fat, decreased body salt, and alterations in the sympathetic drive to the heart (Fleck 1988, 1992).

Despite the evidence to the contrary, there is still a common misconception that resistance training results in hypertension. Hypertension, when it occurs in resistance-trained athletes, is most likely related to essential hypertension, chronic overtraining, use of steroids, large increases in muscle mass, or increases in total body weight (Fleck 1992; Stone et al. 1991).

Double Product. Heart rate times systolic pressure is called the *double product*. It is an estimate of myocardial work and oxygen consumption. Several short-term resistance training studies show the resting double product to decrease significantly (Goldberg, Elliot, and Kuehl 1994; Stone et al. 1991). This indicates a decrease in myocardial oxygen consumption and is normally viewed as a positive adaptation to training.

Stroke Volume. Stroke volume is the amount of blood pumped per beat of the heart. An increase in resting stroke volume is viewed as a positive adaptation to training. Highly resistance-trained males have normal or above normal absolute resting stroke volumes (Effron 1989; Fleck 1988). However, relative to body surface area or lean body mass the resting stroke volume of highly resistance-trained males is not significantly different from normal (Effron 1989; Fleck 1988). Greater than normal absolute stroke volume is caused by a significantly greater diastolic left ventricular diameter, indicating greater filling of the ventricle with blood prior to each beat, and a normal ejection fraction or percentage of blood in the ventricle pumped per beat (Fleck 1988). A short-term training study showed absolute resting stroke volume to be unchanged (Lusiani et al. 1986), indicating that to increase absolute resting stroke volume a long training period, a high training volume, or both are needed.

Lipid Profile. The effect of weight training on the lipid profile is controversial. Resistance-trained male athletes have been reported to have normal, higher, and lower than normal high-density lipoprotein cholesterol (HDL-C), low-density lipoprotein cholesterol (LDL-C), total cholesterol, and total cholesterol–to–HDL-C ratios (Kraemer, Deschenes, and Fleck 1988; Hurley 1989; Stone et al. 1991). Reports on the lipid profile in strength-trained female athletes also show no consensus (Elliot et al. 1987; Morgan et al. 1986). The lipid profile of body builders is similar to that of runners, whereas power lifters have lower HDL-C and higher LDL-C values than runners when body fat, age, and steroid use (steroid use lowers HDL-C concentrations) are considered (Hurley, Seals, Hagberg, et al. 1984; Hurley et al. 1987).

Short-term training studies are also inconclusive. Both positive effects and no effect have been shown in the lipid profile from resistance training (Hurley 1989; Lee et al. 1990; Stone et al. 1991). Although the effect of resistance training on the lipid profile varies, it does appear that resistance training can positively affect this profile. High-volume programs with short rest periods between sets and exercises probably have the most positive effect on the lipid profile.

Cardiac Wall Thickness. Increased ventricular wall thicknesses are an adaptation to the intermittent elevated blood pressures during resistance training (Effron 1989). Echocardiographic and MRI techniques both show highly resistance-trained athletes to have greater than normal absolute posterior left ventricular and intraventricular septum wall thicknesses (Fleck 1988; Fleck, Henke, and Wilson 1989; Spirits et al. 1994). In general, no significant differences from normal are present, however, if these wall thicknesses are expressed relative to body surface area or lean body mass (Fleck 1988). The caliber of the athlete appears to have some impact on ventricular wall thicknesses. Meta-analysis (a statistical procedure in which data from different studies can be analyzed and compared) indicates absolute intraventricular septum but not posterior left ventricular wall thickness to be greater in national- and international-caliber athletes than in recreational resistance trainers (Fleck 1988). Short-term training studies also show resistance training to result in either an increase in ventricular wall thickness or to have no effect (Effron 1989; Fleck 1988). An example of an MRI used to determine various dimensions and thicknesses is shown in figure 7.8.

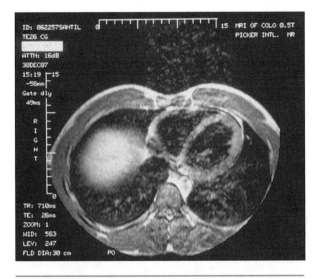

Fig. 7.8 Magnetic resonance image of left ventricle (circular chamber with thick walls) and right ventricle (triangular chamber). Courtesy of Dr. Fleck's laboratory.

Whether or not an increase in left ventricular wall thickness occurs probably depends on differences in the training performed. The highest blood pressures during a set to concentric failure occur during the last few repetitions (Fleck and Dean 1987; MacDougall et al. 1985; Sale et al. 1994). Therefore, it is possible that for left ventricular wall thickness to increase maximally it is necessary to carry sets to concentric failure. Exercises involving large muscle masses, such as leg presses, have been reported to produce a higher blood pressure response than exercises involving smaller muscle masses (MacDougall et al. 1985). This indicates that the exercises performed may also have an impact on increases in ventricular wall thicknesses.

It appears that resistance training can result in increased left ventricular wall thickness but that it is not a necessary consequence of all resistance training programs. The intermittent elevated blood pressure during weight training is the stimulus for

an increase in left ventricular wall thickness. Factors related to increased left ventricular wall thickness include the caliber of the athlete, whether or not sets are carried to concentric failure, and the size of the muscle mass involved in the exercises.

Heart Chamber Dimensions. An increase in left ventricular chamber size or volume is an indication of volume overload on the heart, as occurs in endurance athletes. The majority of short-term training studies and studies on highly strength-trained males show resistance training to have little or no impact on absolute left ventricular internal dimensions, an indicator of chamber size (Effron 1989; Fleck 1988; Stone et al. 1991). This is true whether systolic or diastolic chamber dimensions are examined.

It has been reported that at rest body builders but not weight lifters have greater than normal absolute left ventricular end-diastolic and systolic volumes (Deligiannis, Zahopoulou, and Mandroukas 1988), which indicates that high-volume programs may have a greater impact than low-volume programs on ventricular volume. If the left ventricular volumes are examined relative to body surface area or lean body mass, however, neither the body builders nor the weight lifters were significantly different from normal.

Deligiannis, Zahopoulou, and Mandroukas (1988) also reported that at rest the right ventricular internal dimension of body builders but not of weight lifters is greater than normal in absolute and in relative terms to body surface area and lean body mass. The finding that weight lifters do not have greater than normal right ventricular internal dimensions is supported by another study showing this to be true in junior elite Olympic-style weight lifters (Fleck, Henke, and Wilson 1989). The left atrial internal dimension of both body builders and weight lifters is greater than normal in absolute terms and relative to body surface area and lean body mass (Deligiannis, Zahopoulou, and Mandroukas 1988). Body builders also have a significantly greater left atrial internal dimension than weight lifters (Deligiannis, Zahopoulou, and Mandroukas 1988).

It appears resistance training can result in an increase in both ventricular and atrial volumes. However, no difference from normal is generally apparent when examined relative to body surface area or lean body mass. It does appear that high-volume body building programs may have the greatest potential to affect cardiac chamber sizes.

Left Ventricular Mass. An increase in ventricular

mass can be brought about by an increase in either wall thickness or chamber size. The majority of studies on highly resistance-trained athletes and of short-term training studies show absolute left ventricular mass, like left ventricular wall thickness, to be greater than normal (Fleck 1988; Fleck, Henke, and Wilson 1989; Stone et al. 1991). However, the difference is greatly reduced or nonexistent relative to body surface area or lean body mass. Some data indicate that national- and international-caliber athletes have a greater left ventricular mass as well as wall thickness than athletes of lesser caliber (Effron 1989; Fleck 1988).

Both body builders and weight lifters have a significantly greater than normal absolute left ventricular mass; however, they are not significantly different from each other (Deligiannis, Zahopoulou, and Mandroukas 1988). Body builders and weight lifters both also have significantly greater than normal left ventricular wall thicknesses. However, only body builders have a significantly greater than normal left ventricular end-diastolic dimension (Deligiannis, Zahopoulou, and Mandroukas 1988). Thus, in body builders the increased left ventricular mass is caused by both greater left ventricular wall thickness and chamber size, whereas in weight lifters the increase is caused for the most part only by a greater than normal wall thickness.

Absolute left ventricular mass can be increased by resistance training. The increased mass can be caused by an increase both in wall thickness and chamber size and may also be related to the type of program performed.

Cardiac Function. Abnormalities in systolic and diastolic function are associated with cardiac hypertrophy caused by hypertension and valvular heart disease. The majority of studies show that the common measures of systolic function—percentage fractional shortening, ejection fraction, and velocity of circumferential shortening—are unaffected by resistance training (Fleck 1988, 1992). However, it has also been reported that percentage fractional shortening is significantly greater in strength-trained athletes than in normal subjects (Colan, Sanders, McPherson, and Borrow 1985) and that short-term training significantly increases percentage fractional shortening (Kanakis and Hickson 1980), indicating an increase in systolic function.

Power lifters, who have significantly greater absolute and relative (to body surface area) left ventricular mass, have been reported to have normal and even enhanced measures of diastolic function (peak rate of chamber enlargement and atrial peak filling rate) (Colan et al. 1985; Pearson et al. 1986). Use of anabolic steroids has been reported to be detrimental (Pearson et al. 1986) or to have no effect (P.D. Thompson et al. 1992) on measures of diastolic function. Differences in the results of these two reports may be related to length of use and type of anabolic steroid used.

A limited number of studies have examined the effect of resistance training on cardiac function. It appears that, in general, resistance training has no effect or even a possible positive effect on some measures of systolic and diastolic function.

Acute Cardiovascular Responses

The acute response to resistance training refers to what happens during one set of an exercise. Study of the acute response has centered around the blood pressure, heart rate, stroke volume, cardiac output, and intrathoracic pressure responses during the concentric and eccentric phase of an exercise.

Heart Rate and Blood Pressure. Heart rate and blood pressure increase substantially during dynamic resistance training (Fleck 1992; Stone et al. 1991). This is true for machine, free-weight, and isokinetic exercise (Fleck and Dean 1987; Sale et al. 1994; Sale et al. 1993; Scharf et al. 1994), although the peak blood pressure response is higher during weight training in which both a concentric and eccentric phase occur than in concentric-only isokinetic training (Sale et al. 1993). The increases in blood pressure and heart rate can be large: Peak blood pressures of 320/250 mmHg and a heart rate of 170 beats per minute were reported for a two-legged leg press at 95% of 1 RM during a set to voluntary concentric failure in which a Valsalva maneuver was performed (MacDougall et al. 1985). However, heart rate and blood pressure responses are also substantial even when an attempt is made to limit the performance of a Valsalva maneuver (Fleck and Dean 1987).

The peak blood pressure and heart rate responses normally occur during the last several repetitions of a set to voluntary concentric failure (Fleck 1992; MacDougall et al. 1985; Sale et al. 1994) and are higher during sets at submaximal resistances to voluntary failure than during sets using 1-RM resistances (Sale et al. 1993). In dynamic resistance training, higher blood pressures but not heart rates occur during the concentric than during the eccentric portion of a repetition (Falkel, Fleck, and Murray 1992; MacDougall et al. 1985; Miles et al. 1987). In addition, the blood pressure response in-

TABLE 7.4
Acute Cardiovascular Responses to Resistance Exercise

	Phase of repetition	
	Eccentric	Concentric
Heart rate	+	+
Blood pressure		
Diastolic	+	+
Systolic	+	+
Intrathoracic pressure	+	+
Stroke volume	+	No change
Cardiac output	+	+ or no change

+ = increased

creases with the active muscle mass, but the response is not linear (Fleck 1988; Stone et al. 1991; table 7.4).

Stroke Volume and Cardiac Output. Stroke volume (determined by electrical impedance) is not elevated significantly above resting values during the concentric phase of resistance training exercise either when attempts are made to limit the performance of a Valsalva maneuver (Miles et al. 1987) or with the performance of a Valsalva maneuver (Falkel, Fleck, and Murray 1992). However, during the eccentric phase both without (Miles et al. 1987) and with a Valsalva maneuver (Falkel, Fleck, and Murray 1992) stroke volume is significantly increased above resting values and is significantly greater than during the concentric phase of a repetition.

During both the concentric and eccentric phases of a repetition, cardiac output can be elevated above resting values. During the eccentric phase of a squat, cardiac output can reach approximately 20 L, while during the concentric phase of a repetition it may reach only approximately 15 L (Falkel, Fleck, and Murray 1992). However, during an exercise involving a smaller muscle mass, such as the knee extension, cardiac output may be elevated above resting values only during the eccentric phase of repetition. This difference between the eccentric and concentric phases can result in no significant change from resting values in mean cardiac output and stroke volume for the entire set of an exercise involving a small muscle mass (Miles et al. 1987).

Heart rate is not significantly different between the concentric and eccentric phases of a repetition (Falkel, Fleck, and Murray 1992; MacDougall et al. 1985; Miles et al. 1987), whereas stroke volume is significantly greater during the eccentric than during the concentric phase of a repetition (Falkel, Fleck, and Murray 1992; Miles et al. 1987). Therefore, the greater cardiac output during the eccentric as compared to the concentric phase of a repetition is caused solely by the increase in stroke volume.

Intrathoracic Pressure. Intrathoracic pressure increases while performing resistance training exercise (Falkel, Fleck, and Murray 1992; MacDougall et al. 1985; Sale et al. 1994). This increase may have a protective function for the cerebral blood vessels (MacDougall et al. 1985). Any change in intrathoracic pressure is transmitted to the cerebral spinal fluid, which results in the cerebral spinal pressure matching the intrathoracic pressure. Therefore, any increase in blood pressure during resistance training is paralleled by an increase in intrathoracic pressure and cerebral spinal pressure. The increased cerebral spinal fluid pressure reduces the transmural pressure (difference between pressure inside vs. outside of a vessel) in the cerebral blood vessels, protecting them from damage caused by the increase in blood pressure.

Mechanisms of the Pressor Response. Several hypotheses have been advanced concerning possible mechanisms of the pressor response during weight training. An increase in cardiac output can result in an increase in blood pressure. However, mean cardiac output may not be elevated during resistance training exercise (Miles et al. 1987), and a significant inverse relationship between cardiac output and systolic and diastolic blood pressures has been shown (Fleck, Falkel, et al. 1989). Thus, an increase in cardiac output may not be a major contributor to the increase in blood pressure. In fact, the increase in blood pressure may actually limit cardiac output.

Increased intramuscular pressure can increase total peripheral resistance and occlude blood flow, resulting in increased blood pressure. Intramuscular pressure during static muscle actions can be quite high (Edwards, Hill, and McDonnell 1972). There is substantial intramuscular variability, but even during static muscular actions that are moderate in nature (40% to 60% of maximum) blood flow can be occluded. During the concentric phase of a repetition the intramuscular pressure is probably greater than during the eccentric phase. Thus, the differences in intramuscular pressure between the eccentric and concentric phases of a repetition and their effect on total peripheral pressure and blood flow probably contribute to the greater blood pressures during the concentric than during the eccentric phase of a repetition (Miles et al. 1987).

Increased intrathoracic pressure is classically thought to limit venous return to the heart and so to limit stroke volume and cardiac output. It has been hypothesized that intrathoracic pressure has an impact on stroke volume and cardiac output during resistance training (Falkel, Fleck, and Murray 1992; Fleck 1988). Intrathoracic pressure does have a significant inverse correlation to stroke volume and cardiac output and a significant positive correlation to the systolic and diastolic blood pressure response during resistance training (Fleck, Falkel, et al. 1989). These correlations indicate that intrathoracic pressure does indeed limit stroke volume and cardiac output during resistance training. They also indicate that intrathoracic pressure is related to the blood pressure response.

Blood pressures and heart rates are higher during sets carried to voluntary concentric failure at approximately 70% to 85% of the maximal weight possible than during one repetition at 100% of the maximal weight possible (Fleck and Dean 1987; MacDougall et al. 1985; Sale et al. 1994). Sets performed to voluntary concentric failure with approximately 70% to 85% of 1 RM are probably of sufficient duration and resistance to allow all factors contributing to an increase in blood pressure and heart rate to occur, whereas sets performed with heavier or lighter resistances are insufficient in either duration or intensity to allow all factors to contribute to the pressor response.

Chronic Cardiovascular Adaptations During Exercise

Traditional cardiovascular training results in adaptations that allow the performance of a given submaximal workload with less cardiovascular stress. This has also recently been demonstrated for resistance training (table 7.5).

Heart Rate, Blood Pressure, and Double Product. Several studies have clearly demonstrated that resistance training can reduce cardiovascular stress during resistance training and other exercise tasks. Male body builders have lower maximal intra-arterial systolic and diastolic blood pressures and maximal heart rates during sets to voluntary concentric fatigue at 50%, 70%, 80%,

TABLE 7.5 Chronic Cardiovascular Adaptations During Resistance Exercise	
Heart rate	–
Blood pressure	
Diastolic	– or no change
Systolic	– or no change
Double product	–
Stroke volume	+ or no change
Cardiac output	+ or no change
$\dot{V}O_2$peak	+ or no change

– = decreased, + = increased

90%, and 100% of 1 RM than sedentary males and novice (6-9 mo of training) resistance-trained males (Fleck and Dean 1987). The body builders in this study were stronger than the other subjects, so they had a lower pressor response not only at the same relative workload, but also at greater absolute workloads. Body builders also have lower heart rates and double products but not blood pressures during arm ergometry at the same absolute workload than medical students (Colliander and Tesch 1988). In addition, body builders have a lower heart rate at the same relative workload (% 1 RM) than power lifters during resistance training exercises (Falkel, Fleck, and Murray 1992). This indicates that high-volume programs may have the greatest impact on the pressor response during resistance training.

Short-term training studies also demonstrate cardiovascular adaptations during the performance of exercise tasks. Training studies 12 to 16 wk in length have shown that the heart rate, blood pressure, and double product can all decrease during bicycle ergometry, treadmill walking, and treadmill walking holding hand weights (Blessing et al. 1987; Goldberg, Elliot, and Kuehl 1988, 1994). Short-term training studies also demonstrate significant decreases in the blood pressure and heart rate response during isometric work (Goldberg, Elliot, and Kuehl 1994) and in both young adults (Sale et al. 1994) and in 66-yr-old adults (McCartney et al. 1993) during dynamic resistance training at the same absolute resistance. However, after training at the same relative resistance (% 1 RM) the blood pressure response is elevated (Sale et al. 1994). Resistance training can clearly result in adaptations that allow a lower pressor response and lower myocardial oxygen consumption, as indicated by the double product, during a variety of exercise tasks.

Stroke Volume and Cardiac Output. Weight lifters' cardiac output can increase up to 30 L/min, with stroke volume increasing up to 150 to 200 ml immediately after resistance training exercise, whereas untrained people show no significant change (Stone et al. 1991). Body builders' peak stroke volume and cardiac output are significantly greater than those of power lifters during sets to voluntary concentric failure at various percentages of 1 RM of both the knee-extension and squat exercises (Falkel, Fleck, and Murray 1992). The body builders' greater cardiac output and stroke volume were evident during both the concentric and eccentric phases of both exercises and may have been caused by the body builders performing a more limited Valsalva maneuver, resulting in a smaller elevation of intrathoracic pressure. These results indicate that the type of resistance training program may affect the magnitude of any adaptation that results in the ability to maintain cardiac output during activity.

Pressor Response During Activity. The factors that affect acute or chronic blood pressure, stroke volume, and cardiac output response during activity are similar. Decreases in blood pressure during activity result in a decreased afterload on the left ventricle, which in turn results in increased cardiac output and decreased myocardial oxygen consumption. Changes in all these variables during activity have been demonstrated, as previously described.

Increases in intrathoracic pressure can decrease venous return to the heart, resulting in a decreased stroke volume and a buildup of blood in the systemic circulation, and therefore in increased blood pressure. Intrathoracic pressure is inversely correlated to cardiac output and blood pressure (Fleck, Falkel et al. 1989), indicating that an increase in intrathoracic pressure decreases cardiac output and stroke volume. Peak esophageal pressure, an indicator of intrathoracic pressure, normally occurs during the last several repetitions of a set and has been shown to either increase or not change at the same relative resistance after a period of resistance training (Sale et al. 1994). Esophageal pressure does not change during the first repetition of a set at the same relative resistance after a period of resistance training (Sale et al. 1994). This study indicates that at the same absolute resistance (same absolute resistance after training is now a smaller percent of

MVMA compared to pretraining) a reduction in intrathoracic pressure during the first repetitions of a set after training may allow stroke volume and cardiac output to increase compared to pretraining. However, intrathoracic pressure during the last repetitions of a set is unaffected by training, and therefore does not affect stroke volume or cardiac output compared to pretraining values.

Peak Oxygen Consumption. Peak oxygen consumption ($\dot{V}O_2$ peak) on a treadmill or bicycle ergometer is considered an indicator of cardiovascular fitness. $\dot{V}O_2$ peak is normally not considered to be significantly affected by heavy resistance training. The $\dot{V}O_2$ peak of competitive Olympic weight lifters, power lifters, and body builders ranges from 41 to 55 ml $\cdot$ kg^{-1} $\cdot$ L^{-1} (Kraemer, Fleck, and Deschenes 1988; Saltin and Åstrand 1967). These are average to moderately above average values for $\dot{V}O_2$ peak. This indicates it is possible that resistance training can increase $\dot{V}O_2$ peak, but not all programs may bring about an increase in $\dot{V}O_2$ peak.

Some insight into the type of programs that result in the greatest increase in $\dot{V}O_2$ peak can be gained by examining the results of short-term training studies. Traditional heavy resistance training using heavy resistances for a few number of repetitions per set and long rest periods results in small increases or no change in $\dot{V}O_2$ peak (Fahey and Brown 1973; Gettman and Pollock 1981; Lee et al. 1990). An Olympic-style weight-lifting program 7 wk in length can result in moderate gains in absolute $\dot{V}O_2$ peak (9%) and $\dot{V}O_2$ peak relative to body weight (8%) (Stone, Wilson, Blessing, and Rozenek 1983). In this study the first 5 wk of training consisted of three to five sets of 10 repetitions each of each exercise, rest periods between sets and exercises of 3.5 to 4.0 min, and two training sessions per day 3 d/wk. Vertical jumps were performed 2 d/wk for five sets of 10 repetitions each. Most of the gain in $\dot{V}O_2$ peak occurred during the first 5 wk of the program. Training during the next 2 wk was identical to the first 5 wk, except three sets of five repetitions each were performed. This 2-wk period of training resulted in no further gain in $\dot{V}O_2$ peak.

Circuit weight training consists of performing sets of exercises of 12 to 15 repetitions at 40% to 60% of 1 RM with short rest periods of 15 to 30 s between exercises. This type of training results in gains in $\dot{V}O_2$ peak of 4% in men and 8% in women in 8 to 20 wk of training (Gettman and Pollock 1981).

For physical conditioning to elicit changes in $\dot{V}O_2$

peak, heart rate must be maintained for a minimum of 20 min at a heart rate of at least 60% of maximum (American College of Sports Medicine 1990). The rest periods allowed during resistance training allow the heart rate to decrease below the 60% of maximum level. This is one of the reasons many resistance training programs do not result in a significant increase in $\dot{V}O_2$ peak. This information indicates that a resistance training program designed to increase $\dot{V}O_2$ peak should consist of a high volume of training and relatively short rest periods between sets and exercises.

The maximal increase in $\dot{V}O_2$ peak brought about by resistance training is substantially less than the 15% to 20% increases associated with traditional endurance-oriented running, cycling, or swimming programs. Although resistance training can increase $\dot{V}O_2$ peak, it is possible to increase $\dot{V}O_2$ peak to a greater extent with a traditional endurance training program. Therefore, if a major goal of a training program is to increase $\dot{V}O_2$ peak, some form of endurance training should be included in the program.

BODY COMPOSITIONAL CHANGES

Body compositional changes occur in short-term (6- to 24-wk) resistance training programs. Table 7.6 depicts the changes in body composition caused by various training programs. The body's mass is normally divided into fat and lean mass when examining body composition. *Lean body mass* (LBM), also called *fat-free mass,* is what a person's body would weigh if no fat were present. *Fat weight* is the weight of fat contained in the body. Total body weight equals LBM plus fat weight. For the purpose of comparison, fat weight is frequently expressed as a percentage of total body weight or percent body fat (% fat). For example, if a 100-kg athlete's body is 15% fat, that athlete's LBM, fat weight, and total body weight are related as follows:

$$\text{Fat weight} = 0.15 \times 100 \text{ kg}$$
$$= 15 \text{ kg}$$

$$\text{LBM} = \text{total body weight} - \text{fat weight}$$
$$= 100 \text{ kg} - 15 \text{ kg}$$
$$= 85 \text{ kg}$$

Ideally a strength training program should increase LBM and decrease fat weight and percent fat. Increases in LBM normally are viewed as mirroring increases in muscle tissue weight. Table 7.6 indicates that strength training induces decreases in percent fat and increases in LBM. Total body weight, for the most part, shows small increases over short training periods. This occurs in both males and females using DCER, variable resistance (VR), and isokinetic (IK) training with programs involving a variety of combinations of exercises, sets, and repetitions. Because of the variation in the numbers of sets, repetitions, and exercises and relatively small body compositional changes, it is impossible to reach concrete conclusions concerning which program is optimal for decreasing percent fat and increasing LBM.

The largest increases in LBM are a little greater than 3 kg (6.6 lb) in 10 wk of training. This translates into an LBM increase of 0.3 kg/wk (0.66 lb/wk). Though some coaches desire huge gains in body weight for their athletes during the off-season, large weight gains are impossible if the added body weight is to be muscle mass.

Table 7.7 summarizes the results of studies investigating percent fat in body builders and Olympic and power lifters. Average percent fat of these highly resistance-trained males ranged from 8.3% to 12.2%, whereas female body builders demonstrated an average of 13.2% to 20.4%. All these values are lower than the average percent fat of college-age males (14% to 16%) and females (20% to 24%). Highly resistance-trained athletes are therefore leaner than average individuals of the same age.

It should be noted, however, that the average percent fat of all the depicted groups of male athletes is above the essential fat level of 6% (Sinning 1974). Essential fat is the fat necessary to allow the body to function normally. It is not possible to have 0% fat. Fat stores are needed to pad the heart, kidneys, and other vital organs; they also serve as structural components of membranes and as fuel stores for energy. Female body builders' average percent fat of 13.2% is very close to the lower limit of female essential fat of 13% to 22% (Frisch and McArthur 1974). Women's essential fat levels may need to be higher than men's to ensure normal functioning of the reproductive cycle (Frisch and McArthur 1974). As many men and women approach essential fat levels, they become lethargic and moody. Essential fat levels, therefore, are not to be viewed as ideal or target fat levels for athletes.

BIOENERGETIC ADAPTATIONS

Increases in the activity of an energy source's enzymes can lead to more ATP production and

TABLE 7.6

Changes in Body Composition Based on Type of Training

Reference	Gender	Type of training	Length of training (wk)	Days of training per week	Sets and repetitions	Number of exercises	Total weight (kg)	LBM (kg)	% fat
Withers 1970	F	DCER	10	3	40%-55% 1 RM/30 s	10	+0.1	+1.3	−1.8
Withers 1970	M	DCER	20	3	40%-55% 1 RM/30 s	10	+0.7	+1.7	−1.5
Fahey and Brown 1973	M	DCER	9	3	2 exercises 5 × 5 2 exercises 3 × 5 1 exercise 5 × 1-2	5	+0.5	+1.4	−1.0
C.H. Brown and Wilmore 1974	F	DCER	24	3	8 wk = 1 × 10, 8, 7, 6, 5, 4 16 wk = 1 × 10, 6, 5, 4, 3	4	−0.4	+1.0	−2.1
Mayhew and Gross 1974	F	DCER	9	3	2 × 10	11	+0.4	+1.5	−1.3
Misner et al. 1974	M	DCER	8	3	1 × 3-8	10	+1.0	+3.1	−2.9
Peterson 1975	M	VR	6	3	1 × 10-12	20	–	−0.8	+0.6
Coleman 1977	M	DCER	10	3	2 × 8-10 RM	11	+1.7	+2.4	−9.1
Coleman 1977	M	VR	10	3	1 × 10-12 RM	11	+1.8	+2.0	−9.3
Gettman et al. 1978	M	IK (60°/s)	10	3	3 × 10-15	7	−1.9	+3.2	−2.5
Gettman et al. 1978	M	IK (120°/s)	10	3	3 × 10-15	7	+0.3	+1.0	−0.9
Wilmore et al. 1978	F	DCER	10	2	2 × 7-16	8	−0.1	+1.1	−1.9
Wilmore et al. 1978	M	DCER	10	2	2 × 7-16	8	+0.3	+1.2	−1.3
Gettman et al. 1979	M	DCER	20	3	50% 1 RM, 6 wk = 2 × 10-20 14 wk = 2 × 15	10	+0.5	+1.8	−1.7
Gettman et al. 1979	M	IK	8	3	4 wk = 1 × 10 at 60°/s 4 wk = 1 × 15 at 90°/s	9	+0.3	+1.0	−0.9
Gettman, Culter, and Strathman 1980	M	VR	20	3	2 × 12	9	−0.1	+1.6	−1.9
Gettman, Culter, and Strathman 1980	M	IK (60°/s)	20	3	2 × 12	10	−0.6	+2.1	−2.8

(continued)

TABLE 7.6
(continued)

Reference	Gender	Type of training	Length of training (wk)	Days of training per week	Sets and repetitions	Number of exercises	Changes based on type of training		
							Total weight (kg)	LBM (kg)	% fat
Hurley, Seals, Ehsani, et al. 1984	M	VR	16	3-4	1 × 8-12 RM	14	+1.6	+1.9	−0.8
Hunter 1985	F	DCER	7	3	3 × 7-10	7	−0.9	+0.3	−1.5
Hunter 1985	F	DCER	7	4	2 × 7-10	7	+0.7	+0.7	−0.5
Hunter 1985	M	DCER	7	3	3 × 7-10	7	+0.6	+0.5	−0.2
Hunter 1985	M	DCER	7	4	2 × 7-10	7	0	+0.5	−0.9
Crist et al. 1988	M & F	DCER	6	5	—	—	+1.0	+2.0	−3.0
Bauer, Thayer, and Baras 1990	M & F	SSC	10	3	4-7 × 20 s	—	0	+1.0	−3.0
Staron et al. 1991	F	DCER	20	2	1 d/wk, 3 × 6-8 RM 1 d/wk, 3 × 10-12 RM	3	+2.0	+6.0	−4.0
Staron et al. 1989	F	DCER	18	2	3 × 6-8	4	0	+1.0	−1.0
Pierce, Rozenek, and Stone 1993	M	DCER	8	3	3 wk, 3 × 10 RM 3 wk, 3 × 5 RM 2 wk, 3 × 10 RM	10	+1.0	+1.0	−4.0
Staron et al. 1994	M	DCER	8	2	M: 2 warm-up, 3 × 6-8 RM F: 2 warm-up, 3 × 10-12 RM	3	+0.7	+1.8	−2.1
Staron et al. 1994	F	DCER	8	2	M: 2 warm-up, 3 × 6-8 RM F: 2 warm-up, 3 × 10-12 RM	3	+1.3	+2.4	−2.9

DCER = dynamic constant external resistance

VR = variable resistance

SSC = stretch-shortening cycle

IK = isokinetic

RM = repetition maximum

TABLE 7.7
Percent Fat of Advanced Strength-Trained Athletes

Reference	Caliber of athletes	% fat
Men		
Fahey, Akka, and Rolph 1975	OL, national & international	12.2
Tanner 1964	OL, national & international	10.0
Sprynarova and Parizkova 1971	OL, national & international	9.8
Fry, Stone, Thrush, and Fleck 1995	OL, national & international	8.9
Fahey, Akka, and Rolph 1975	PL, national & international	15.6
Katch et al. 1980	OL and PL, national & international	9.7
Katch et al. 1980	BB, national	9.3
Zruback 1972	BB, national	6.6
Fahey, Akka, and Rolph 1975	BB, national & international	8.4
Pipes 1979	BB, national & international	8.3
Women		
Freedson et al. 1983	BB, national & international	13.2
Alway 1994	BB, national & international	13.8
Alway 1994	BB, national	18.7
Stoessel et al. 1991	OL, national & international	20.4

OL = Olympic lifters
PL = power lifters
BB = body builders

utilization per unit of time, which in turn could lead to increases in physical performance. Enzyme activity of the ATP-PC energy source (e.g., creatine phosphokinase and myokinase activity) has been shown to increase in humans because of isokinetic training (Costill et al. 1979) and in rats because of isometric training (Exner, Staudte, and Pette 1973). Costill and colleagues used two training regimens for the legs in their isokinetic study. The enzymes associated with the ATP-PC energy source showed significant increases of approximately 12% in the leg trained with 30-s bouts and insignificant changes in the leg trained with 6-s bouts. According to these findings, enzymatic changes associated with the ATP-PC energy source are linked to the duration of the exercise bouts; the changes do not take place with exercise bouts of 6 s or less. However, little or no change in enzymes associated with the ATP-PC energy source (creatine phosphokinase and myokinase) has been observed from resistance training (Tesch 1992a), which emphasizes the point

that the type of program will affect the enzymatic adaptations.

Costill and colleagues (1979) also reported significant increases in phosphofructokinase (PFK), an enzyme associated with the lactic acid energy source, of 7% and 18%, respectively, in the 6-s-trained and 30-s-trained legs. Neither leg showed a significant increase in a second enzyme, lactate dehydrogenase, associated with the lactic acid energy source. The enzymes PFK and lactate dehydrogenase have been shown to be unaffected by heavy resistance exercise training (Houston et al. 1983; Komi et al. 1982; Tesch 1987; Tesch, Thorsson, and Colliander 1990; Thorstensson et al. 1976). It appears that the type of lifting protocol affects the adaptations of all the enzymes associated with the lactic acid energy source, as it does those associated with the ATP-PC energy source.

Increases in the activity of enzymes associated with aerobic metabolism have been reported with isokinetic training in humans (Costill et al. 1979), with isometric training in humans (G. Grimby et al. 1973), and with isometric training in rats (Exner, Staudte, and Pette 1973). Enzymatic changes associated with the aerobic energy source may also depend on the duration of individual exercise bouts (Costill et al. 1979). However, enzymes involved with aerobic metabolism obtained from pooled samples of weight-trained muscle fibers have not demonstrated increased activity (Tesch 1992a). Body builders using high-volume programs, short rest periods between sets and exercises, and moderate-intensity training resistances have been shown to have higher citrate synthase activity in Type II fibers than other types of lifters who train with heavier loads and longer rest periods between sets (Tesch 1992b). Again, the type of program may influence the magnitude of enzyme changes in the muscle.

An enzyme associated with all three energy sources, myosin ATPase, demonstrated only minor changes in pooled muscle fibers (Tesch 1992a). The fact that various types of myosin ATPase exist and are altered with strength training may indicate that the type of myosin ATPase is more important than the absolute concentration change.

Enzymatic changes that are associated with any of the three energy sources depend on the duration of individual sets rather than the total amount of work performed. For practical application, normal heavy resistance programs have a minimal effect on enzyme activities. However, a training program that calls for resistances that are tolerable for at least 30 s will most likely effect increases in the activity of enzymes.

Muscle Substrate Stores

One adaptation that can lead to increased physical performance is an increase in the fuel available to the three energy sources. In humans it has been demonstrated that after 5 mo of strength training the resting intramuscular concentrations of PC and ATP are elevated 22% and 18%, respectively (MacDougall et al. 1977), although this finding is not supported by other studies (Tesch 1992a). The concept that PC and ATP stores are not increased by performing resistance training is supported by a finding of normal concentrations of PC and ATP in athletes who show a significant amount of muscular hypertrophy (Tesch, Thorsson, and Colliander 1990).

A 66% increase in intramuscular glycogen stores was shown after resistance training for 5 mo (MacDougall et al. 1977). However, another study failed to show a change in muscle glycogen content with resistance training (Tesch, Thorsson, and Colliander 1990). It has also been shown that blood glucose levels do not change significantly during resistance training sessions (Kraemer et al. 1990; Keul, Haralambie, Bruder, and Gottstein 1978), which indicates that the supply of glucose to muscle does not limit the performance of resistance training. Whether or not increases in PC and ATP occur with resistance training may depend on pretraining status, muscle group examined, and type of program performed. However, it is clear that skeletal muscle glycogen content can increase from resistance training and that blood glucose concentrations do not decrease during resistance training. This finding indicates that, at least during one training session, fuel availability for the lactic acid energy source is not a limiting factor to performance.

The aerobic energy source uses glycogen (carbohydrates), triglycerides (fats), and some protein to produce ATP. It has already been stated that intramuscular glycogen stores can be increased by strength training. The enhancement of triglyceride stores in muscles with resistance training remains equivocal, because increases have been observed in the triceps muscle of the arm but not in the quadriceps muscle after training (Tesch 1992a). Thus, there may be differences in the response of different muscle groups in terms of triglyceride stores. Although dietary practices and type of program may affect triglyceride concentrations, because most resistance training programs are anaerobic in nature, it can be speculated that intramuscular concentrations of triglyceride are minimally affected by resistance training.

Myoglobin Content

Myoglobin content in the muscle following strength training may decrease (Tesch 1992a). It therefore has been postulated that long-term strength training may depress myoglobin content and consequently the ability of the muscle fibers to extract oxygen. Again, the initial state of training as well as the specific type of program that is used may influence the effect of resistance training on myoglobin content.

Capillary Supply

An increased number of capillaries in a muscle helps support metabolism by increasing the potential blood supply to the muscle and contributes to total muscle size. Improved capillarization has been observed with resistance training of untrained subjects (Frontera et al. 1988; Hather, Mason, and Dudley 1991; Staron et al. 1989; Tesch, Thorsson, and Colliander 1990). Hather, Mason, and Dudley (1991) demonstrated that with different types of training (i.e., different combinations of concentric and eccentric muscle actions) capillaries per unit area and per fiber increased significantly in response to heavy resistance training even with an increase in fiber areas. As does the selective hypertrophy of Type II fibers, the increase of capillaries appears to be linked to the intensity and volume of resistance training. However, the time course of changes in capillary density appears to be slow, as studies have shown that 6 to 12 wk may not stimulate capillary growth beyond normal untrained levels (Tesch 1992a; Tesch, Hjort, and Balldin 1983; Tesch, Thorsson, and Colliander 1990).

It has been shown that power lifters and weight lifters exhibit no change in the number of capillaries per muscle fiber, because of muscle hypertrophy. However, these same athletes show a decrease in capillary density (i.e., the number of capillaries per cross-sectional area of tissue) when compared to nonathletic individuals (Tesch, Thorsson, and Kaiser 1984). It has been proposed that the training performed by body builders induces increased capillarization (Schantz 1982). Thus, high-intensity, low-volume strength training actually decreases capillary density, whereas low-intensity, high-volume strength training may have the opposite effect of increasing capillary density. An increase in capillary density may facilitate the performance of low-intensity weight training by increasing the blood supply to the active muscle. The short rest periods used by body builders during their workouts result in large increases in blood lactate concentrations, from resting concentrations of 1 to 2 mmol/L to greater than 20 mmol/L (Kraemer, Noble, Clark, and Culver 1987). A higher capillary density may increase the ability to remove lactate from the muscle to the blood, thereby allowing better tolerance to training under such high lactate conditions (Kraemer, Noble, Clark, and Culver 1987). This idea is supported by data demonstrating that body builders can use heavier resistance under the same lactate conditions than power lifters can use (Kraemer, Noble, Clark, and Culver 1987). These data suggest that greater clearance and buffering took place to allow the superior performance by the body builders in the lifting protocol. Because blood lactate concentrations observed with heavy resistance protocols used by power lifters and weight lifters are rarely above 4 mmol/L, the physi-

ological stimulus to increase capillarization may not be as great as with the higher lactate concentrations found due to body-building type programs.

Capillarization can increase with resistance training. However, the time required for this adaptation to take place can be longer than 12 wk. An increase in the total number of capillaries can be masked by muscle hypertrophy and may result in no change in number of capillaries per fiber area. A high-volume program may cause capillarization to occur, whereas a low-volume program will not.

Mitochondrial Density

Few studies have examined the effect of resistance training on mitochondrial density. In a fashion similar to capillaries per muscle fiber, mitochondrial density has been shown to decrease with resistance training because of the dilution effects of muscle fiber hypertrophy (MacDougall et al. 1979). The observation of decreased mitochondrial density is consistent with the minimal demands for oxidative metabolism placed on the musculature during most resistance training programs. The effect of resistance training on mitochondrial density requires further study.

ENDOCRINE SYSTEM ADAPTATIONS

The endocrine system helps an organism in adapting to its environment. This fact is very important to both the acute response and the chronic adaptations associated with resistance training. A specific stimulus causes the release into the blood of a chemical messenger, or hormone, targeted for specific tissue cells. The hormone travels in the blood to the target cell (e.g., muscle), where it interacts and signals a change or adaptation.

One example of hormonal action is the basic endocrine reflex: a feedback system that maintains a specific homeostatic level of a particular substance. For example, blood glucose levels are maintained by a negative feedback system. Elevation of blood glucose levels after eating a candy bar stimulates the pancreas to secrete the hormone insulin. Insulin causes the cells to increase the uptake of glucose from the blood, resulting in decreased blood glucose concentration. The lower blood glucose concentration produces a negative feedback on the cells of the pancreas; that is, it causes the pancreas to reduce the amount of insulin secreted.

Over time this feedback system brings the blood glucose concentration back to normal.

Hormones can also be released inside the cell itself for interaction with that cell. This is called an *autocrine* hormonal action. In addition, a hormone can be released from one cell to interact with another cell and never enter the circulatory system. This is called a *paracrine* hormonal action. Thus, there are a number of ways for hormones to interact with the cells of the body. Each of these mechanisms is involved with adaptations of the body to resistance training (Kraemer 1992a, 1992b).

Both the mechanisms of various hormones' actions and the actions themselves are diverse (Kraemer 1988, 1992a, 1992b, 1994; Norris 1980). Hormones can affect almost every physiological function in the body. Cellular transport, enzyme synthesis, cell growth, protein synthesis, cell metabolism, and reproductive function are just a few physiological events that are mediated in part by hormonal actions. The close association of hormones to the nervous system makes the neuroendocrine system potentially one of the most important physiological systems related to resistance training adaptations.

The endocrine system plays an important support function for adaptational mechanisms that ultimately lead to enhanced muscular force production (Kraemer 1988, 1992b; Kraemer et al. 1992; Kraemer, Gordon et al. 1991). The primary mechanisms through which hormones mediate changes are related to their metabolic or tropic effects on nerve and muscle cells. It is well established that anabolic hormones (e.g., testosterone, insulin, growth hormone) play various roles in enhancing tissue growth and development. In addition, gender differences (i.e., testosterone responses) in these hormonal concentrations and responses to exercise have been demonstrated (Kraemer et al. 1993). The key sequence of events is related to the effective stimulation of an endocrine, paracrine, or autocrine endogenous response by the exercise protocol. These signals must then be received by the receptor mechanisms of the target tissues. The alteration

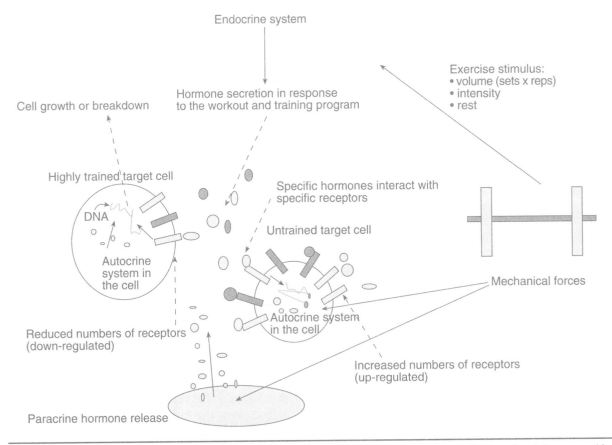

Fig. 7.9 Endocrine interactions with cells. The resistance exercise stimulates the body's endocrine glands to respond by releasing hormones. These hormones interact with receptors. Signals initiated by the hormones—which come from the endocrine, paracrine, or autocrine sources—interact with the cell's DNA, resulting in the hormone's signals for either more protein synthesis or a reduction in a specific protein.

of (typically protein) metabolism and the molecular mechanisms associated with cell transport phenomena must then be translated to enhance synthesis of, reduce degradation of, or augment the cell's functional structure or secretory products, leading to enhanced muscle mass or improved force production. Figure 7.9 reviews some of the basic interactions of the endocrine system with target tissues.

In studies by Kraemer and colleagues (Kraemer, Fleck, Dziados, et al. 1993; Kraemer, Gordon, et al. 1991; Kraemer, Marchitelli, et al. 1990) it was determined that acute resistance exercise can increase circulating concentrations of hormones, but that hormones are differentially sensitive to different types of acute program variables. For example, the highest growth hormone, beta-endorphin, and cortisol concentrations were observed when short-rest (1 min), 10-RM, multiple (3) sets of exercises were performed. Testosterone appears responsive to a high-intensity, long-rest (3 min), 5-RM resistance exercise protocol as well as to the 10-RM, short-rest protocol. This series of studies showed that both rest period length and the intensity of the resistance exercise can affect the magnitude of the hormonal response to a workout. It appears that the following factors determine whether anabolic

hormone concentrations increase with a resistance exercise workout (Kraemer 1988, 1992a, 1992b):

- Amount of muscle mass recruited
- Intensity of the workout
- Amount of rest between sets and exercises
- Volume of total work
- Training level of the individual

Besides the anabolic function of hormones, many hormones help to meet the metabolic demands of strenuous exercise. Regulation of blood glucose levels, glycogen storage, and mineral metabolism are all mediated via hormonal actions. Table 7.8 provides a summary of the major hormones and their actions. A myriad of interactions occur among hormones and hormonal factors; the complexity of the neuroendocrine system has just started to be understood. Endocrine function is highly integrated with nutritional status, nutritional intake, training status, and other external factors (e.g., stress, sleep, disease) that affect the remodeling and repair processes of the body. The effects of resistance training on acute and chronic hormonal responses require more detailed study. The challenge is to link physiological responses to

TABLE 7.8
Selected Hormones of the Endocrine System and Their Actions

Endocrine gland	Hormone	Some actions
Testes	Testosterone	Stimulates development and maintenance of male sex characteristics, growth, and increased protein anabolism
Anterior pituitary	Growth hormones	Stimulate the release of insulin-like growth factors I and II, protein synthesis, growth, and organic metabolism
	Adrenocorticotropin (ACTH)	Stimulates glucocorticoids' release in adrenal cortex
	Thyroid-stimulating hormone (TSH)	Stimulates thyroid hormone synthesis and secretion
	Follicle-stimulating hormone (FSH)	Stimulates growth of follicles in ovary and of seminiferous tubules in testes, ovum and sperm production
	Luteinizing hormone (LH)	Stimulates ovulation and secretion of sex hormones in ovaries and testes
	Prolactin (LTH)	Stimulates milk production in mammary glands; maintains corpora lutea; and stimulates secretion of progesterone

(continued)

TABLE 7.8
(continued)

Endocrine gland	Hormone	Some actions
Anterior pituitary	Melanocyte-stimulating hormone	Stimulates melanocytes, which contain the dark pigment melanin
Posterior pituitary	Antidiuretic hormone (ADH)	Increases contraction of smooth muscle and reabsorption of water by kidneys
	Oxytocin	Stimulates uterine contractions and release of milk by mammary glands
Adrenal cortex	Glucocorticoids (cortisol, cortisone, etc.)	Inhibits or retards amino acid incorporation into proteins; stimulates conversion of proteins into carbohydrates; maintains normal blood sugar level; conserves glucose; promotes metabolism of fat
	Mineralocorticoids (aldosterone, desoxycorticosterone, etc.)	Increases or decreases sodium-potassium metabolism; increases body fluid
Adrenal medulla	Epinephrine	Increases cardiac output; increases blood sugar, glycogen breakdown, and fat mobilization
	Norepinephrine	Similar to epinephrine, plus constriction of blood vessels
Thyroid	Thyroxine	Stimulates oxidative metabolism in mitochondria and cell growth
	Calcitonin	Reduces blood calcium phosphate levels
Pancreas	Insulin	Glycogen storage and glucose absorption
	Glucagon	Increases blood glucose levels
Ovaries	Estrogens	Develops female sex characteristics; exerts systemic effects, such as growth and maturation of long bones
	Progesterone	Develops female sex characteristics; maintains pregnancy; develops mammary glands
Parathyroids	Parathormone	Increases blood calcium; decreases blood phosphate

chronic adaptations such as muscle hypertrophy and strength.

It is apparent that the endocrine system plays a major role in adaptational responses of skeletal muscle. A study by Staron and co-workers (1994) demonstrated that serum testosterone concentrations increased in the first 6 wk of training and then returned to pretraining values. During this time significant changes in the quality of muscle protein took place (i.e., type of myosin ATPase). Thus, hormones may be a part of the process whereby protein synthesis or reduced degradation is mediated in some training phases then returns to resting values after a training adaptation is completed until needed again.

How paracrine and autocrine changes are affected by heavy resistance training remains unknown because of methodological difficulties in determining the small changes in cells or in various intercellular spaces. Furthermore, research has been limited to those hormone forms that can be detected with an antibody assay (immunoreactive molecular forms), thus eliminating the various forms which are not immunoreactive (e.g., some types of growth hormone). Finally, our understanding of how receptors on target tissues translate the endocrine message is just starting to develop (Deschenes et al. 1994). Each receptor can be differentially regulated in various fiber types in response to different exercise regimens (Bricourt et al. 1994; Deschenes et al. 1994). These responses at the target level of the cell (e.g., muscle, nerve) determine whether a hormonal message is realized. If the receptors are down-regulated, they will not interact with the hormone; if they are up-regulated, they will interact with the hormone. Therefore, quantity of hormone may not be as important as quantity of receptors in the cells.

SUMMARY

Physiological adaptations are the goals of every resistance training program. The information in this chapter shows that the specificity of the resistance training program is vital for the specific adaptations desired. In the next chapter we will see how some of these adaptations are affected without training or with detraining.

SELECTED READINGS

Fleck, S.J. 1988. Cardiovascular adaptations to resistance training. *Medicine and Science in Sports and Exercise* 20:S146-51.

Fleck, S.J. 1992. Cardiovascular response to strength training. In *Strength and power in sport*, ed. P.V. Komi, 305-15. Oxford: Blackwell Scientific.

Knuttgen, H.G., and Kraemer, W.J. 1987. Terminology and measurement in exercise performance. *Journal of Applied Sport Science Research* 1:1-10.

Kraemer, W.J. 1990. Physiological and cellular effects of exercise training. In *Sports-induced inflammation*, eds. W.B. Leadbetter, J.A. Buckwalter, and S.L. Gordon, 659-76. Park Ridge, IL: American Academy of Orthopaedic Surgeons.

Kraemer, W.J. 1992. Endocrine responses and adaptations to strength training. In *Strength and power in sport*, ed. P.V. Komi, 291-304. Oxford: Blackwell Scientific.

Kraemer, W.J. 1992. Hormonal mechanisms related to the expression of muscular strength and power. In *Strength and power in sport*, ed. P.V. Komi, 64-76. Oxford: Blackwell Scientific.

Kraemer, W.J. 1994. General adaptations to resistance and endurance training programs. In *Essentials of strength and conditioning*, ed. T.R. Baechle, 127-50. Champaign, IL: Human Kinetics.

Kraemer, W.J. 1994. Neuroendocrine responses to resistance exercise. In *Essentials of strength and conditioning*, ed. T.R. Baechle, 86-107. Champaign, IL: Human Kinetics.

Kraemer, W.J. 1994. The physiological basis for strength training in mid-life. In *Sports and exercise in midlife*, ed. S.L. Gordon, 413-33. Park Ridge, IL: American Academy of Orthopaedic Surgeons.

Kraemer, W.J., and Daniels, W.L. 1986. Physiological effects of training. In *Sports physical therapy*, ed. D.B. Bernhardt, 29-53. New York: Churchill Livingston.

Kraemer, W.J.; Deschenes, M.R.; and Fleck, S.J. 1988. Physiological adaptations to resistance training implications for athletic conditioning. *Sports Medicine* 6:246-56.

Kraemer, W.J.; Fleck, S.J.; and Deschenes, M. 1988. A review: Factors in exercise prescription of resistance training. *National Strength and Conditioning Association Journal* 10:36-41.

Kraemer, W.J.; Fleck, S.J.; and Evans, W.J. 1996. Strength and power training: Physiological mechanisms of adaptation. In *Exercise and sport sciences reviews*, ed. J.D. Holloszy, vol. 24, 363-397. Baltimore: Williams and Wilkins.

Kraemer, W.J., and Fry, A.C. 1995. Strength testing: Development and evaluation of methodology. In *Physiological assessment of human fitness*, eds. P. Maud and C. Foster, 115-38. Champaign, IL: Human Kinetics.

Kraemer, W.J., and Koziris, L.P. 1994. Olympic weightlifting and power lifting. In *Physiology and nutrition for competitive sport*, eds. D.R. Lamb, H.G. Knuttgen, and R. Murray, 1-54. Carmel, IN: Cooper.

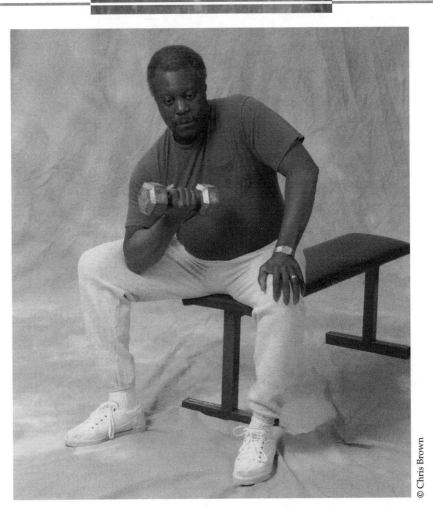

© Chris Brown

CHAPTER 8

Detraining

Cessation of resistance training or reduction of training volume, intensity, or frequency results in a period of detraining. Detraining is a deconditioning process that affects performance by diminishing physiological capacity. Resistance training may be stopped or reduced because of injury or as a planned part of the yearly training cycle, as may occur during many in-season programs. An understanding of detraining will facilitate the design of optimal resistance training programs for improving performance and maintaining strength or power during periods when resistance training is reduced.

CESSATION OF RESISTANCE TRAINING

Early studies indicated that when training ceases completely or is drastically reduced, strength declines but at a slower rate than the rate at which strength increased due to training (McMorris and Elkins 1954; Morehouse 1967; Rasch 1971; Rasch and Morehouse 1957; Waldman and Stull 1969). In most instances, complete cessation of resistance training results in an immediate decline of strength (table 8.1). For example, squat ability of Olympic-style weight lifters shows a decline of approximately 10% in a 4-wk period after cessation of weight training (figure 8.1). After a period of training, active males showed a slight increase in isometric force during a 2-wk detraining period (figure 8.2). In general, a short detraining period results in a decrease in strength, although the magnitude of the decrease in strength varies. The strength decrease during short periods of detraining will result in a strength level after detraining that is still greater than pretrained levels (table 8.1).

Longer periods of detraining (up to 30 wk) also result in a decrease of strength (table 8.1); in general, strength after the detraining period is still greater than it was before beginning resistance training. Ishida, Moritani, and Itoh (1990) reported

relatively quick decreases in strength during a detraining period followed by a slower decline in strength. It has also been reported that maximal isometric force declines at the same rate (0.3% per day) at which it was gained with isokinetic training (Narici et al. 1989).

Collectively the information available on both short (2 wk to 4 wk) and longer periods of detraining indicates that in general strength decreases do occur but that the loss is quite variable in magnitude. The rate of strength loss may depend in part on the length of the training period prior to detraining, the type of strength test used (e.g., bench press, eccentric, concentric), and the specific muscle group examined.

Normal resistance training (concentric and eccentric actions) may result in a slower loss of strength during 4 wk of detraining than concentric-only training (Dudley et al. 1991). Normal resistance training and concentric-only training consisted of three sets of 10 to 12 repetitions at a 10- to 12-RM resistance. Double-volume concentric training consisted of six sets of 10 to 12 repetitions at the normal 10- to 12-RM resistance. During double-volume concentric training the total number of concentric-only muscle actions was therefore equal to the total number of concentric and eccentric actions performed during the normal resistance training. Concentric-only regimens consisted of lifting the weight but never lowering the weight. The leg

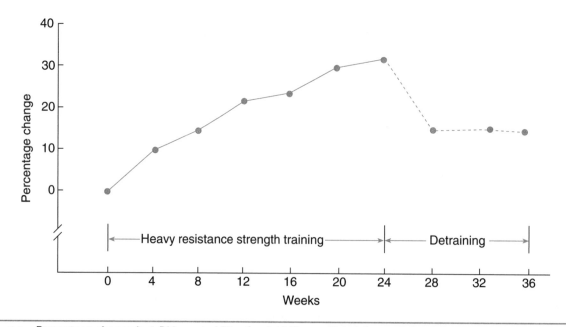

Fig. 8.1 Percentage change in 1-RM squat ability of weight lifters with training and detraining.

Adapted, by permission, from K. Häkkinen and P.V. Komi, 1985, "Changes in electrical and mechanical behavior of leg extensor muscles during heavy resistance strength training," *Scandinavian Journal of Sports Science* 7:55-64. © 1985 Munksgaard International Publishers Ltd., Copenhagen, Denmark.

TABLE 8.1
Strength and Power Changes With Detraining

Reference	Subjects	Length of training (wk)	Type of training	D/wk	Sets/reps	Length of detraining (wk)	Type of strength test	% above pretrained Trained	% above pretrained Detrained
Hortobágyi et al. 1993	Power lifters & football players	8.1 yr	Weight lifting	3.4	2-5/1-12	2	1-RM squat 1-RM bench press	? ?	-1.7 -0.9
Dudley et al. 1991	Males	19	Leg press, knee extension	2	4-5/6-12	4	3-RM leg press 3-RM knee extension	26* 29*	20 20
Häkkinen et al. 1989	Male strength athletes	10.5	Weight lifting	3.5	(70%-100% 1 RM)	2	Maximal isometric knee extension	8*	5
	Males	10.5	Weight lifting	3.5	(70%-100% 1 RM)	2	Maximal isometric knee extension	13*	15
	Females	10.5	Weight lifting	3.5	(70%-100% 1 RM)	2	Maximal isometric knee extension	19*	18
Narici et al. 1989	Males	8.6	Isokinetic, 120°/s	4	6/10	5.7	Isometric	21*	3 wk = 10 5.7 wk = 4
Häkkinen and Komi 1983	Males	16*	Squat	3	15 reps, 80%-100% 1 RM; 5 reps eccentrically, 100%-120% 1 RM	8	Isometric squat	30*	19*
Ishida et al. 1990	Males	8	Calf raise	3	3/15, 70% 1 RM	8	Isometric	32*	4 wk = 20 8 wk = 16
Blimkie et al. 1992	Boys	20		3	3/10-12 RM	8	Bench press Leg press Isometric knee extension Isometric elbow flexion	35* 22* 21* 31*	34 17 14 30
Häkkinen, Alén, and Komi 1985	Males	24	Squat	3	18-30 reps, 70%-100% 1 RM, 3-5 reps eccentrically, 100%-120% 1 RM	12	Isometric squat	27*	12*

(continued)

TABLE 8.1
(continued)

Reference	Subjects	Length of training (wk)	Type of training	D/wk	Sets/reps	Length of detraining (wk)	Type of strength test	% above pretrained	
								Trained	Detrained
Häkkinen and Komi 1985a	Males	24	Squat	3	18-30 reps, 70%-100% 1 RM, 3-5 reps eccentrically, 100%-120% 1 RM	12	1-RM squat	30*	15*
Houston et al. 1983	Males	10	Leg press, knee extension	4	3/10 RM	12	Knee extension, 0-270°/s	39-60	4 wk = 29-52 12 wk = 15-29*
Häkkinen and Komi 1985b	Males	24	Jump training with 10%-60% of 1-RM squat	3	100-200 jumps/ session	12	Isometric squat	6.9*	2.6*
Staron et al. 1991	Females	20	Leg press, squat, knee extension	2	3/6-8 RM one session, 3/10-12 RM one session	30-32	1-RM squat 1-RM leg press 1-RM knee extension	67* 148* 70*	45* 105* 61

* = significantly different from pretrained

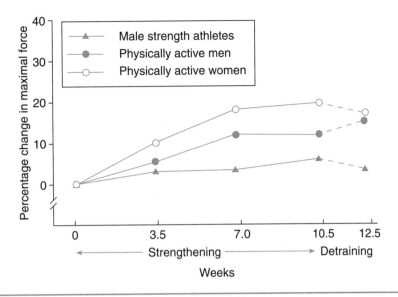

Fig. 8.2 Percentage change in maximal isometric force with training and detraining.

Reprinted from *Journal of Biomechanics*, Volume 8, K. Häkkinen, A. Pakarinen, P.V. Komi, T. Ryushi, and H. Kauhanen, "Neuromuscular adaptations and hormone balance in strength athletes, physically active males, and females during intensive strength training," 889-94, Copyright 1989, with kind permission from Elsevier Science Ltd, The Boulevard, Langford Lane, Kidlington OX5 1GB, UK.

press and knee extension were the only exercises performed, and training was performed 3 d/wk for 19 wk.

A 3-RM leg press and knee extension were used to evaluate strength after the training and detraining periods. Strength increases for both exercises were tested both with concentric-only actions and with normal concentric and eccentric actions. All groups improved significantly in concentric-only leg press ability (figure 8.3).

After the detraining period the normal resistance training and double concentric training resulted in greater retention of strength than the concentric-only training (figure 8.3). In addition, the normal

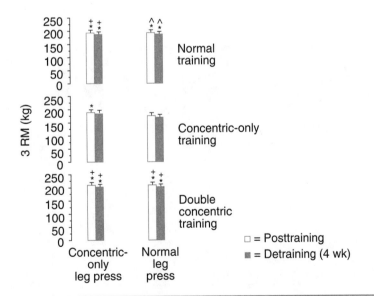

Fig. 8.3 Changes in 3-RM leg press with normal resistance training, concentric-only training, and double-volume concentric training. * = increase over pretraining; + = greater increase than concentric-only group; ^ = increase greater than concentric-only and double concentric groups.

Adapted, by permission, from G.A. Dudley, P.A. Tesch, B.J. Miller, and P. Buchanan, 1991, "Importance of eccentric actions in performance adaptations to resistance training," *Aviation, Space, and Environmental Medicine* 62:543-50.

resistance training resulted in a smaller loss of strength than the double concentric training. The knee-extension strength followed a similar pattern. This information indicates that normal resistance training results in greater strength retention during detraining than concentric-only training, even when the volume of concentric-only training is doubled.

REDUCTION OF TRAINING VOLUME

An early study (Berger 1962b) indicated that strength could be improved over a 6-wk detraining period using only one set of 1 RM and training only 1 d/wk. This early study indicated that strength can be maintained with a program consisting of reduced training frequency and volume of exercise.

A study using various jumping and stretch-shortening cycle drills three times per week for 16 wk showed an increase in isometric leg strength of 28% (Häkkinen et al. 1990). After 8 wk of performing the same type of training session at a reduced frequency of only one time per week, isometric strength had decreased to 6% above pretraining. This was a nonsignificant decrease, however, and a great deal of individual variation in the response to the detraining period occurred.

Reducing training frequency for 12 wk after 10 to 18 wk of training may not have an effect on

isometric strength and training weight used for 7 to 10 repetitions at a 7 to 10 RM (Graves et al. 1988). A training session consisted of one set of 7 to 10 knee extensions with resistances of 7 to 10 RM. Training was performed either two or three times per week and was reduced to two, one, or no training sessions per week. All training frequencies significantly increased isometric strength and training resistance used (table 8.2). After the 12 wk of reduced training frequencies, training ceased and a significant decline in strength ensued. In another study (Tucci et al. 1992) 12 wk of reduced training after 10 to 12 wk of variable-resistance or isometric training did not change isometric back strength at seven angles of back extension. Training was performed one to three times per week and consisted of either two sets of 8 to 12 repetitions of back extensions at an 8- to 12-RM resistance, two sets of isometric back extensions, or one set of each type of exercise. During detraining, frequency was reduced to either one session every 2 wk, one session every 4 wk, or no training at all. Training resulted in significant increases in isometric back extension strength at all seven angles tested (+8% to +60%). Detraining frequencies of one session once every 2 or 4 wk resulted in nonsignificant decreases in isometric strength from posttraining values (+1% to −13%). No training at all during the 12-wk detraining period resulted in significant decreases from posttraining values at all seven back angles (−6% to −14%). These studies indicate that re-

TABLE 8.2
Changes in Average Knee-Extension Strength After 10-18 wk of Training Followed by 12 wk of Detraining

Training/detraining frequency (d/wk)	Isometric force (% above pretraining)		Training weight (% above pretraining)	
	Trained	Detrained	Trained	Detrained
3/2	27*	23*	64*	65*
3/1	20*	20*	59*	59*
2/1	17*	15*	47*	40*+
3-2/0	18*	6*+	40*	—

* Significantly greater than pretraining

+ Significantly less than posttraining

Note. Data from J.E. Graves et al., 1988, "Effect of reduced training frequency on muscular strength," *International Journal of Sports Medicine* 9:316-19.

duced training can maintain strength levels in a variety of muscle groups if training intensity is maintained at a high level, but that no training at all results in loss of strength.

EFFECTS ON MOTOR PERFORMANCE

The effect of detraining on motor performance has received much less attention than its effect on strength. After 24 wk of heavy resistance training three times per week, vertical jump ability increased 13% (Häkkinen and Komi 1985a). Training consisted primarily of squat-type movements using 70% to 100% of 1 RM. Twelve weeks of detraining resulted in a decrease in vertical jump ability, but it was still 2% above the pretraining value. Another study showed that 24 wk of stretch-shortening cycle training increased vertical jump ability 17%; after 12 wk of detraining vertical jump ability had decreased but was still 10% above the pretraining value (Häkkinen and Komi 1985b). Training consisted of various jumps with and without added weight. During both of these studies squat-jump ability (jump with no countermovement) also decreased during the detraining period. Two weeks of detraining in strength-trained athletes (power lifters and football players) resulted in nonsignificant increases in vertical jump (2.3%) and squat-jump (3.6%) ability (Hortobágyi et al. 1993).

It appears that short-term detraining periods may not significantly affect vertical jump ability but that longer periods of detraining do result in decreased vertical jump ability. Whether the vertical jump results can be generalized to other types of motor performance is unknown, but this is an attractive hypothesis. Data from Thorstensson (1977) suggest that performance of complex skills involving strength components (e.g., vertical jump) may decline if these skills are not included in the training program. Thus, if the goal of an in-season program is to maintain motor performance, the

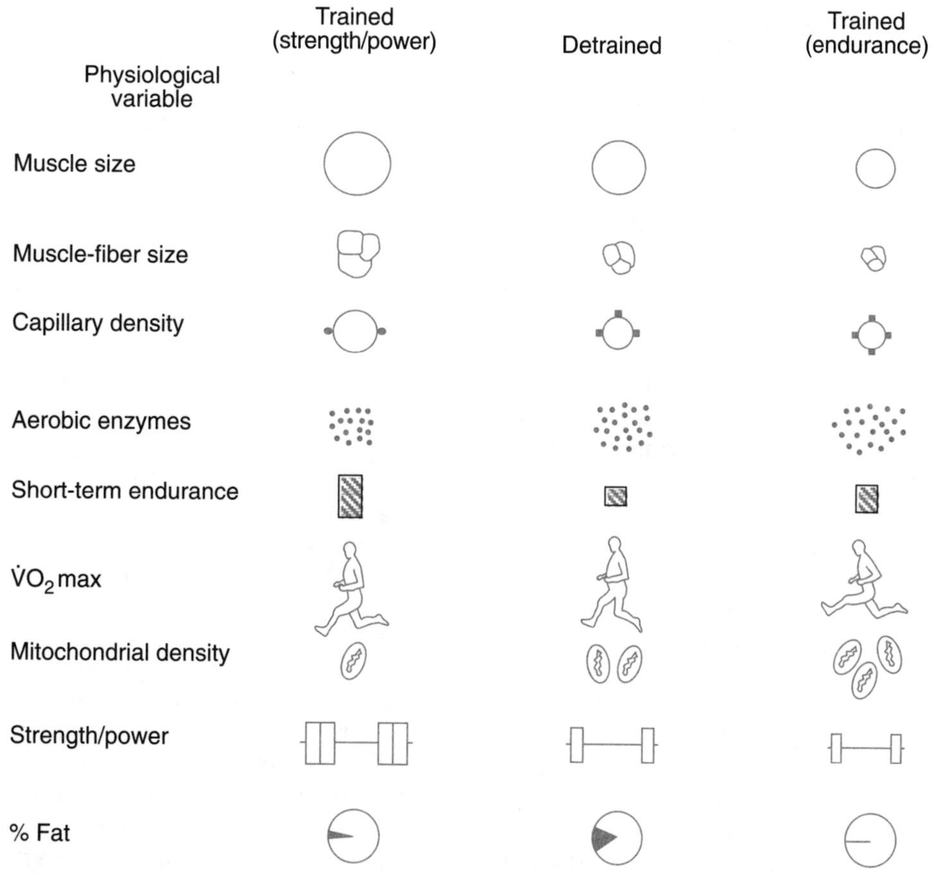

Fig. 8.4 General effects of detraining.

motor performance task should be included in the training program. The general effects of detraining are shown in figure 8.4.

MECHANISMS OF STRENGTH LOSS

As with strength gains during training, there are several possible mechanisms that could result in strength and power changes during periods of detraining. Knowledge of these mechanisms will help the practitioner design better in-season programs.

Electromyographic (EMG) changes during muscular actions after training and detraining indicate changes in motor unit firing rate and motor unit synchronization. EMG changes have been followed during detraining periods ranging from 2 to 12 wk. No change or a decrease in EMG activity and no change or a decrease in strength/power measurements during short periods of detraining have been observed (Häkkinen et al. 1990; Häkkinen and Komi 1985a, 1986; Häkkinen, Komi, and Alén 1985; Hortobágyi et al. 1993; Narici et al. 1989). When decreases in EMG activity occur, they have shown significant correlations to decreases in strength (Häkkinen, Alén, and Komi 1985; Häkkinen and Komi 1985b, 1986). However, decreases in EMG activity of some muscles (vastus lateralis) but not others (vastus medialis, rectus femoris) have also been observed (Häkkinen, Alén, and Komi 1985). This EMG information indicates that the initial strength loss during the first several weeks of detraining, when it does occur, is caused in part by neural mechanisms, with muscle atrophy contributing to further strength loss as the detraining continues (Häkkinen and Komi 1983).

Training adaptations of muscle fiber are discussed extensively in chapter 7. However, few studies have examined the effects of detraining on cellular-level variables. In general, during periods of detraining any adaptations that occurred from training regress toward the untrained or pretrained state. During short periods (2-8 wk) of detraining in males, Type I and Type II fiber area may decrease compared with the trained state (Häkkinen, Komi, and Alén 1985; Häkkinen, Komi, and Tesch 1981; Hather et al. 1992; Hortobágyi et al. 1993) or may stay the same (Hather et al. 1992; Hortobágyi et al. 1993). In males, the Type II-to-Type I fiber area ratio has been reported to decrease during periods of detraining (Häkkinen, Komi, and Tesch

1981; Hather et al. 1992)—indicating a selective atrophy of Type II fibers—or to remain unchanged compared to the trained state (Hather et al. 1992).

In females nonsignificant decreases in Type I fiber areas accompanied by a significant decrease in the combined areas of Type IIAB and IIB fibers have been observed (Staron et al. 1991). No change in either Type I or II fiber area has also been reported during 8 wk of detraining (Häkkinen et al. 1990); however, this study also showed no increase in fiber area from the stretch-shortening cycle training performed prior to the detraining period.

These studies together indicate that Type II fibers may atrophy to a greater extent than Type I fibers during short periods of detraining in both males and females. This can occur, of course, only if the training induced an increase in fiber area.

During short periods of detraining lean body mass and percent body fat show nonsignificant changes (Häkkinen, Komi, and Alén 1985; Häkkinen, Komi, and Tesch 1981; Häkkinen et al. 1990; Hortobágyi et al. 1993; Staron et al. 1991), whereas muscle cross-sectional areas show either nonsignificant (Häkkinen et al. 1989) or significant decreases (Narici et al. 1989). The lack of a significant change in lean body mass is probably caused by the gross nature of this measurement and the short duration of the detraining periods, whereas the decrease in muscle cross-sectional area supports the data showing decreases in muscle fiber area.

Changes in the blood hormonal profile during detraining could have an impact on strength, body composition, and muscle fiber hypertrophy. During 12 wk of detraining, decreases in the testosterone-cortisol and testosterone–sex-hormone-binding globulin ratios are significantly related to leg-extensor isometric strength decreases (Häkkinen, Pakarinen, Alén, and Komi 1985), but no significant changes in testosterone and free testosterone concentrations in males and females during short periods of detraining have also been reported (Häkkinen et al. 1990, 1989). During two weeks of detraining by strength-trained athletes (American football players and power lifters), growth hormone, testosterone, and the testosterone-cortisol ratio have been reported to increase significantly while cortisol decreased significantly (Hortobágyi et al. 1993). After 2 wk of one training session per day followed by a 1-wk period of reduced training volume, no significant change in testosterone, free testosterone, cortisol, or the testosterone-cortisol ratio occurred (Häkkinen and Pakarinen 1991). However, if the same training volume is performed but divided into two training sessions per day for a 1-wk training period followed by a 1-wk period of reduced training volume, testosterone and the testosterone-cortisol ratio significantly decrease while cortisol significantly increases after the 1-wk reduced training period (Häkkinen and Pakarinen 1991). No significant changes during short periods of detraining have been shown in follicle-stimulating hormone, luteinizing hormone, progesterone, and estradiol (Häkkinen et al. 1990; Häkkinen and Pakarinen 1991; Häkkinen, Pakarinen, Alén, and Komi 1985). The hormone response to detraining periods appears to be quite varied and probably depends on the volume, intensity, and duration of training prior to the detraining period and on the individual's training history.

EFFECT OF MUSCLE ACTION TYPE ON CELLULAR ADAPTATIONS

The previously described studies by Dudley and colleagues (1991) and Hather and colleagues (1992) indicate that normal resistance training and double-volume, concentric-only training result in greater retention of training adaptations during a short (4 wk) detraining period than concentric-only training (see figure 8.3).

All three types of training resulted in an increase in the percentage of Type IIA fibers and a corresponding decrease in Type IIB fibers. These changes were maintained during the detraining period. This could be interpreted to indicate that the concentric portion of resistance training is responsible for the Type II subtype transformations. Alternatively, it could mean that any type of high-intensity resistance training will cause this subtype transformation.

The normal resistance training and the double concentric training resulted in an increase in mean fiber area, but only the normal resistance training resulted in a maintenance of this increase after the detraining period. The concentric-only training resulted in no increase in mean fiber area. Only the normal resistance training resulted in increased fiber areas of both Type I and II fibers and in maintenance of these increases during the detraining period. The double concentric training resulted in an increased size of only the Type II fibers and in maintenance of this increase after detraining. The concentric-only training resulted in no significant size

increase of either the Type I or II fibers. This could be interpreted to indicate that normal resistance training and high-volume training result in the greatest maintenance of fiber size during a short detraining period.

The number of capillaries per fiber was increased by all three types of training and was maintained above pretraining values after the detraining period. However, only the double concentric and concentric-only training resulted in an increase of capillaries per cross-sectional area and maintenance of this increase during detraining. This result was caused in part by a slightly greater fiber size increase with normal resistance training and by a slightly greater increase in capillaries per fiber with double concentric and concentric-only training. This change could indicate that concentric-only training may be appropriate for athletes who need to maintain aerobic fitness capabilities.

IN-SEASON DETRAINING

In-season detraining refers to losses of performance when resistance training is stopped completely or performed at a reduced training volume while another sport-type training is performed. This is a very important issue, but it has received little attention from the sport science community. In a study by D.E. Campbell (1967) isometric elbow-flexion strength increased over spring football practice during which no resistance training was performed, but isometric leg-extension strength significantly decreased. The amount of both weight-bearing activity and leg stress involved in the sport might have contributed to the impaired isometric leg strength performances.

The effects of an alpine ski season (down hill, free style, speed skiing) in elite athletes on knee-extension and -flexion strength and power output have been examined (Koutedakis et al. 1992). Three months into the season isokinetic knee-extension strength at 60°/s decreased significantly (6%) and knee-flexion strength decreased nonsignificantly (7%). After 7 mo knee-extension strength at 60°/s decreased significantly by 14% and knee-flexion strength by 16%. Isokinetic knee-flexion and -extension strength at 180°/s after 3 and 7 mo showed nonsignificant decreases. The skiers demonstrated nonsignificant changes in power output during a 30-s maximal cycling test (Wingate test). Thus, skiers' strength at very slow velocities but not intermediate velocities may be lost during a season.

However, no loss of power output occurs, so the effect on performance may be minimal.

Rowing requires a high strength and aerobic level of conditioning. Rowers after 10 wk of resistance training three times per week demonstrate increased strength (figure 8.5; Bell et al. 1993). Six weeks of resistance training at a reduced frequency of either one or two times per week resulted in either no significant change or an increase in strength (figure 8.5). All training sessions consisted of approximately three sets of each of the six exercises shown in figure 8.5 at an intensity of approximately 75% of maximal. Rowing was performed throughout both the initial and the reduced frequency portions of resistance training. These results indicate that strength can be maintained or increased for a period of 6 wk in rowers who are also rowing. Rowing itself, however, has a high-strength component, so the applicability of these results to other sports or activities that do not have a high-strength component is questionable.

Another study examined a Division I men's basketball team that performed a 5-wk resistance training program immediately prior to a 20-wk season (J.R. Hoffman et al. 1991). The 5-wk program resulted in a significant increase in 1-RM squat of 18%, whereas nonsignificant changes in 1-RM bench press (4%), 27-m sprint time (2%), and vertical jump ability (no change) occurred. During the 20-wk basketball season, no resistance training was performed. One-RM bench press, 1-RM squat, and vertical jump ability all showed nonsignificant changes during the 20-wk season (–1% to +5%), whereas 27-m sprint ability declined significantly (3%). This study indicates that most measures of fitness can be maintained during the course of a college basketball season without an in-season resistance training program and that playing basketball and the associated drills with training may maintain fitness levels. An important consideration in the interpretation of this study is that the preseason training program did not cause

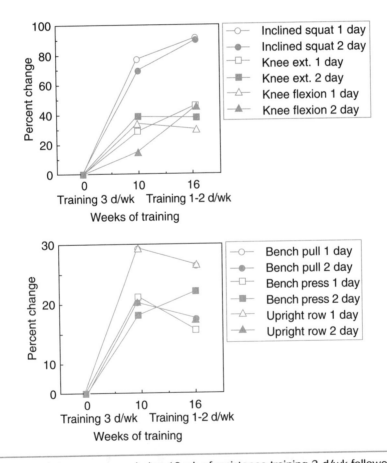

Fig. 8.5   Changes in strength in oarswomen during 10 wk of resistance training 3 d/wk followed by 6 wk of resistance training 1 or 2 d/wk.

Adapted, by permission, from G.J. Bell, D.G. Syrotuik, K. Attwood, and H.A. Quinney, 1993, "Maintenance of strength gains while performing endurance training in oarswomen," *Journal of Applied Physiology* 18:104-15.

a significant change in three of the four tests. However, all the aforementioned studies indicate that, at least for the sports examined, normal training for that sport without resistance training may maintain fitness levels of athletes for a short period of time.

IN-SEASON RESISTANCE PROGRAMS

The goal of an in-season resistance program is to further increase or at least maintain strength and power. Unpublished data by Kraemer support the concept that reduced training frequencies can maintain strength levels during a playing season. Sixty-eight college football players performed a 1 RM on three separate occasions: preseason, midseason, and postseason. All athletes trained two times per week during the 14-wk season. The in-season program is presented in table 8.3.

Each player completed winter and summer resistance training programs, lifting on 4 to 5 d/wk, with a much larger training volume and more ex-

ercises than the in-season program. The entire group exhibited no significant decreases in 1 RM for any of the exercises tested during the in-season program (figure 8.6). A separate evaluation of backs and linemen produced similar results.

TABLE 8.3 14-wk In-Season Training Program for College Football Players	
Exercise	**Reps/set**
Bench press	8, 5, 5, 8
Squats	8, 5, 5, 5
Single-leg knee extensions	10, 10
Single-leg knee curls	10, 10
Military press	8, 8, 8
Power cleans	8, 8, 8

Note. 2-min rest period between sets and exercises. Training frequency was 2× per week.

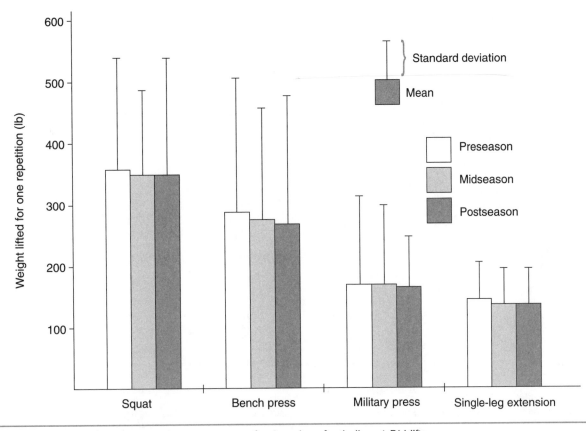

Fig. 8.6　Results of in-season resistance program for American football on 1-RM lifts.

During a 22-wk basketball season in which resistance training was performed one to two times per week, the vertical jump ability of female basketball players increased significantly by 6% (Häkkinen 1993a). Maximal isometric leg-extension force remained unchanged. The in-season training consisted of one to two lower-extremity exercises per session and three to eight repetitions per set at 30% to 80% of maximal. A total of 20 to 30 repetitions per training session were performed. In addition, once every 2 wk a jump training session was performed, consisting of 100 to 150 total jumps of various horizontal and vertical types. This in-season program maintained strength and increased vertical jumping ability.

Collectively these studies indicate that in-season programs can maintain or increase strength and power during a season. In addition, in some sports that have an inherent high-strength component, short periods without in-season resistance training can be tolerated with little or no decrease in strength.

LONG DETRAINING PERIODS

Long periods of detraining have received very little attention from the sport science community. However, two case studies have been performed. Table 8.4 depicts the effects of 7 mo of detraining and dieting on an elite power lifter (Staron, Hagerman, and Hikida 1981). The individual performed no resistance training during this period. The data from this study suggest that detraining results in a physiological shift from a strength profile to an improved aerobic profile. Three observations reflected this shift: the improvement of maximal oxygen consumption ($\dot{V}O_2$max), increased mitochondrial density, and improved oxidative enzyme profile of the muscle fibers. These changes occurred

TABLE 8.4
Physiological Changes After 7 mo of Detraining

Variable	Trained	Detrained
Height (cm)	170.0	170.0
Weight (kg)	121.5	94.0
% body fat	25.2	14.8
Thigh girth (cm)	82.5	66.5
Blood pressure (systolic/diastolic)	146/96	137/76
$\dot{V}O_2$max (ml $\cdot$ kg^{-1} $\cdot$ min^{-1})	32.6	49.1
Maximal heart rate	200	198
% volume of mitochondria		
Slow-twitch	3.04	4.41
Fast-twitch	1.76	2.46
Fiber type (%)		
SO	31.2	38.1
FG	53.2	34.7
FOG	15.6	27.2
Cross-sectional area (μm²)		
SO	5625	3855
FG	8539	5075
FOG	9618	5835

SO = slow oxidative (smaller than fast-twitch fibers and smaller than FOG fibers)

FG = fast glycolytic

FOG = fast oxidative glycolytic

Reprinted from *Journal of Neurological Sciences*, 51 R.S. Staron, F.C. Hagerman, and R.S. Hikida, "The effects of detraining on an elite power lifter," 247-57, 1981 with kind permission of Elsevier Science-NL, Sara Burgerhartstraat 25, 1055 KV Amsterdam, The Netherlands.

without any aerobic training stimulus during the 7-mo detraining period. The large weight loss (27.5 kg) and reduction in body fat during this period may account for some of these changes. The decrease in muscle fiber area contributed to the decrease in thigh girth. These observations are consistent with changes normally attributed to muscle atrophy.

A second study examined two males who performed resistance training for 8 wk and then detrained for 5 mo (Thorstensson 1977). The initial training period consisted of various exercises for the leg extensors and weighted and unweighted jumping exercises. After the initial training period one subject performed resistance training at a reduced volume 2 to 3 d/wk and did not perform any jumping exercises. The other subject performed no training at all for the 5-mo detraining period. The subject who trained at a reduced volume during the detraining period showed the following changes after detraining compared with immediate posttraining values: increased 1-RM squat ability, increased isokinetic torque at 60°/s and faster (but not at slower) velocities of movement, decreased isometric leg-extension force, and decreased vertical jump and horizontal jump ability. However, all measures were still above pretraining values. The subject who performed no training during the detraining period showed decreases in all of the preceding measures, with only 1-RM squat ability still greater than the pretraining value after the detraining period. Lean body mass continued to increase in the subject who trained at a reduced volume but decreased to slightly below pretrained levels in the subject who performed no training. The Type II-to-Type I fiber area ratio decreased in both subjects during the detraining period but was still above pretraining values for both subjects.

After 5 mo of detraining virtually all increases in strength and muscle mass from an 8-wk resistance training program are lost if no resistance training is performed. However, resistance training at a reduced volume for 5 mo can maintain or even increase gains in strength and muscle mass after an 8-wk resistance training program.

DETRAINING THE BULKED-UP ATHLETE

Little attention has been given to detraining the bulked-up athlete. Through resistance training many athletes gain substantial amounts of body weight. These weight gains are related to the increased muscle mass necessary for successful participation in sports such as American football, throwing events in athletics, and power lifting.

After an athletic career, chronic detraining leads to potential health and fitness problems. Obesity and a sedentary lifestyle often contribute to an increased risk of cardiovascular disease (Kraemer 1983a). Many athletes who exercise to increase muscle mass and strength do not know how to exercise for health and recreation using other types of training (e.g., aerobic training, circuit weight training). The retired athlete needs to start training again with new objectives and to examine dietary habits in order to avoid large weight gains.

Some studies have shown that, compared with nonathletes, former athletes have an advantage in cardiovascular fitness (Fardy et al. 1976). This advantage did not exist in a comparison of former athletes with nonathletes who engaged in strenuous leisure-time activities. One study (Paffenbarger et al. 1984) concluded that postcollege physical activity is more important than participation in college athletics in predicting low coronary artery disease. Few data exist with regard to specific athletic subgroups and lifelong health. However, a survey study of Finnish former world-class athletes concluded that athletes do have a longer than normal life expectancy and hypothesized that recreational aerobic activity and infrequent smoking after athletic retirement may explain the longer life expectancy (Fogelholm, Kaprio, and Sarna 1994). It might also be speculated that athletes who require substantial body weight gains during their sport careers are at the greatest risk for cardiovascular diseases (CD). To reduce this risk, retired athletes require the proper exercise prescription, along with diet and weight control.

The exercise program of a retired strength-trained athlete must recognize that resistance training can still be enjoyed but should reflect new training needs and goals. The modifications include lighter resistances (e.g., 10 to 12 RM) and shorter rest periods between sets and exercises to induce a higher caloric expenditure during the workout. Healthy detraining of the resistance-trained athlete necessitates aerobic exercise programs for improving cardiovascular function and reducing body weight. As the retired athletes age, a primary goal should be to reduce CD risk.

Table 8.5 lists the CD risk factors. When individuals have all four primary risk factors, the

TABLE 8.5
Cardiovascular Disease Risk Factors

Primary risk factors	Secondary risk factors
	Changeable
Smoking	Obesity
Elevated blood lipids	Diabetes
High LDL-cholesterol	Stress
Low HDL-cholesterol	
High triglycerides	*Unchangeable*
High blood pressure (hypertension)	Heredity (family history)
Physical inactivity	Male gender
	Advancing age

danger of heart attack is five times greater than when none are present (Fox and Mathews 1981). Management of these risk factors helps to reduce the risk of CD. It is easy to perform a risk-factor analysis; this procedure has been described extensively (Kraemer 1983a; Wilmore and Costill 1994).

Despite the fact that a strong genetic link is thought to be responsible for CD, former athletes should continue an active lifestyle with new goals and objectives for their training programs. The role of teachers and coaches is to educate students and athletes about lifelong health and fitness, exposing them to types of training other than heavy resistance training. Frequently, it is possible to implement different programs either during certain periods of the training cycle or as a supplement to the regular exercise prescription. This adds variety to the program and also contributes to a healthy transition for athletes whose careers end after high school, college, or professional participation in sports. It is up to the conditioning professionals to help athletes make a transition from competitive sports to lifetime sports and exercise for health.

SUMMARY

Research has not yet indicated the exact resistance, volume, frequency of resistance training, or the type of program needed to maintain the training gains achieved by an individual. In-season programs are probably as specific as the strength development prescription. Studies do, however, in-

dicate that to maintain strength gains or to slow strength loss during a detraining period the intensity should be maintained, but the volume and frequency of training can be reduced. All the material presented in parts I and II of this book is applicable to any population. In part III considerations for designing programs for women, children, aging individuals, and the weight-lifting sports are explored.

SELECTED READINGS

Bell, G.J.; Syrotuik, D.G.; Attwood, K.; and Quinney, H.A. 1993. Maintenance of strength gains while performing endurance training in oarswomen. *Journal of Applied Physiology* 18:104-15.

Häkkinen, K. 1993. Changes in physical fitness profile in female basketball players during the competitive season including explosive type strength training. *Journal of Sports Medicine and Physical Fitness* 33:19-26.

Häkkinen, K.; Pakarinen, A.; Komi, P.V.; Ryushi, T.; and Kauhanen, H. 1989. Neuromuscular adaptations and hormone balance in strength athletes, physically active males, and females during intensive strength training. In *Proceedings of the XII International Congress of Biomechanics*, no. 8, eds. R.J. Gregor, R.F. Zernicke, and W.C. Whiting, 889-94. Champaign, IL: Human Kinetics.

Hather, B.M.; Tesch, P.A.; Buchanan, P.; and Dudley, G.A. 1992. Influence of eccentric actions on skeletal muscle adaptations to resistance training. *Acta Physiologica Scandinavica* 143:177-85.

Hoffman, J.R.; Fry, A.C.; Howard, R.; Maresh, C.M.; and Kraemer, W.J. 1991. Strength, speed, and endurance changes during the course of a Division I basketball season. *Journal of Applied Sport Science Research* 5:144-49.

Hortobágyi, T.; Houmard, J.A.; Stevenson, J.R.; Fraser, D.D.; Johns, R.A.; and Israel, R.G. 1993. The effects of detraining on power athletes. *Medicine and Science in Sports and Exercise* 25:929-35.

Koutedakis, Y.; Boreham, C.; Kabitsis, C.; and Sharp, N.C.C. 1992. Seasonal deterioration of selected physiological variables in elite male skiers. *International Journal of Sports Medicine* 13:548-51.

Staron, R.S.; Leonardi, M.J.; Karapondo, D.L.; Malicky, E.S.; Falkel, J.E.; Hagerman, F.C.; and Hikida, R.S. 1991. Strength and skeletal muscle adaptations in heavy-resistance-trained women after detraining and retraining. *Journal of Applied Physiology* 70:631-40.

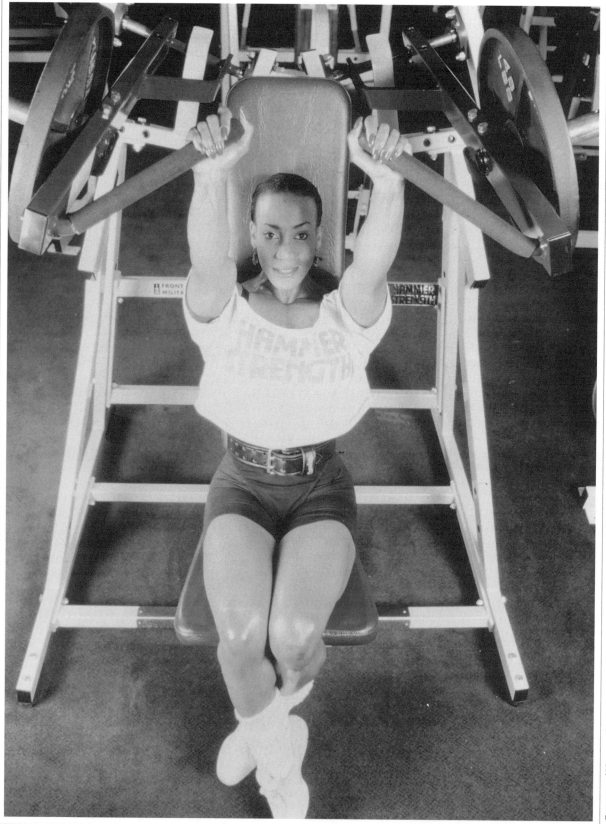

PART III

RESISTANCE TRAINING AND SPECIAL POPULATIONS

Young male athletes are no longer the only individuals who resistance train; women, children, and seniors are all discovering the benefits of resistance training. Chapter 9 discusses research on gender differences and examines special considerations for female athletes and for women in general who engage in resistance training. Chapter 10 explores resistance training for children, along with safety issues unique to younger resistance trainers. Chapter 11 discusses resistance training for seniors and the potential to enhance strength and power, which enhances quality of life. Finally, chapter 12 looks at the traditional resistance training sports—Olympic weight lifting, power lifting, and body building—and at how these sports have shaped concepts and understanding of resistance training.

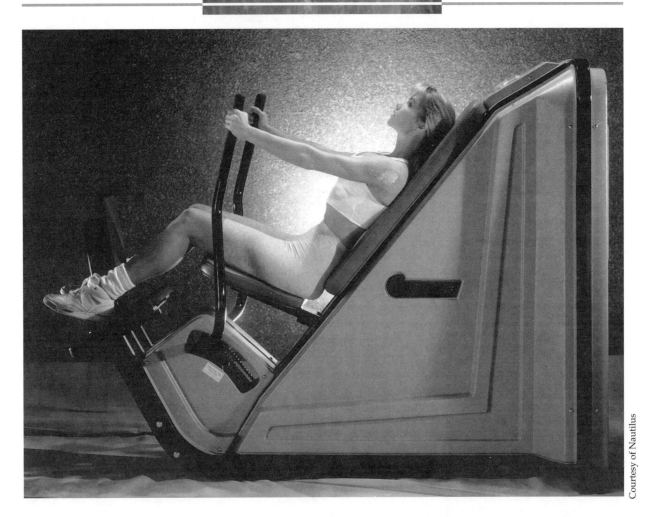

Courtesy of Nautilus

CHAPTER 9

Women and Resistance Training

More and more women are performing resistance training as part of their physical conditioning programs. An increasing number of female athletes also are using resistance training to improve performance in a sport. This is evident by the great number of resistance training facilities available to women, the number of female high school and college athletes performing resistance training, and the increasing popularity of female body-building, power-lifting, and Olympic-style weight-lifting contests. This chapter examines areas of interest concerning women and resistance training and common misconceptions about women and resistance training.

183

GENDER DIFFERENCES IN ABSOLUTE STRENGTH

The average woman's maximal mean total body strength is 63.5% of the average man's; women's isometric upper-body strength averages 55.8% of men's; women's isometric lower-body strength averages 71.9% of men's (Laubach 1976). The large variation in strength between the genders is a result of the large number of different single-joint (e.g., elbow extension, shoulder flexion, hip extension) and multiple-joint (e.g., squat, bench press, shoulder press) movements possible with both the upper and lower body and differences in muscle mass distribution in various parts of the body. Other comparisons (table 9.1) also indicate that large variations in a woman's strength as compared to a man's occur in 1-RM, isometric, concentric isokinetic, and eccentric isokinetic strength of various movements or exercises. The large variation shown in table 9.1 is caused in part by different types of maximal strength tests. As an example, women's 1-RM knee-extension strength on a machine is only 50% that of men; however, women's concentric peak torque at 90°/s is 78% that of men. Table 9.1 and isometric data (Cureton et al. 1988; Hudson 1978) indicate that absolute (body weight not considered) lower-body strength of women is closer in general to that of men than is absolute upper-body strength.

This gender difference in 1-RM strength exists even when competitive power lifters' world records are compared for the same approximate weight class (Kraemer and Koziris 1994). For example, the 1991 world records in the collegiate 53-kg body-weight class of the Drug-Free Power Lifting Association for women were 142.8 kg for squat; 72.6 kg for bench press; 156.8 kg for deadlift; for men in the 52-kg body-weight class corresponding records were 183 kg for squat; 115.9 kg for bench press; 192.8 kg for deadlift.

GENDER DIFFERENCES IN RELATIVE STRENGTH

Body size may partly explain differences in strength between the genders. Wilmore (1974) reported that women's 1-RM bench press is 37% that of men. If the bench press is expressed relative to body weight or lean body mass, women are 46% and 55%, respectively, as strong as men. Women's maximal isometric force in a leg press movement is 73% that of men. But if leg press strength is expressed relative to body weight and lean body mass, women are 92% and 106% as strong as men.

These data indicate that women's upper-body strength is less than that of men both absolutely and relative to total body weight or lean body mass. However, when leg strength is expressed relative to body weight, strength differences between the

TABLE 9.1
Absolute Strength Differences by Gender

Reference	Movement or exercise	Type of test	Female (% of male)
Cureton et al. 1988	Elbow extension	1 RM with free weights	42
Cureton et al. 1988	Elbow flexion	1 RM with machine	53
Cureton et al. 1988	Knee flexion	1 RM with machine	54
Cureton et al. 1988	Knee extension	1 RM with machine	50
Wilmore 1974	Leg press	Maximal isometric	73
Wilmore 1974	Elbow flexion	1 RM with machine	52
Wilmore 1974	Bench press	1 RM with machine	37
Wilmore 1974	Grip	Maximal isometric	57
Maughton et al. 1986	Knee extension	Maximal isometric	68
Maughton et al. 1986	Elbow flexion	1 RM with machine	46

Reference	Movement or exercise	Type of test	Female (% of male)
Ryushi et al. 1988	Knee extension	1 RM with machine	58
Ryushi et al. 1988	Knee extension	Maximal isometric	73
Miller et al. 1992	Elbow flexion	1 RM with machine	69
Miller et al. 1992	Knee extension	1 RM with machine	62
Miller et al. 1992	Knee extension	Maximal isometric	52
Davies, Greenwood, and Jones 1988	Grip	Maximal isometric	60
Clarke 1986	Grip	Maximal isometric	62
Colliander and Tesch 1989	Knee extension	Concentric isokinetic peak torque:	
		60°/s	64
		90°/s	62
		150°/s	60
Colliander and Tesch 1989	Knee flexion	Eccentric isokinetic peak torque:	
		60°/s	64
		90°/s	62
		150°/s	62
Colliander and Tesch 1989	Knee extension	Eccentric isokinetic peak torque:	
		60°/s	69
		90°/s	78
		150°/s	76
Borges and Essen-Gustavsson 1989	Knee extension	Concentric isokinetic peak torque:	
		12°/s	78
		90°/s	78
		150°/s	72
Borges and Essen-Gustavsson 1989	Knee extension	Maximal isometric	70
Hayward et al. 1986	Shoulder flexion	Concentric isokinetic peak torque:	
		60°/s	64
Hayward et al. 1986	Knee extension	Concentric isokinetic peak torque:	
		60°/s	68
Falkel et al. 1985	Elbow flexion	Concentric isokinetic peak torque:	
		30°/s	56
Falkel et al. 1985	Elbow extension	Concentric isokinetic peak torque:	
		30°/s	63
Falkel et al. 1985	Knee extension	Concentric isokinetic peak torque:	
		30°/s	68
Falkel et al. 1985	Knee flexion	Concentric isokinetic peak torque:	
		30°/s	66

genders are greatly reduced. When leg strength is expressed relative to lean body mass, women may actually be stronger than men.

Other data support the concept that lower-body but not upper-body strength is equal in men and women when expressed relative to body weight or lean body mass. Women's absolute isokinetic bench press and leg press strength is 50% and 74% that of men, respectively (T. Hoffman, Stauffer, and Jackson 1979). When adjusted for height and lean body mass, women's bench press strength is 74% that of men, but women's leg press strength is 104% that of men.

It has also been reported that women's concentric isokinetic peak torque at 30°/s for elbow extension, knee extension, and knee flexion but not for elbow flexion is equal to men's when expressed relative to lean body mass (Falkel et al. 1985). This study matched the genders for absolute (not relative to body weight) aerobic fitness (maximal oxygen consumption). Thus, the women tested were quite aerobically fit compared to other women, but the men tested were of only average aerobic fitness compared to other men. This might explain the parity in three out of four strength measures in this study.

Concentric isokinetic peak torque at 60°/s for shoulder flexion and knee extension was also reported to be not significantly different between the genders when expressed relative to lean body mass (Hayward et al. 1986). However, the absolute concentric isokinetic peak torques of female basketball and volleyball players during the bench press and leg press were 71% and 50% of the average male's and relative to lean body mass were 75% and 56% of the average male's (Morrow and Hosler 1981), which indicates that female athletes' upper- and lower-body strength relative to lean body mass both were less than the average male.

Eccentric isokinetic peak torque relative to lean body mass may be more similar between the genders than concentric isokinetic peak torque (Colliander and Tesch 1989). Women's concentric isokinetic peak torque relative to lean body mass of the quadriceps and hamstrings at 60°/s, 90°/s, and 150°/s averaged 81% of men's (table 9.2). But women's eccentric isokinetic peak torque relative to lean body mass at these same velocities averages 93% of men's. These data indicate that women's lower-body eccentric strength relative to lean body mass is almost equal to men's, whereas concentric strength is not. This may be because women are able to use stored elastic energy to a greater extent than men and because women are

TABLE 9.2
Women's and Men's Quadriceps and Hamstrings Eccentric and Concentric Isokinetic Peak Torque

	Percentage of women's strength to men's, relative to body mass	
	Eccentric	Concentric
Quadriceps		
60°/s	90	83
90°/s	102	81
150°/s	99	77
Hamstrings		
60°/s	84	84
90°/s	90	80
150°/s	92	81

Note. Adapted, by permission, from E.B. Colliander and P.A. Tesch, 1989, "Bilateral eccentric and concentric torque of quadriceps and hamstring muscles in females and males," *European Journal of Applied Physiology* 59:230.

not able to recruit as many of their motor units during concentric muscle actions as during eccentric actions. Whatever the reason, women may be better at performing eccentric than concentric muscle actions.

Women's 1-RM knee extension and elbow flexion have been reported to be 80% and 70% of men's when expressed relative to lean body mass (Miller et al. 1992). However, when expressed relative to the muscle's cross-sectional area, no significant difference exists between the genders' knee extension or elbow flexion (Miller et al. 1992). Women's 1-RM and maximal-isometric-force for knee extension have also been reported to be 74% and 92% of men's when expressed relative to muscle cross-sectional area (Ryushi et al. 1988). The 1 RM, but not the maximal isometric force, was significantly different between the genders.

In summary, the majority of evidence indicates that the average woman's absolute upper- and lower-body strength is not as great as the average man's. However, a large range exists when comparing absolute strength (figure 9.1; table 9.1). This large range is in part caused by the large number of movements possible with both the upper and lower body and by different testing methods (e.g., isokinetic, isometric). When strength is expressed relative to lean body mass or muscle cross-sectional area, the difference in strength between the genders in many, but not all, instances disappears. Ec-

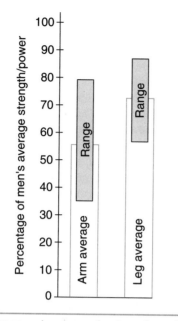

Fig. 9.1 Range and average of various dynamic strength measurements of the average woman compared with those of the average man.

Adapted, by permission, from L.L. Lauback, 1976, "Comparative muscular strength of men and women: A review of the literature," *Aviation, Space and Environmental Medicine* 47:534-42.

centric strength relative to lean body mass may be more similar between the genders than concentric strength. Lower-body strength more often than upper-body strength is approximately equal between the genders when expressed relative to lean body mass or muscle cross-sectional area.

GENDER DIFFERENCES IN POWER OUTPUT

Power output in many sports or activities is a major determinant of success. One such event is the snatch lift. Comparisons of international-caliber Olympic weight lifters indicate that for the complete pull phase of the lift women's power output relative to total body weight is 65% of men's (Garhammer 1989). Maximal vertical jump and standing long jump ability are also in large part determined by power output. The average woman has been reported to have 54% to 73% of the maximal vertical jump and 75% of the maximal standing long jump of the average male (Colliander and Tesch 1990b; B.N. Davies, Greenwood, and Jones 1988; Maud and Shultz 1986; Mayhew and Salm 1990). For the standing long jump this translates to the average woman generating approximately 63% of the power generated

by the average man (B.N. Davies, Greenwood, and Jones 1988).

This gender difference in power exists even when competitive weight lifter's world records are compared for the same approximate weight class (Kraemer and Koziris 1994). For example, in the open age category in Olympic weight lifting for the 52-kg (115-lb) body-weight class, the 1992 world records for women were 108 kg (238 lb) in the clean and jerk and 72.5 kg (160 lb) in the snatch, while for men the records were 155.5 kg (343 lb) in the clean and jerk and 120.5 kg (266 lb) in the snatch.

When vertical jump ability is expressed relative to lean body mass, only small (0% to 5.5%) differences between the genders are apparent (Maud and Shultz 1986; Mayhew and Salm 1990). This indicates that differences in lean body mass may account for the differences in vertical jump ability between the genders. However, power generated by women during the standing long jump per unit of lean leg volume is significantly less than that generated by men (B.N. Davies, Greenwood, and Jones 1988). Cycling short-sprint ability (30-s Wingate test) is not significantly different (2.5%) between the genders if expressed relative to lean body mass (Maud and Shultz 1986). If lean body mass is accounted for, women's running, short sprints, and maximal stair-climbing ability (Margaria-Kalamen test) are 77% and 84% to 87%, respectively of men's (Maud and Shultz 1986; Mayhew and Salm 1990). Accounting for differences in lean body mass between the genders does not appear to explain lower power outputs and differences in performance in all power-type tests.

Although the data are not consistent, they do raise the question of why women may generate less power per unit volume of muscle. One possible reason is differences in muscle fiber type; however, there is no consistent evidence that muscle fiber type varies by gender within a particular muscle. It is also not certain how variations in muscle fiber type may affect performance. Power at faster velocities of movement would be affected if women's force-velocity curve were different from men's. However, it appears that the drop-off in force as the velocity of movement increases is similar in both genders (Alway, Stray-Gundersen, Grumbt, and Gonyea 1990) and that peak velocity during knee extension is not different between the genders (Houston, Norman, and Froese 1988).

The rate of force development could affect power output. It appears that the skeletal muscle's rate of force development is slower for the average woman than for the average man (Komi and Karlsson 1978;

Ryushi et al. 1988). Thus, women's smaller skeletal muscle power output as compared with men's may in part be caused by a slower rate of force development.

TRAINING EFFECTS

Does resistance training produce the same training effects in women as it does in men? Some people believe that women's adaptations to resistance training are less than men's and therefore that women benefit less from resistance training than men (Wells 1978). Research to date, however, indicates that resistance training is at least as beneficial, if not more so, for women as for men.

Women's $\dot{V}O_2$ peak increases 8% on the average as a result of 8- to 20-wk circuit weight training programs, while men's increases an average of 5% over the same time period (Gettman and Pollock 1981). The average woman's endurance capabilities therefore increase more than those of the average man because of circuit weight training. The greater gains in $\dot{V}O_2$ peak by women may be partly accounted for by men's higher cardiovascular fitness levels prior to the onset of the circuit weight training programs.

Body compositional changes are a goal of some resistance training programs for women as well as for men. Increases in lean body mass and decreases in percent body fat from short-term (8- to 20-wk) resistance training programs are of the same magnitude in women as they are in men (table 7.6). Muscle fiber hypertrophy of Type I (slow-twitch) and the two major Type II (Types IIA and IIB) fibers can occur in women who perform resistance training (Staron et al. 1989, 1991). In addition, the transition of the myosin heavy chains from Type IIB to Type IIAB to Type IIA (quality of protein) starts to take place within a couple of workouts in women, which is faster than observed in men (Staron et al. 1994). Increased muscle cross-sectional area determined by computerized tomography from isometric (B.N. Davies, Greenwood, and Jones 1988) and from DCER training (Cureton et al. 1988) are of the same magnitude in both genders. Thus, it appears that body composition and fiber type changes from resistance training occur equally in both genders or possibly faster in women.

When performing the identical resistance training program, women gain strength at the same rate or faster than men (Cureton et al. 1988; Wilmore 1974; Wilmore et al. 1978). Over the course of a 10-wk (figure 9.2) and a 16-wk (figure 9.3) resistance training program, women gained strength at a rate equal to or greater than men. Greater absolute increases may be demonstrated by men, but relative increases (% increases) can be the same or greater in women than in men.

Some initial evidence indicates that women's strength gains may plateau after 3 to 5 mo of training and may not progress as well as men's after

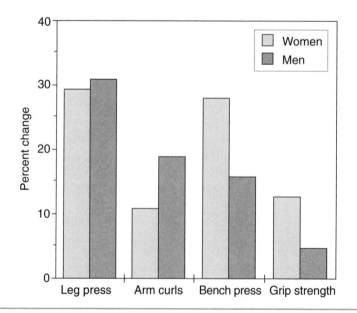

Fig. 9.2 Male and female strength changes from a 10-wk resistance training program.

Data from J.H. Wilmore, 1974, "Alterations in strength, body composition, and anthropometric measurements consequent to a 10-week weight training program," *Medicine and Science in Sports* 6:133-38.

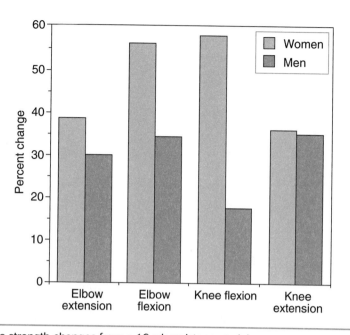

Fig. 9.3   Male and female strength changes from a 16-wk resistance training program.
Data from K.J. Cureton, M.A. Collins, D.W. Hill, and F.M. McElhannon, 1988, "Muscle hypertrophy in men and women," *Medicine and Science in Sports and Exercise* 20:338-44.

this time (Häkkinen et al. 1989; Häkkinen 1993a). This difference might be more pronounced in the upper body, where women's absolute muscle mass is less than men's. Hormonal output from training is different in women and men (Kraemer, Gordon, et al. 1991). The women's plateau in strength gains may represent a shift in physiological strategies (neural or hypertrophic) that the body uses to adapt to result in strength gains. Alternatively, it could represent a type of staleness because periodized training has not been employed in studies on women to date (Kraemer unpublished data).

MISCONCEPTIONS ABOUT WOMEN AND RESISTANCE TRAINING

A common misconception is that women's resistance training programs need to be different than men's. As previously discussed, comparisons of men and women who used identical resistance training programs demonstrate that women make the same, if not greater, gains in strength as men. This indicates that programs for women do not have to be different from those for men. The muscle groups that need to be strong or powerful to be successful in a particular sport or activity are the same for both genders. The goal of a resistance training program is to increase strength or power

of the muscles needed for success in an activity, regardless of the athlete's gender.

In general, the upper body shows the greatest difference in strength between the genders, as previously discussed. It has been proposed that this is because women tend to have a lower proportion of their lean body mass in their upper bodies (Miller et al. 1992). Thus, emphasizing development of women's upper-body lean body mass may be warranted in sports in which upper-body strength is a limiting factor of performance. This does not mean that a program to develop lean body mass in the upper body will be different for men and for women, but that women may benefit from having such a program constitute a greater portion of their total training volume.

Muscle of both genders has the same physiological characteristics and therefore responds to training in the same manner. Muscle's force output is directly related to the muscle's cross-sectional area (figure 9.4; Alway, Stray-Gundersen, Grumbt, and Gonyea 1990; Ikai and Fukunaga 1970; Miller et al. 1992). A significant amount of individual variation exists between cross-sectional area and force output. This appears to be true at all velocities of movement (Alway, Stray-Gundersen, Grumbt, and Gonyea 1990). However, there is some indication that maximal isometric force per cross-sectional area (Ryushi et al. 1988), maximal isometric force per unit volume of muscle (B.N. Davies, Greenwood,

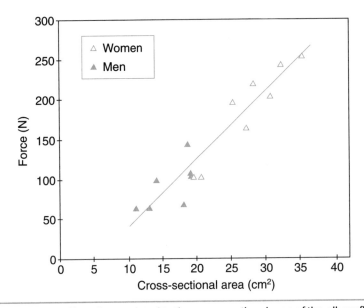

Fig. 9.4   Elbow flexor strength is significantly correlated to the cross-sectional area of the elbow flexors ($r = .95$) in a group composed of both genders.

Adapted, by permission, from A.E.J. Miller, J.D. MacDougall, M.A. Tarnopolsky, and D.G. Sale, 1992, "Gender differences in strength and muscle fiber characteristics," *European Journal of Applied Physiology* 66:254-62.

and Jones 1988), and 1-RM weight per cross-sectional area (Ryushi et al. 1988) are lower in women's muscles than in men's. Possible reasons for this potential difference in force output per cross-sectional area are the same as those previously discussed for possible differences in strength relative to lean body mass. Even if force output per cross-sectional area of muscle were different between the genders, it would have no impact on program design.

In general, both genders have the same percentage of Type I and II fibers in a particular muscle (Drinkwater 1984); however, fiber composition may vary from muscle to muscle. Although it has been reported that on average a man's vastus lateralis muscle has a greater percentage (62% vs. 50%) of Type II fibers than a woman's (Miller et al. 1992). In general, differences are apparent in fiber size between the genders; untrained women have smaller Type I and II fibers than untrained males (Drinkwater 1984; Miller et al. 1992; Ryushi et al. 1988). Cross-sectional areas of an untrained women's Type I and II fibers are 68% and 71%, respectively, of an untrained man's (Drinkwater 1984). These differences in fiber size appear also in strength athletes. Female strength athletes have 66% and 71% of the Type I and II fiber areas of their male counterparts (Drinkwater 1984).

Differences in fiber size are also apparent in the Type II subtypes: Women's Type IIA and IIB fibers are significantly smaller than males (Ryushi et al.

1988). It has been suggested that this difference in fiber size is not caused by a difference in physical activity but is an innate difference between the genders (Miller et al. 1992).

Muscle cross-sectional area is a product of the muscle fiber size and the number of muscle fibers. It is generally accepted that women have smaller muscle fiber areas than men. However, comparisons of the estimated number of fibers in a muscle are inconclusive. The number of muscle fibers in the average woman's biceps brachii has been reported to be less than (Sale et al. 1987) or the same as (Miller et al. 1992) the average man's. Female body builders have been reported to have the same number of muscle fibers in the biceps brachii as male body builders (Alway, Grumbt, Gonyea, and Stray-Gundersen 1989). Women's tibialis anterior has also been reported to have fewer muscle fibers than men's (Henriksson-Larsen 1985). Another study showed that women's triceps brachii and vastus lateralis have the same number of muscle fibers as men's (Schantz et al. 1983, 1981). Thus, no conclusive answer is available to the question of whether the number of muscle fibers within a muscle is different between the genders.

There is some evidence indicating that the concentration of certain aerobic and anaerobic enzymes in muscle may be different between the genders. It has been reported that the concentrations of one aerobic (citrate synthase) and one anaerobic (creatine phosphokinase) enzyme are greater in men's than in women's muscle, whereas other aerobic (3-OH-acyl CoA dehydrogenase) and anaerobic (lactate dehydrogenase, myokinase) enzyme concentrations are not different between the genders (Borges and Essen-Gustavsson 1989). The majority of evidence suggests that there is no difference in enzyme concentrations (Drinkwater 1984).

One difference between male and female muscle may be the amount of fat within the muscle. Female muscle has a greater amount of fat between the fascicles (bundles) than male muscle (Miller et al. 1992; Prince, Hikida, and Hagerman 1977). This does not affect the trainability of the muscle tissue, however.

Many people do not perform resistance training because they are afraid they will become muscle-bound (a reference to the lack of flexibility sometimes associated with improper resistance training technique or program design). This fear is unfounded because resistance training can increase flexibility in both genders. Women and men increased flexibility by 6% and 8%, respectively, in the sit-and-reach test (a common measure of lower-back and hamstring flexibility) during 10 wk of resistance training (Wilmore et al. 1978). Resistance training either has no effect or a positive effect on flexibility (see chapter 4). This appears to be true for both genders.

Men at rest normally have 10 times the testosterone concentrations of women (Wright 1980). This may account for the larger increases in muscle hypertrophy in men than in women. Other hormones, such as growth hormone and cortisol, however, could also have an effect on muscle growth and hypertrophy. In addition, low concentrations of a hormone do not necessarily mean that the hormone does not have an active role in controlling a body function or process such as growth.

Women's resting serum testosterone concentration remained unchanged during an 8-wk resistance training program (Hetrick and Wilmore 1979). Another study found no relationship between blood testosterone concentrations and strength in college-age women (Fahey et al. 1976). However, more recently it has been shown that during a 16-wk resistance training program, although women's resting serum testosterone concentrations did not change significantly, individual mean serum levels of both total and free testosterone correlated significantly with changes in muscle force production (Häkkinen et al. 1990). This indicates that small individual changes of testosterone concentrations due to training may affect the muscles' force capabilities in women.

Women's serum testosterone concentrations (figure 9.5) did not change significantly during one resistance training session (Kraemer, Gordon, et al.

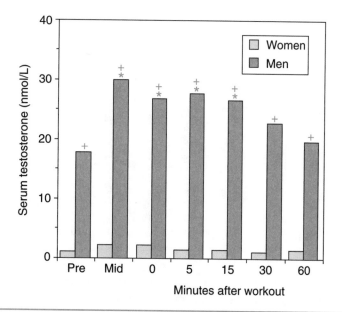

Fig. 9.5 Serum testosterone concentrations in men and women caused by performing the same resistance training session of three sets of eight exercises at 10 RM with 1-min rest between sets and exercises.

* = significantly different from preexercise value of same gender, + = significantly different from female value at the same time point.

Adapted, by permission, from W.J. Kraemer et al., 1991, "Endogenous anabolic hormonal and growth factor responses to heavy resistance exercise in males and females," *International Journal of Sports Medicine* 12:231.

1991; Kraemer et al. 1993), whereas men's serum testosterone concentrations did increase significantly from performance of the same resistance training session (Kraemer, Gordon, et al. 1991; Kraemer et al. 1990). However, both women's and men's serum growth hormone increased significantly (figure 9.6) from the same resistance training session (Kraemer, Gordon, et al. 1991). Hormones other than testosterone (e.g., growth hormone) play a role in adaptations to resistance training. This may be especially true for women.

Some women do not perform heavy resistance training because they believe that their muscles will hypertrophy and that they subsequently may look less feminine. The average woman's muscles do not, however, hypertrophy excessively. This is good news for a woman who does not want an increase in muscle size, but bad news for a woman who wants increased muscle size, like a woman body builder. The greatest increase in various body circumferences in women from 10 wk (Wilmore 1974), 12 wk (Boyer 1990), or 20 wk (Staron et al. 1991) of training was 0.6, 0.4, and 0.6 cm, respectively. Such increases in circumference are virtually unnoticeable. With a 10-wk program hip, thigh, and abdomen circumferences actually decreased 0.2 to 0.7 cm. During three different 12-wk programs abdomen circumference decreased 0.2 to 1.1 cm (Boyer

1990). The finding that resistance training in women results in no change or small changes in body circumferences is supported by other studies (Capen, Bright, and Line 1961; Häkkinen et al. 1989; Wells, Jokl, and Bohanen 1973). Body circumferences do not change as a result of the combination of small increases in muscle mass (see table 7.6) and decreases in adipose tissue in the limb or body part (Mayhew and Gross 1974). Muscle tissue is denser than adipose tissue, so an increase in muscle mass accompanied by a decrease in adipose tissue will result in no change or a slight decrease in body circumferences. The 10-, 12-, and 16-wk training studies discussed earlier all demonstrated decreases in skinfold thicknesses. The lack of increases or even small decreases in body circumferences is good news for women who want increased strength or the firm look of trained muscle without increased body circumferences.

Some women do develop a large amount of hypertrophy from resistance training. After a 6-mo resistance training program a group of female athletes exhibited an increase of 37% in upper-body strength and increases of 3.5, 1.1, and 0.9 cm (5%, 4%, and 2%) in shoulder girth, upper-arm circumference, and thigh circumference, respectively (Brown and Wilmore 1974). Larger increases in lean body mass and limb circumferences than normal

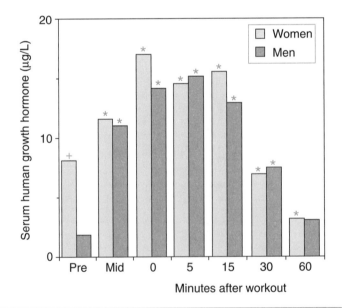

Fig. 9.6   Serum growth hormone concentrations in men and women caused by performing the same resistance training session of three sets of eight exercises at a 10 RM with 1-min rest between sets and exercises.

* = significantly different from preexercise value of same gender, + = significantly different from female value at the same time point.

Adapted, by permission, from W.J. Kraemer et al., 1991, "Endogenous anabolic hormonal and growth factor responses to heavy resistance exercise in males and females," *International Journal of Sports Medicine* 12:232.

in some women are probably caused by several factors, including

- higher than normal resting testosterone, growth hormone, or other hormone levels;
- greater hormonal response than normal to the performance of resistance training;
- lower than normal estrogen-to-testosterone ratio;
- genetic disposition to develop a large muscle mass; and
- ability to perform more intense resistance training program.

In general, however, the beliefs that women will become excessively hypertrophied, that resistance training programs for women must be different from those for men, and that resistance training will result in a decrease in flexibility are unfounded.

ENDOCRINE SYSTEM ADAPTATIONS TO PHYSICAL TRAINING

Some women engaged in physical training, including resistance training, experience variations in their menstrual cycles. Common irregularities experienced by women performing physical training include shortening of the luteal (postovulatory) phase to less than 10 d; lack of ovulation (release of an egg); oligomenorrhea, an irregular menstrual cycle in women who previously had a normal menstrual pattern or a cycle with more than 36 d between menstrual flows; secondary amenorrhea, the absence of menstruation for 180 d or more in women who previously menstruated regularly; and dysmenorrhea, pain during menstruation. Research concerning the frequency of these irregularities in women who perform resistance training is limited. The physiological mechanisms responsible for development of menstrual irregularities are presently not fully defined. Differences in menstrual cycle patterns among women can be considerable; it can therefore be difficult to determine what is a regular, as opposed to an irregular, menstrual cycle for a particular woman. The majority of menstrual irregularities return to normal with a reduction or cessation of training, so there is no long-term negative effect from physical training on women's reproductive systems.

Oligomenorrhea and Secondary Amenorrhea

Oligomenorrhea and secondary amenorrhea have been reported to be more common in women engaged in vigorous physical activity (DeSouza and Metzger 1991; Gray and Dale 1984; Loucks and Horvath 1985; Prior, Vigna, and McKay 1992). Out of 199 Olympic-style weight lifters of an average age of 16 yr, 25% reported having irregular menses; only three of these athletes aged 13 to 15 had not yet begun to menstruate (Liu, Liu, and Qin 1987). The prevalence of oligomenorrhea and secondary amenorrhea in women not taking oral contraceptives was 20% and 2%, respectively, in a group of recreational resistance trainers; 71% and 14%, respectively, in a group of women who had competed in at least one body-building contest; and 9% and 4% in a group of sedentary women (Walberg and Johnston 1991). Thirty-three percent of women who competed in a body-building contest and did not take oral contraceptives reported oligomenorrhea or secondary amenorrhea (Elliot and Goldberg 1983). The limited data indicate that women who perform resistance training may be at greater risk than normal of acquiring menstrual cycle irregularities.

In distance runners, greater training distance, intensity, frequency, and duration of training season have all been implicated as factors that increase the risk of menstrual irregularities (Cameron, Wark, and Telford 1992; Gray and Dale 1984; Loucks and Horvath 1985). Athletes who train for long periods of time (daily or over years) at high intensities are therefore at greater risk of experiencing oligomenorrhea or secondary amenorrhea. In women who do not use oral contraceptives the incidence of either oligomenorrhea or amenorrhea in recreational resistance trainers is 22%, whereas it is 85% in competitive body builders (Walberg and Johnston 1991). Thus, it also appears to be true for resistance training that greater training intensity or volume results in greater risk of menstrual irregularities. However, not all athletes performing high-volume, high-intensity training will experience menstrual irregularities.

Aspects of reproductive history and maturity have also been associated with menstrual irregularities. The incidence of amenorrhea is higher in younger than in older women. One study reported that 85% of runners experiencing secondary amenorrhea were under 30 yr of age (Speroff and Redwine 1980). It has been proposed that physical training at an early age delays menarche and that late menarche is associated with a greater chance of experiencing amenorrhea (Gray and Dale 1984; Loucks and Horvath 1985). A previous pregnancy has been associated with a decreased risk of amenorrhea (Loucks and Horvath 1985). The mechanisms by which any of these factors affect menstrual cycle irregularities have not, however, been fully elucidated.

Psychological stress, which can be a part of training and competing, has also been associated with amenorrhea (Loucks and Horvath 1985). Psychological stress may cause changes in various neurotransmitters that regulate the reproductive system, though the exact mechanisms have not been fully determined.

Bone Density

Physical activity in women can result in increased bone density (Dalsky et al. 1988; De Cree, Vermeulen, and Ostyn 1991; Jacobson et al. 1984). Menstrual dysfunction, however, may result in decreases in bone density and increased risk of osteoporosis (Cameron, Wark, and Telford 1992; De Cree, Vermeulen, and Ostyn 1991; Nyburgh et al. 1993). Age at menarche and duration of menstrual dysfunction have both been correlated with reduced lumbar vertebrae bone density compared to normal values (Cameron, Wark, and Telford 1992). In addition, athletes who were amenorrheic and who then regained menses for 15 mo showed an increase in bone density, whereas athletes who did not regain menses showed no change or a continued loss of bone density (Cameron, Wark, and Telford 1992). Young amenorrheic women may therefore be losing bone mass at a point in their lives when bone mass should be increasing. However, amenorrheic athletes do have greater bone densities than amenorrheic nonathletes (Cameron, Wark, and Telford 1992). It appears that amenorrhea may be associated with a decrease in bone density and mass but that physical activity may partially slow the loss of bone mass caused by amenorrhea. Highly trained women, however, appear to have a greater than normal risk for menstrual problems (as previously discussed) and therefore may also be at risk for osteoporosis.

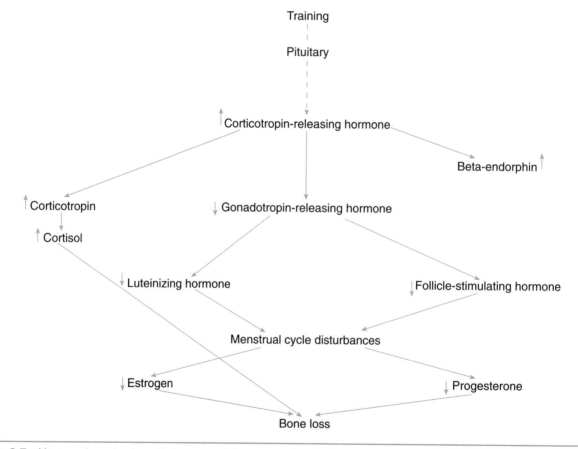

Fig. 9.7   Hormonal mechanisms that may result in menstrual cycle disturbances and bone loss.

The loss of bone mass may occur predominantly during the first 3 to 4 yr of amenorrhea (Cann et al. 1984). Decreased bone density and bone mass can occur both in the lumbar spine, composed predominately of trabecular bone (Cameron, Wark, and Telford 1992; Prior, Vigna, and McKay 1992), and in the axial skeleton, composed primarily of cortical bone (Nyburgh et al. 1993). It therefore appears that the entire skeletal system of amenorrheic women, including amenorrheic athletes, may experience a decrease in bone density.

Hormonal Mechanisms

The hormonal mechanisms that control menstrual cycle irregularities and bone loss are not completely defined. Presently it is believed that stressors—such as physical stress from training, mental stress, and dietary deficiencies—that may result in menstrual cycle disturbances act through a common pathway (Prior, Vigna, and McKay 1992). The stressors cause an increase in corticotropin-releasing hormone from the hypothalamus (figure 9.7), causing a decrease in gonadotropin-releasing hormone, which in turn results in a decrease in the pituitary hormones, luteinizing hormone, and follicle-stimulating hormone. The decrease in the pituitary hormones results in menstrual cycle disturbances. Menstrual cycle disturbances result in decreases in the ovarian hormones progesterone and estrogen, which in turn result in decreased bone density.

Decreased concentrations of the ovarian hormones estrogen and progesterone are the hormonal factors most frequently associated with osteoporosis and bone loss. It has been suggested that estrogen may reduce bone reabsorption (bone loss) but that it has little impact on bone formation, resulting in a net loss of bone (Cameron, Wark, and Telford 1992; De Cree, Vermeulen, and Ostyn 1991). However, no estrogen receptors have been found in bone (Nutik and Cruess 1974), leaving in doubt whether estrogen has a direct effect on bone loss. It is possible that estrogen has an indirect effect on bone by acting through another hormone (De Cree, Vermeulen, and Ostyn 1991). Progesterone does promote bone formation, especially cortical bone, and therefore a decrease in progesterone may result in a net decrease in bone mass.

Because of the complicated interactions of hormones with each other, many hormones may act to increase the bone loss related to physical training and menstrual cycle disturbances. Corticotropin-releasing hormone also stimulates corticotropin release from the anterior pituitary, which

stimulates cortisol release from the adrenal cortex and may result in bone loss and be related to menstrual cycle disturbances (Prior, Vigna, and McKay 1992; DeSouza and Metzger 1991). Increased beta-endorphin may also be associated with menstrual cycle disturbances (Cameron, Wark, and Telford 1992; Prior, Vigna, and McKay 1992; De Cree, Vermeulen, and Ostyn 1991). Increases in beta-endorphin have been shown to occur in women in response to resistance training, especially when accompanied by a negative caloric balance, and this could be responsible in part for menstrual cycle disturbances in women performing resistance training (Walberg-Rankin, Franke, and Gwazdauskas 1992). Many other hormones, such as growth hormone, testosterone, estradiol, insulin, and calcitonin, are also probably involved with menstrual cycle disturbances and bone loss in active women (Cameron, Wark, and Telford 1992; Prior, Vigna, and McKay 1992).

Dysmenorrhea and Premenstrual Symptoms

One of the first adaptations to an exercise program is a decrease in normal premenstrual symptoms (Prior, Vigna, and McKay 1992), such as breast enlargement, appetite cravings, bloating, and mood changes. Active, athletic women have fewer problems with premenstrual symptoms than sedentary women (Prior, Vigna, and McKay 1992). If training is decreased, however, premenstrual symptoms may increase, especially if weight gain is concurrent with the decrease in training (Prior, Vigna, and McKay 1992). When training is decreased for athletes who have excessive premenstrual symptoms, it should not be decreased abruptly and an attempt should be made to avoid large weight gains.

Dysmenorrhea, or abdominal pain with menstruation, may increase with an increase in premenstrual symptoms (Prior, Vigna, and McKay 1992). Dysmenorrhea is reported by 60% to 70% of adult women, and it increases with chronological and gynecological age (Brooks-Gunn and Rubb 1983; Widholm 1979). Like premenstrual symptoms, dysmenorrhea occurs less frequently and is less severe in athletes than in the general population (Dale, Gerlach, and Wilhite 1979; Timonen and Procope 1971).

Increased production of the hormone prostaglandin is associated with uterine cramping and is thought to be the cause of dysmenorrhea (Dawood 1983). The reduced frequency and severity of premenstrual and dysmenorrheic symptoms in athletes could be caused by differences in hormonal concentrations or a higher pain threshold in athletes. In either case it appears that physical training decreases the incidence of premenstrual symptoms and dysmenorrhea. Treatment strategies for athletes with premenstrual symptoms and dysmenorrhea are reviewed by Prior, Vigna, and McKay (1992).

Performance and Menstrual Problems

Isokinetic strength is not different at three points in the menstrual cycle in normally menstruating women (Dibrizzo, Fort, and Brown 1988); other reports, however, indicate that the best physical performance probably occurs between the immediate postmenstrual period and the 15th day of the menstrual cycle (Allsen, Parsons, and Bryce 1977; Doolittle and Engebretsen 1972). Premenstrual symptoms or dysmenorrhea could have a detrimental effect on athletic performance, and some researchers recommend using oral contraceptives or progesterone injections to control the occurrence of menses and avoiding competition while menstruating (Liu, Liu, and Qin 1987). However, Olympic medal-winning performances have taken place during all portions of the menstrual cycle. The effect of the menstrual cycle on performance is therefore unclear and is probably very specific to the individual. Oligomenorrhea or secondary amenorrhea should have no effect on performance. Participation in physical training and athletic events during menstruation should not be discouraged and has no detrimental effect on health.

GENERAL NEEDS ANALYSIS

The needs analysis for a woman in a particular sport or for general strength is conducted using the outline presented in chapter 5. What it takes to be successful in a particular sport is dictated by the sport and not by the gender of the participant. A training program for a particular sport is based on the requirements for successful participation in that sport and the athlete's individual weaknesses, training history, and injury history. The process of designing a resistance training program for a sport or activity is essentially the same for either gender. Because of the absolute strength differences between the genders, the major difference between programs for men and for women is the amount of resistance used for particular exercises.

For sports or activities that require upper-body strength and power, the needs analysis must take into account women's absolutely and relatively weaker upper-body musculature compared with men's. Women's generally smaller upper-body muscle mass may limit their performance in sports requiring upper-body strength or power. The training program for such sports or activities therefore should stress upper-body exercises to try to increase total upper-body strength and power. This can be accomplished by adding one or two upper-body exercises and/or one or two extra sets.

Most women's weaker upper-body musculature also causes problems in the performance of structural exercises such as power cleans and squats. In this type of exercise women may find it very difficult or impossible for their upper bodies to support the resistances their lower bodies can tolerate. Incorrect form for these exercises to allow the individual to lift greater resistances should not be tolerated. Sacrificing form can cause injury to the lifter. Instead, the program should stress assistance exercises to strengthen the upper-body musculature.

SUMMARY

Although women's absolute strength is less than men's, the difference is greatly reduced if compared on a total body weight or lean body mass basis. This is especiaaly true for the lower body where no strength difference on a lean body mass basis between the genders has been shown. Women's adaptations to a resistance training program are of the same magnitude or even slightly greater than men's for some variables. This means that, in general, resistance training programs for women do not need to be different than those for men, except that the absolute resistance used will be less. Menstrual irregularities may be more prevalent in women performing strenuous resistance activity, as compared to the normal population. However, menstrual irregularities normally cease once strenuous resistance training is stopped. Resistance training can result in many of the fitness characteristics desired by many women of a fit appearance and increased strength and power for daily and sport activities.

SELECTED READINGS

Colliander, E.B., and Tesch, P.A. 1990. Responses to eccentric and concentric resistance training in females and males. *Acta Physiologica Scandinavica* 141:49-156.

De Cree, C.; Vermeulen, A.; and Ostyn, M. 1991. Are high-performance young women athletes doomed to become low-performance old wives? A reconsideration of the increased risk of osteoporosis in amenorrheic women. *Journal of Sports Medicine and Physical Fitness* 31:108-14.

Drinkwater, B.L. 1984. Women and exercise: Physiological aspects. In *Exercise and sport science reviews*, ed. R.L. Terjung, 21-52. Lexington, KY: MAL Callamore Press.

Häkkinen, K.; Pakarinen, A.; Komi, P.V.; Ryushi, T.; and Kauhanen, H. 1989. Neuromuscular adaptations and hormone balance in strength athletes, physically active males and females during intensive strength training. In *Proceedings of the XII International Congress of Biomechanics*, no. 8, eds. R.J. Gregor, R.F. Zernicke, and W.C. Whiting, 889-94. Champaign, IL: Human Kinetics.

Kraemer, W.J.; Fleck, S.J.; Dziados, J.E.; Harman, E.A.; Marchitelli, L.J.; Gordon, S.E.; Mello, R.; Frykman, P.N.; Koziris, L.P.; and Triplett, N.T. 1993. Changes in hormonal concentrations following different heavy resistance exercise protocols in women. *Journal of Applied Physiology* 75:594-604.

Laubach, L.L. 1976. Comparative muscular strength of men and women: A review of the literature. *Aviation, Space and Environmental Medicine* 47:534-42.

Mayhew, J.L., and Salm, P.C. 1990. Gender differences in anaerobic power tests. *European Journal of Applied Physiology* 60:133-38.

Miller, A.E.J.; MacDougall, J.D.; Tarnopolsky, M.A.; and Sale, D.G. 1992. Gender differences in strength and muscle fiber characteristics. *European Journal of Applied Physiology* 66:254-62.

Nyburgh, K.H.; Bachrach, L.K.; Lewis, B.; Kent, K.; and Marcus, R. 1993. Low bone mineral density at axial and appendicular sites in amenorrheic athletes. *Medicine and Science in Sports and Exercise* 25:1197-1202.

Prior, J.C.; Vigna, Y.M.; and McKay, D.W. 1992. Reproduction for the athletic female: New understandings of physiology and management. *Sports Medicine* 14:190-99.

Staron, R.S.; Karapondo, D.L.; Kraemer, W.J.; Fry, A.C.; Gordon, S.E.; Falkel, J.E.; Hagerman, F.C.; and Hikida, R.S. 1994. Skeletal muscle adaptations during the early phase of heavy-resistance training in men and women. *Journal of Applied Physiology* 76:1247-55.

Walberg, J.L., and Johnston, C.S. 1991. Menstrual function and eating behavior in female recreational weight lifters and competitive body builders. *Medicine and Science in Sports and Exercise* 23:30-36.

Walberg-Rankin, J.; Franke, W.D.; and Gwazdauskas, F.C. 1992. Response of beta-endorphin and estradiol to resistance exercise in females during energy balance and energy restriction. *International Journal of Sports Medicine* 13:542-47.

CHAPTER 10

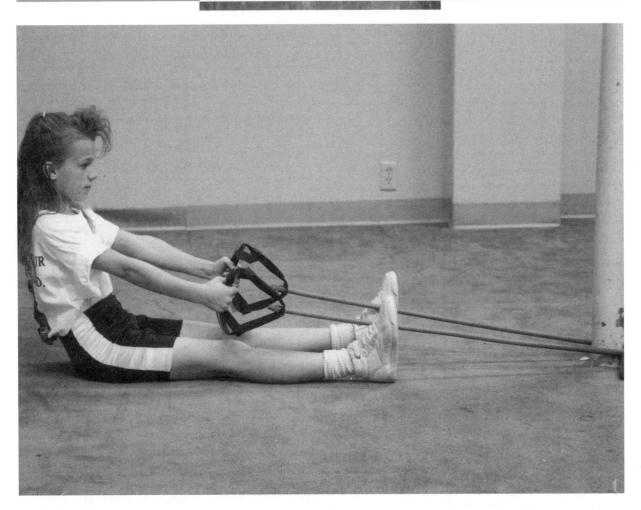

Children and Resistance Training

Over the past 10 years resistance training for children has gained acceptance and popularity among educational, medical, and scientific professionals, but it is a controversial subject. Can resistance training cause strength gains in children? Does resistance training actually harm children's skeletal systems? These two questions are at the heart of the controversy. A factor that complicates this issue is that children are constantly maturing. What is not appropriate for a prepubescent (for males, prior to growth spurt; for females, prior to first menstruation) may be appropriate for a pubescent. The answers to these questions and other serious concerns harbored by parents, teachers, coaches, and scientific and medical professionals are obscured by many misconceptions and misunderstandings about resistance training, its dangers, and how it can be adapted for young people (Hamil 1994; Kraemer and Fleck 1993).

The information in this chapter, especially that concerning skeletal injuries, stresses the difference between resistance training and the sports of weight lifting, power lifting, and body building. Resistance training involves the individualized prescription and performance of exercises in an attempt to make a child stronger and more powerful. Resistance training does not have to involve the use of maximal or near-maximal resistances. The risk of injuries from weight lifting in children may not be as dramatic as perceived (Hamil 1994). Nevertheless, in weight lifting or power lifting the object is to lift as much as possible for one repetition of a particular competitive exercise. Training for these sports consequently does require lifting maximal or near-maximal resistances. Most children would benefit from resistance training programs to help enhance physical fitness and sport performance or to reduce the probability of injury during sport and recreational activities. Paradoxically, many competitive sporting activities children participate in carry much greater risk of injury than resistance training. The benefits of a properly designed and supervised resistance training program appear to outweigh the risks (Hamil 1994).

The National Strength and Conditioning Association, the American Orthopaedic Society for Sports Medicine, and the American Academy of Pediatrics all suggest that children can benefit from participation in a properly prescribed and supervised resistance training program. The major benefits include:

- Increased muscular strength and local muscular endurance (i.e., the ability of a muscle or muscles to perform multiple repetitions against a given resistance)
- Decreased injuries in sports and recreational activities
- Improved performance capacity in sports and recreational activities

Although professionals have supported the use of resistance exercise programs for children, they have cautioned parents, teachers, and coaches about the need for proper program design, competent supervision, and correct teaching of exercise techniques. These areas are paramount for safe and effective resistance training programs for children. Some of the benefits (e.g., performance enhancement in preadolescence) (Blimkie 1993) need further study to verify anecdotal and clinical impressions. However, greater understanding has started to diminish the unrealistic fears about children and resistance training.

STRENGTH GAINS

Much research on the topic over the past several years has demonstrated equivocally that strength gains in children occur with resistance training when compared with children who do not perform resistance training (Faigenbaum 1993; Kraemer, Fry, et al. 1989; Blimkie 1989, 1993; Sale 1989). In the late 1970s opponents of resistance training for children argued that little if any gains in strength or muscle hypertrophy (beyond that caused by normal growth) could be achieved in prepubescents because of their immature hormonal systems (Legwold 1982). This argument appeared to be supported by the first studies, which were unable to demonstrate strength gains in children after a resistance training program (Vrijens 1978). The lack of strength changes found by various studies over the years may have been caused by poorly designed resistance training programs or poor experimental designs. Building on previous scientific studies, more recent investigations provide evidence showing that muscular strength improvements are indeed possible in children, including prepubescents (Blimkie 1989; Freedson, Ward, and Rippe 1990; Sale 1989; table 10.1).

The research clearly demonstrates that resistance training of prepubescent boys and girls can cause significant increases in strength (table 10.1). These studies indicate that strength gains in boys and girls occur from performing resistance training over a wide range of ages. In addition, many of the studies state that no injuries occurred from the resistance training programs.

Hormonal changes may have an effect on strength increases and muscle hypertrophy. Serum testosterone concentrations do not increase in prepubescent boys from exercise as they do in adult men. In fact, 14- to 17-yr-old male Olympic weight lifters with less than 2 yr of training experience did not show an increase in serum testosterone after a training session, while weight lifters with more than 2 yr of experience did show an increase in serum testosterone after a training session (Kraemer et al. 1992). Training experience therefore may have an impact on the hormonal response to training in young male athletes.

Serum testosterone concentrations in adult women are not typically affected by resistance training (Kraemer et al. 1993). Therefore, the line

TABLE 10.1
Strength Training Studies in Prepubescent Children

Reference	Age or grade	Gender	Training mode	Testing mode	Duration (wk)	Frequency (per wk)	Control group	Strength increase
Hetherington 1976	Grade 5	M	Isometric	Isometric	6-8	2-5	Yes	No
Vrijens 1978	10.4	M	Weights	Isometric	8	3	No	No
Nielson et al. 1980	7-19	F	Isometric	Isometric	5	3	Yes	Yes
Baumgartner and Wood 1984	Grades 3-6	M, F	Calisthenics	Calisthenics	12	3	Yes	Yes
Clarke et al. 1984	7-9	M	Wrestling	Isometric, Calisthenics	12	3	Yes	Yes
McGovern 1984[a]	Grades 4-6	M, F	Weights	Weights	12	3	Yes	Yes
Servidio et al. 1985[a]	11.9	M	Weights	Isokinetic	8	3	Yes	Yes
Pfeiffer and Francis 1986	8-11	M	Weights	Isokinetic	8	3	Yes	Yes
Sewall and Micheli 1986	10-11	M, F	Weights, Pneumatic	Isometric	9	3	Yes	Yes
Weltman et al. 1986	6-11	M	Hydraulic	Isokinetic	14	3	Yes	Yes
Funato et al. 1987	6-11	M, F	Isometric	Isometric, Isokinetic	12	3	Yes	Yes
Sailors and Berg 1987	12.6	M	Weights	Weights	8	3	Yes	Yes
Siegal et al. 1989	8.4	M, F	Weights, Calisthenics	Isometric, Calisthenics	12	3	Yes	Yes
Ramsay et al. 1990	9-11	M	Weights	Weights, Isokinetic, Isometric	20	3	Yes	Yes
Williams 1991[a]	10.5	M	Weights	Isometric, Calisthenics	8	3	Yes	Yes
Brown et al. 1992[a]	Tanner 1-2[b]	M, F	Weights	Weights	12	3	Yes	Yes
Westcott 1992	10.5	M, F	Weights	Weights	7	3	No	Yes
Fukunaga, Funato, and Ikegawa 1992	Grades 1, 3, 5	M, F	Isometric	Isometric, Isokinetic	12	3	Yes	Yes
Faigenbaum et al. 1993	10.8	M, F	Weights	Weights	8	2	Yes	Yes

[a] Abstract
[b] Refers to Tanner stages 1 and 2 of sexual maturation

Adapted, by permission, from Faigenbaum, A. *National Strength and Conditioning Association Journal* (1993) 15(5):20-29 (table 1) Strength Training: A Guide for Teachers and Coaches.

of reasoning that if resistance training does not result in increased testosterone concentrations, strength gains do not occur would indicate that women would not benefit from resistance training. Research shows this is not the case: Women *do* experience strength gains and muscle hypertrophy from resistance training. Figure 10.1 shows the changes in serum testosterone levels in prepubescent children after an exercise bout. Neural factors and other hormones are responsible for increased strength and hypertrophy in women (see chapter 9) and may also play a role in strength increases in prepubescent boys and girls.

The need for continuous training may be an important factor when prepubescents participate in resistance training. It is interesting to note that growth rates in prepubescents are so great that without continued training any strength advantage caused by training disappears quickly. After a summer of no training the advantage in strength achieved by resistance training is lost as nontraining children naturally become stronger and previously trained children detrain just like adults (Blimkie 1993). These data suggest that continued training may be necessary to gain and keep increased muscle strength in the prepubescent child.

MUSCLE HYPERTROPHY

What is the cause of strength improvements in children? To date, scientific evidence indicates that neural adaptations produce the majority of strength gains observed in children (Ramsay et al. 1990). Therefore, by improving the functional ability of the nervous system rather than by dramatically increasing muscle size, children make gains in muscular strength. This appears to be the case at least for resistance training programs lasting 6 mo or less. What happens over longer periods of time remains unknown. However, hypertrophy is more difficult to achieve in children, especially in prepubescents, than in adults.

It appears that enhanced growth of muscle in response to resistance training may start after adolescence, when male and female adult hormonal profiles start to emerge (Kraemer and Fleck 1993). In males, the influence of testosterone on muscle size and strength starting at puberty without any training is dramatic. It appears that after puberty the ability of resistance training to enhance muscular hypertrophy beyond normal growth begins to occur. However, Fukunaga, Funato, and Ikegawa (1992) examined 51 first-, third-, and fifth-grade students who resistance trained for 12 wk. Training consisted of three maximal sustained isometric actions of elbow flexion for 10 s twice a day, 3 d/wk. A control group of 47 students did not participate in the training program. Ultrasonic methods were used to measure muscle and bone cross-sectional area. Following the resistance training program a significant increase in muscle and bone cross-sectional area was observed in the training

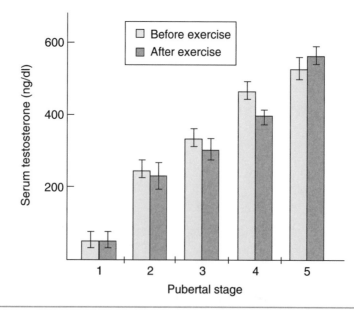

Fig. 10.1   Serum testosterone levels before and after an exercise bout in prepubescent children. Pubertal stages 1 through 5 refer to the maturity of the individual, with 1 being immature and 5 fully mature.

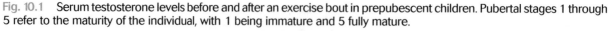

Adapted, by permission, from T.D. Fahey, A. DelValle-Zuris, G. Oehlsen, M. Trieb, and J. Seymour, 1979, "Pubertal stage differences in hormonal and hematological responses to maximal exercise in males," *Journal of Applied Physiology* 46:825.

group. The control group demonstrated an increase in fat area. The muscle size increase was only 50% of that which the researchers had observed in adults, and the magnitude of increase in muscle cross-sectional area was significantly correlated with skeletal age. Isokinetic strength remained unchanged with training, which points to the importance of muscle action specificity in training, even in children. Other study data indicate that muscle size gains may be possible in younger children. Figure 10.2 presents a group of physiological variables that ultimately contribute to the ability of the body to exhibit strength (Kraemer, Fry, et al. 1989). Dramatic progress in each of the variables is observed during a child's adolescent phase of development. This indicates that physiological age will affect the magnitude of strength increases from resistance training in children.

It is important to note that, although increases in quantity of muscle (i.e., hypertrophy) may not occur in children of all ages, many other changes in the muscle, nerve, and connective tissue of children suggest an increase in the quality of muscle tissue and the neuromuscular unit. Changes in muscle protein (myosin forms) recruitment patterns and in connective tissue could contribute to the improvement in strength, sport performance, and injury prevention. Knowing that increases in muscle mass beyond normal growth are not pos-

sible in younger children, it is even more important that muscle hypertrophy not be a goal of their training programs. Increased muscle mass can be a concern for younger boys especially, who still physically can't achieve large muscle mass increases beyond normal growth but see older boys (16- or 17-yr-old) who have better-defined, larger muscles. It is a mistake for a young boy to believe that merely by starting to lift weights he will have the muscle size and physique he desires in a few months. As the child grows older and goes through puberty, increases in muscle size, especially in males, become more biologically feasible. Only after a child has entered adolescence, usually at about 14 yr or later, do size gains become a viable objective. However, because of the differences in maturation rates among children, care must be taken to individually evaluate this goal, especially for young men and women who are 14 to 15 yr of age.

BONE DEVELOPMENT

Children's bone development may be enhanced with resistance exercise. Resistance training increases muscle strain, strain rate, and compression, which are all important stimuli to bone modeling (Conroy et al. 1992).

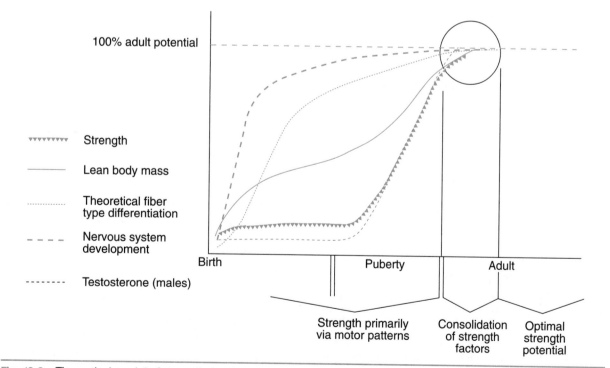

Fig. 10.2   Theoretical model of strength development factors in males.

Adapted, by permission, from W.J. Kraemer, A.C. Fry, P.N. Frykman, B. Conroy, and J. Hoffman, 1989, "Resistance training and youth," *Pediatric Exercise Science* 1 (4):336-50.

Increased bone density via resistance training may be one of the primary mediating factors involved in empirical observations that resistance training prevents injury in young athletes (Hejna et al. 1982). In a study by Conroy and colleagues (1993) young, elite, junior Olympic weight lifters demonstrated bone density values that were greater than age- and weight-matched controls. In addition, bone densities of the back, hip, and femur were significantly correlated with strength in squat and competitive lifts. Thus, increased bone density may be an adaptation needed to tolerate the stresses encountered during heavy resistance training.

CONCERNS ABOUT INJURY

Resistance training helps prevent injuries in adults. There is also some evidence that resistance training helps to prevent injuries in adolescent athletes (Hejna et al. 1982) and that stronger athletes may be less susceptible to certain types of injury (Moskwa and Nicholas 1989). The possibility of acute and chronic injuries to children's growth cartilage, however, is a valid concern (Dalton 1992; Markiewitz and Andrish 1992). A resistance training program for children therefore should not focus primarily on lifting maximal or near-maximal amounts of resistance. Furthermore, proper technique must always be stressed, because most injuries in resistance exercise are related to improper exercise technique. Also, children need time to adapt to the stress of resistance training, and some children find it difficult to train or don't enjoy training at a particular age. Interest, growth, maturity, and understanding all influence the child's view of exercise training and proper safety precautions.

GROWTH CARTILAGE DAMAGE

In addition to the possibility of the types of injury that occur in adults, the prepubescent child is subject to growth cartilage injury. Growth cartilage is located at three sites: the epiphyseal plate, or growth plate; the epiphysis, or joint surface; and the apophyseal insertion, or tendon insertion (figure 10.3). The long bones of the body grow in length from the epiphyseal plates located at each end of the long bones. Normally, because of hormonal changes, these epiphyseal plates ossify after puberty. Once ossified, growth of the long bones is

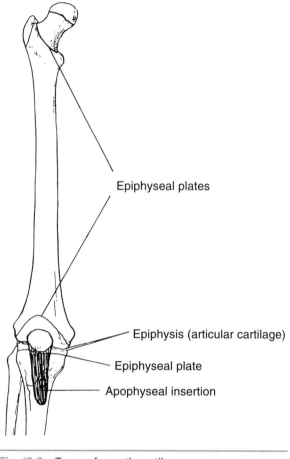

Fig. 10.3   Types of growth cartilage.

no longer possible. Thus, an increase in the height of an individual is also no longer possible. The epiphysis acts as a shock absorber between the bones that form a joint. Damage to this cartilage may lead to a rough articular surface and subsequent pain during movement of the joint. The growth cartilage at apophyseal insertions of major muscle-tendon-bone units ensures a solid connection between the tendon and bone. Damage to the growth cartilage here may cause pain and also increase the chance of separation between the tendon and bone. All three growth cartilage sites are more susceptible to injury during the adolescent growth spurt because of other factors, such as increased muscle tightness across joints.

ACUTE INJURIES

Acute injury refers to a single trauma causing an injury. Acute injuries to the skeletal system, such as growth cartilage damage or bone fractures, are very rare during weight training.

Muscle Strains

The most common acute injury risk for prepubescent weight trainers, as for adults, is muscle strain. Strains are often the result of not warming up properly before a training session. Several sets of an exercise should be performed before the true training sets of a workout. Another common cause of muscle strain is attempting to lift too much weight for a given number of repetitions. Children should be instructed that the number of repetitions per set is a guideline and that it is acceptable to perform less than that number of repetitions.

Epiphyseal Plate Fractures

Cases of epiphyseal plate fractures in prepubescent weight trainers have been reported (Grumbs et al. 1982; Rowe 1979; Ryan and Salciccioli 1976). The epiphyseal plate is prone to fracture in children because it has not yet ossified and does not have the structural strength of mature adult bone. All these case reports involved overhead lifts (e.g., overhead press, clean and jerk) with near-maximal resistances. These case reports reveal two precautions for prepubescent programs. First, maximal or near-maximal lifts (1 RM) should not be stressed for prepubescent weight trainers, especially in unsupervised settings. Second, because improper form is a contributing factor to any injury, proper form of all exercises (particularly overhead lifts) should be emphasized to young resistance trainees.

Fractures

Peak fracture incidence in boys occurs between the ages of 12 and 14 yr and precedes the age of peak height increase, or growth spurt (Blimkie 1993). It appears that the increased fracture rate is caused by a lag in cortical bone thickness and mineralization to linear bone growth (Blimkie 1993). Therefore, controlling the resistance used during weight training by boys between the ages of 12 and 14 yr is important. This same line of evidence may apply to girls between the ages of 10 and 13 yr.

Lumbar Back Problems

Acute trauma can cause lumbar back problems in adults as well as children. In resistance training, acute trauma may be caused by lifting maximal or near-maximal resistances and attempting to perform too many repetitions. In many cases back pain is associated with improper form in the squat or deadlift exercises. While performing these exercises, it is essential to keep the back in an upright position and to use the legs as much as possible. This form reduces the torque on the lumbar region, protecting the lower back from excessive stress.

CHRONIC INJURIES

Chronic injury refers to injury caused by repeated microtraumas; another common term for this is overuse injury. Shinsplints and stress fractures are common overuse injuries. Improper technique of resistance training over long periods of time can create overuse injuries (e.g., improper bench press technique can cause shoulder problems).

Growth Cartilage

It is possible to damage all three growth cartilage sites through physical stress. As an example, repeated microtrauma to the shoulder from baseball pitching results in damage to the epiphyseal plate of the humerus. This damage causes pain with shoulder movement and is often called Little League shoulder (Barnett 1985; Torg, Pollack, and Sweterlitsch 1972).

The growth cartilage on the articular surface of prepubescent joints—especially at the ankle, knee, and elbow—is more prone to injury than that of adults. Repeated microtrauma appears to be responsible for many cases of osteochondritis dissecans at the elbow of young baseball pitchers (J.E. Adams 1965; Lipscomb 1975) and at the ankle joint of young runners (Conale and Belding 1980). The growth cartilage at the site of a tendon insertion onto a bone may be related to the pain associated with Osgood-Schlatter disease. Although the cause of Osgood-Schlatter disease is not completely known, there is increasing evidence that it may in part be caused by tiny avulsion fractures (i.e., pulling the tendon from the bone) (Micheli 1983). Similar injuries in adolescents could be related to improper resistance exercise technique.

Lordosis

Repeated microtrauma can cause a compression fracture of the vertebrae (Hensinger 1982), resulting in pain. During the growth spurt many children have a tendency to develop lordosis of the lumbar spine. Lordosis is an anterior bending of the spine, usually accompanied by flexion of the pelvis. Several factors contribute to lordosis, including enhanced growth in the anterior portion of the vertebral bodies and tight hamstrings that cause the hips to assume a flexed position (Micheli 1983). Back pain arising from overstress can be caused by muscle spasm, damage to ligaments, or compression of vertebral disks, all of which could be related to improper exercise technique.

Back problems from resistance training can be minimized by performing exercises that strengthen the abdominal muscles (e.g., crunches) and back musculature (e.g., good-morning exercise, back extensions). Strengthening these areas will help maintain proper exercise technique and reduce stress on the lower back. The resistance used in exercises to strengthen the lower back should be of light to moderate intensity, thus allowing the performance of at least 10 repetitions.

PROGRAMS FOR CHILDREN

The development of a prepubescent resistance training program should follow the same steps as that of a program for adults. However, the following questions also need to be considered before a child begins a resistance training program:

- Is the child psychologically and physically ready to participate in a resistance exercise training program?

- What resistance training program should the child follow?
- Does the child understand the proper lifting techniques for each exercise in the program?
- Do spotters understand the safety spotting techniques for each lift in the program?
- Does the child understand the safety concerns for each piece of equipment used in the program?
- Does the resistance training equipment fit the child properly?
- Does the child have a balanced physical exercise training program (i.e., participate in cardiovascular activities and other sports in addition to resistance training)?

A well-organized and well-supervised basic training program for children need not be any longer than 20 to 60 min per training session, three times per week. As the child gets older, more advanced programs can be developed. Table 10.2 shows a program progression from 5 to 18 yr of age. The resistance training program should be conducted in an atmosphere conducive to both the child's safety and enjoyment. The training environment should send out the right signals about the goals and expectations of the program.

TABLE 10.2
Basic Guidelines for Resistance Exercise Progression for Children

Age (yr)	Considerations
5-7	Introduce child to basic exercises with little or no weight; develop the concept of a training session; teach exercise techniques; progress from body weight calisthenics, partner exercises, and lightly resisted exercises; keep volume low.
8-10	Gradually increase the number of exercises; practice exercise technique for all lifts; start gradual progressive loading of exercises; keep exercises simple; increase volume slowly; carefully monitor tolerance to exercise stress.
11-13	Teach all basic exercise techniques; continue progressive loading of each exercise; emphasize exercise technique; introduce more advanced exercises with little or no resistance.
14-15	Progress to more advanced resistance exercise programs; add sport-specific components; emphasize exercise techniques; increase volume.
16 or older	Entry level into adult programs after all background experience has been gained.

Note. If a child at a particular age level has no previous experience, progression must start at previous levels and move to more advanced levels as exercise tolerance, skill, and understanding permit.

Adapted, by permission, from W.J. Kraemer and S.J. Fleck, 1993, *Strength training for young athletes* (Champaign, IL: Human Kinetics Publishers), 5.

EXERCISE TOLERANCE

To promote proper growth and development, the importance of the child's ability to tolerate the exercise stress cannot be overemphasized. Throughout this text the concepts of individualized exercise prescription, proper supervision, and program monitoring have been discussed. For such methods to work, parents, teachers, and coaches need to communicate with the children regardless of the children's age. Adults should encourage discussion and feedback and should listen to the children's concerns and fears. Most important, trainers need to use common sense and to provide exercise variations, active recovery periods, and rest from training. Trainers must not fall into the trap of believing that more is better.

Suggestions about program design are only very general guidelines. No single best program exists. Children should start with a program that is individually tolerable but that becomes more aggressive as they grow older. Dramatic changes in the tolerance to resistance training programs can reflect the increased maturity of a child. It is important not to overestimate the child's ability to tolerate an exercise or sport program. It is better to start out conservatively rather than to overshoot the child's exercise tolerance and reduce the enjoyment of participation. With the proper principles of resistance training, a program can be designed that reflects the child's developmental stage. Using proper guidelines for program development, a resistance exercise program can be implemented at each stage of development that does not compromise enthusiasm and does not overestimate exercise tolerance. Parents, teachers, and coaches must always remember that they are not the ones for whom the program is developed and that children are free to not participate in an exercise or sport program. It is up to the adults to provide a positive environment that protects and serves the children who participate.

NEEDS ANALYSIS

The needs of each child, like those of adults, are individual. Children need to develop cardiovascular fitness, flexibility, and motor skills as well as strength. A resistance training program should not be so time-consuming as to ignore these other aspects of fitness in a child's development and interfere with a child's play time. A child should not be expected to perform an adult program. Individual determination of goals, acceptability, and physical and psychological tolerance is the key component of the training program. If the parents, teachers, or coaches hear such comments as "I don't want to do this," "This program is too demanding, and I would like to change it," "Some of these exercises are hurting me," "I am just too tired after a workout," or "What other exercises can I learn?" then the program needs to be evaluated and appropriate changes made.

The possible dangers of resistance exercise training are related to inappropriate exercise demands being placed on the child. Although general guidelines can be offered and should be followed, sensitivity to the special needs that arise in each individual situation is needed. The program must be designed for each child's needs, and the proper exercise techniques and safety considerations employed. A properly designed and supervised resistance training program can provide many positive physical and psychological benefits for the child. Perhaps an even more important outcome is the behavioral development of an active lifestyle in a child's younger years. Good exercise behaviors can contribute to better health and well-being over a lifetime.

With the increasing participation of children in a wide variety of youth sports, from football and gymnastics to soccer and track, there is a need for better physical preparation to prevent sport-related injuries. Resistance training appears to have great potential to address this need. Resistance training has great potential for improving children's physical ability to tolerate sport stresses, to improve performance, and to avoid athletic injury.

Another consideration for all children is upper-body strength. It has been shown that upper body strength in both boys and girls is declining (Rupnow 1985). This represents a significant weakness in young boys' and girls' fitness profiles. Upper-body strength limits many sport-specific tasks even at the recreational level. Because of the general lack of strength in the upper body of many prepubescent and pubescent children, exercises for the upper body need to be emphasized in a resistance training program for these groups.

After considering the previously discussed general needs, the needs analysis is further developed by deciding what the major goals of the program are. Some common goals for a resistance training program include the following:

- Increased strength/power of specific muscle groups
- Increased local muscular endurance of specific muscle groups
- Increased motor performance (i.e., increased ability to jump, run, or throw)
- Increased total body weight (age dependent)
- Increased muscle hypertrophy (age dependent)
- Decreased body fat

DEVELOPMENTAL DIFFERENCES

Children differ from each other physically and emotionally. Some children are big, others are smaller. One child may be the fastest base runner. One child may become very upset while another is not really concerned about a missed shot in a game. Physical differences are the result of different genetic potentials and growth rates. It is important for adults to realize that children are not just "little adults." Furthermore, all children of a similar age are not equal physically or emotionally. Understanding some of the basic principles of growth and development will allow more realistic expectations for children. This understanding will also help when developing goals and exercise progressions in resistance training programs. It is important that an exercise program match the physical and emotional level of the child.

There are many aspects of children's growth and development. Development is not based on any single factor, such as height. Many factors influence fitness gains, including genetic potential, nutrition, and sleep.

Maturation has been defined as the progress toward adulthood. The maturation of children involves several areas:

- Physical size
- Bone maturity
- Reproductive maturity
- Emotional maturity

Each of these areas can be clinically evaluated. It is common for the family physician to assess the development of a child in several of these areas. Each individual has a chronological age and a physiological age. The physiological age is the most important and determines the functional capabilities and performance for that person, and physiological age should be considered when developing a resistance program.

INDIVIDUALIZED RESISTANCE TRAINING PROGRAMS

The design of the total conditioning program, as well as of the resistance program, should incorporate the following elements to address the needs of all children:

- Conditioning of all fitness components
- Balanced choice of exercises for upper- and lower-body development
- Balanced choice of exercises for muscles on both sides of each joint
- Use of body part as well as structural exercises

After the needs analysis but before beginning a resistance training program, children, like adults, should be examined by a physician to ensure awareness of any physical problems that need to be considered in the design of the program. For example, if a child has Osgood-Schlatter disease, exercises involving extreme bending of the knee may be contraindicated. The child should begin with a basic resistance training program that exercises all the major muscle groups of the body and muscles around each joint of the body. Warm-up, cool-down, and flexibility exercises should be a part of each session. Additional sport-specific exercises and exercises based on individual need can be added to the program after the child has learned basic lifting techniques. Individualizing a program requires considering the strengths, weaknesses, and goals of each lifter.

No major distinction between boys' and girls' resistance training programs needs to be made. General fitness requires training all major muscle groups. Successful performance of a particular sport skill by adults as well as children depends on the strength and power of particular muscle groups and not the gender of the participant.

SAMPLE PROGRAMS

This section outlines two sample programs: One involves the use of either the child's body weight or another child's body weight as resistance; the other requires some resistance training equipment.

Program Using Body Weight

Table 10.3 outlines a program involving the child's own body weight as resistance. This program can be performed as a circuit, moving from one exercise to the next, or in a set-repetition manner, performing all three sets of an exercise with a rest between sets before moving on to the next exercise. The proper performance of the exercises is shown in figure 10.4.

TABLE 10.3
Resistance Training Program for Children Using Body Weight for Resistance

Exercise	Sets and repetitions
Push-ups	3 × 10-20
Bent-leg sit-ups	3 × 15-30
Parallel squats	3 × 10-20
Self-resistance arm curls	10 actions of 6-s duration
Toe raises	3 × 20-30
Partner-resisted lateral arm raises	10 actions of 6-s duration
Lying back extensions	3 × 10-15

Squats and Sit-Ups. Bent-leg sit-ups are performed lying on the floor. Parallel squats involve squatting until the thigh is parallel to the ground. During this exercise the feet should be kept flat on the floor or as nearly flat as possible. Resistance can be added to these exercises by holding an object, or older children, can use partner squats.

Arm Curls. Self-resistance arm curls are performed by placing the elbow of the exercising arm in a fully extended position with the hand palm up in front of the body, then grasping that arm with the opposite hand. Contract the elbow flexors, resisting with the opposite arm but allowing the exercising arm to fully flex in 6 s. Then apply force with the opposite arm while the exercising arm returns to the fully extended position in 6 s.

Toe Raises. Toe raises are performed by rising as high as possible on the toes. Resistance can be added by holding an object in the hands or doing the exercise with only one leg at a time.

Push-Ups. Push-ups should be varied to include those performed with the hands at shoulder width and those with the hands farther than shoulder-width apart. The latter place a greater stress on the chest muscles, whereas the former stress the shoulder and upper arm to a greater extent. A bent-knee push-up (i.e., knees rather than feet touching the ground) should be used by children who cannot perform a regular push-up.

Back Extensions. Back extensions are performed by lying on the stomach and clasping the hands behind the head. A partner holds the child's legs down by placing his or her hands on the back of the exerciser's legs just above the knees. The exerciser then attempts to raise the chest and shoulders as high as possible in a slow, controlled manner. The chest is then lowered to the ground, and the exercise is repeated.

Arm Raises. Partner-resisted lateral arm raises are begun with the arms at the sides. A partner grasps the arms slightly above the elbows, and the exerciser attempts to raise the arms laterally from the body while the partner resists. The partner allows the arms to reach the horizontal position in 6 s. The partner then applies force as the exerciser returns to the starting position, which should take 6 s.

Program Using Free Weights

Table 10.4 outlines a program involving the use of free weights or resistance training machines, and figure 10.5 shows the exercises. Initially, the resistance

TABLE 10.4
Resistance Training Program for Children Using Equipment

Exercise	Sets and repetitions
Squat or leg press	3 × 10-15
Bench press	3 × 10-15
Knee curls	3 × 10-15
Arm curls	3 × 10-15
Knee extensions	3 × 10-15
Overhead press	3 × 10-15
Bent-leg sit-ups	3 × 15-20
Back extensions	3 × 10-15

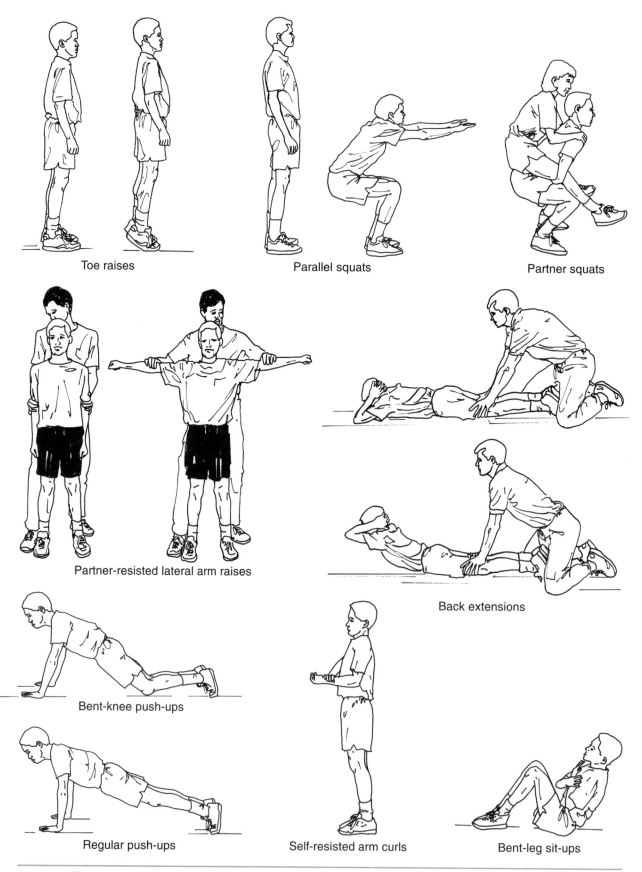

Toe raises

Parallel squats

Partner squats

Partner-resisted lateral arm raises

Back extensions

Bent-knee push-ups

Regular push-ups

Self-resisted arm curls

Bent-leg sit-ups

Fig. 10.4   The proper performance of body-weight exercises.

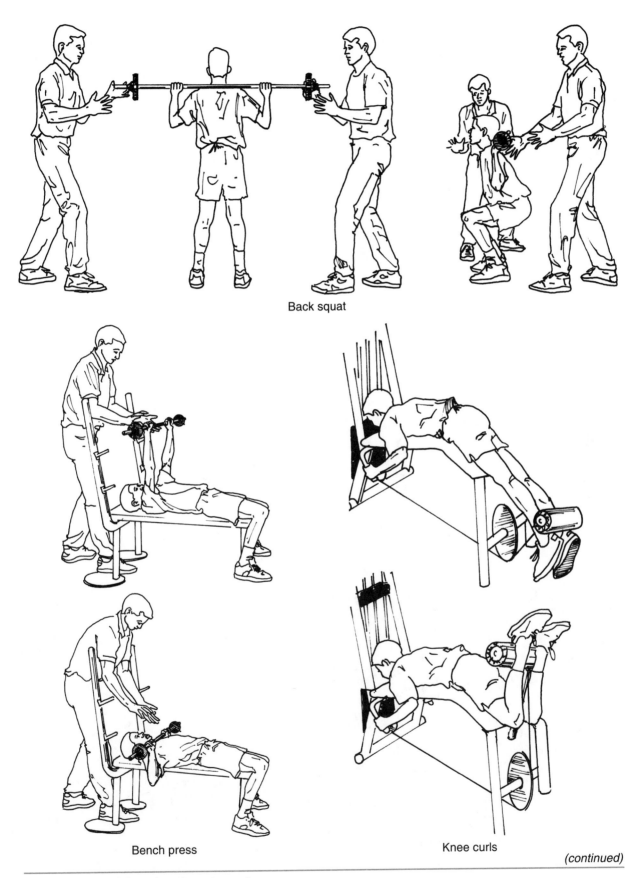

Back squat

Bench press

Knee curls

(continued)

Fig. 10.5 Free-weight and equipment exercises.

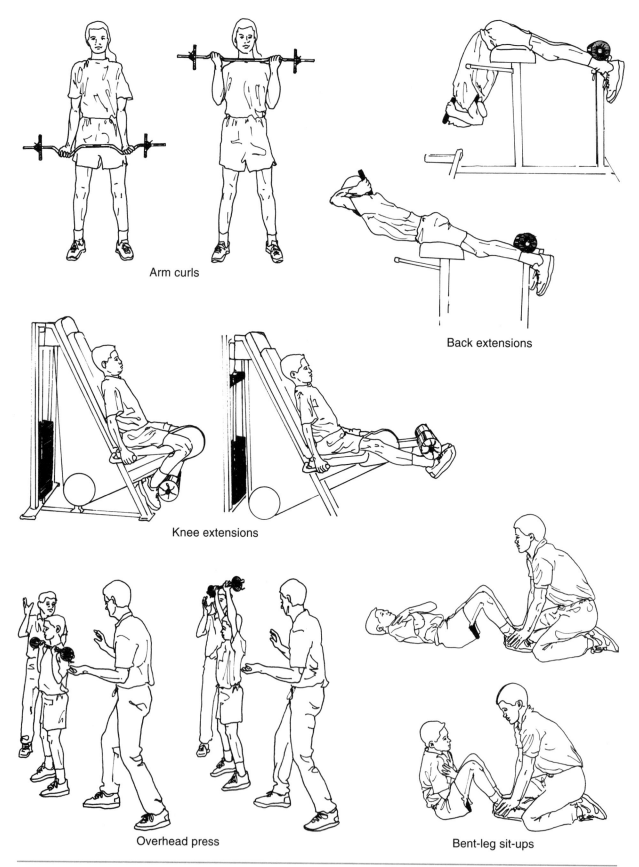

Arm curls

Back extensions

Knee extensions

Overhead press

Bent-leg sit-ups

Fig. 10.5   *(continued)*

used for each exercise should be such that the minimum recommended number of repetitions can be performed. Once the child can perform the maximum number of repetitions, the resistance is increased so that again the minimum number of repetitions can be performed. Form and spotting techniques for all exercises should be continually stressed. The exercises should be performed in a controlled manner to help prevent injury to the trainees caused by losing control of the weights and to prevent damage to the weight stack of a machine or the free weights.

Bench Press. As in the push-ups in the first program, hand spacing in the bench press is varied from shoulder width to wider than shoulder width. This varies the involvement of the shoulder, back of arm, and chest in the exercise.

Sit-Ups. Bent-leg sit-ups are performed lying on the floor as depicted in figure 10.5 or using a sit-up board. Resistance can be increased by holding a weight against the chest if lying on the floor or by increasing the inclination of the board if using a sit-up board.

Back Extensions. Back extensions are performed either with equipment for back extensions or on the floor as described in the previous program. In either case, resistance can be added by holding a weight behind the neck or on the chest.

Knee Extensions and Curls. Knee extensions and knee curls require weight training machines. Care must be taken to ensure that the machines properly fit the child. Arm curls, back squats, and overhead presses are performed using free weights.

COPYING ELITE ATHLETIC PROGRAMS

Programs designed for collegiate or professional athletes should not be performed by prepubescents or pubescents. The ability of older athletes to improve strength using these programs is in part a result of their years of resistance training experience. Often these programs involve lifting very heavy resistances (1-3 RM), which, as previously discussed, may result in injury to prepubescents. Forcing prepubescents or pubescents to perform programs designed for mature, gifted athletes will overstress prepubescents and may result in injury.

PROGRAM CYCLING OR PERIODIZATION

Cycling or periodization is a popular way of varying the training volume and intensity of a workout in adult athletes and is discussed in chapter 5. Periodization and its effects on children or young adults have received little study. It has been demonstrated that use of the traditional periodization model with a high school football team led to greater gains in 1 RM strength and vertical jumping ability than nonperiodized resistance training (Stone, O'Bryant, and Barhanner 1981). However, the use of the traditional periodization model requires the performance of exercises with near-maximal and maximal resistances and therefore may not be applicable for prepubescent individuals. However, variation of a resistance training program can be accomplished within the guidelines of a program for prepubescent individuals (table 10.5). Variation in a program leads to greater and faster gains in strength/power and in local muscular endurance and helps keep the program interesting to the trainees.

TABLE 10.5 Periodization Model and Concepts for Prepubescents		
Training phase	**Sets**	**Repetitions (RM range)**
Base	3	10-15
Strength	3	6-10
Power	2-3	6-8
Peaking	1-2	6-8
Active rest	Physical activity (not necessarily resistance training)	

Adapted, by permission, from W.J. Kraemer and S.J. Fleck, 1993, *Strength training for young athletes* (Champaign, IL: Human Kinetics Publishers), 40.

There are several methods of variation for resistance training, including

- increasing resistance for a particular RM,
- varying the RM used (6-20 RM),
- varying the number of sets (1-3),
- using heavy, moderate, and light training days during a week, and
- varying exercises for the same muscle groups.

PRESENTING THE PROGRAM PHILOSOPHY

For formal programs (e.g., for schools or health clubs) the program philosophy needs to be expressed in the environment. This means that the signs, wall charts, and handouts need to send the right signals to the child. This is especially important when both adults and children are training in the same facility. The program philosophy can be promoted with the following methods.

1. Post age-related instructions for children next to the adult guidelines, for example:

Training Day Schedule		
	Adult	Child (15 and under)
Heavy day:	100% of 3-5 RM	100% of 8-10 RM
Moderate day:	90% of 3-5 RM	90% of 8-10 RM
Light day:	85% of 3-5 RM	85% of 8-10 RM

2. Use posters and pictures that depict children (both boys and girls) and promote proper expectations from resistance training.

3. Use charts, contests, and awards to promote the principles that children need to concentrate on, such as training consistency charts and awards, exercise technique contests and awards, "total conditioning" fitness awards focusing on other aspects of progress in other components of physical fitness (e.g., endurance runs, flexibility), fitness preparation awards prior to a sports season, and in-season program awards over a sports season.

It is important that the environment, exercise programs, and awards reflect the program philosophy. Since children learn in different ways, it is important that these messages are sent in all forms of communication, including oral, written, audio, and pictorial media. Make communication clear and appropriate for children so that they are neither intimidated nor confused about what to expect.

EQUIPMENT MODIFICATION

More individualized help is required when working with children than with adults. Organi-

zational problems can be encountered that may not be present when training adults. For example, each exercise station must have pads and blocks if necessary to modify the equipment to fit the children (e.g., blocks to set chest height to the bar height in a machine bench press), or equipment such as dumbbells must be available to perform an alternate exercise when a machine does not fit or cannot provide the proper resistance for some children in a group (e.g., dumbbell bench press instead of machine bench press). Each child must also know how to set up the modification for each exercise if needed (e.g., how to place pads in the correct position). It will also be necessary to change the equipment modifications as the child grows. It is therefore necessary to check equipment for proper fit as frequently as every month.

Modifications needed to make the equipment fit each child can cause organizational problems, but they can be solved. Two solutions to this problem are to have each needed modification on each child's workout card or to have an adult make the equipment modification for the child. Although effective, these solutions may be somewhat impractical with a large group of children. If timed workouts (specific exercise periods and rest periods) are used, the time needed for equipment modifications must be considered, especially when a whole group of children are training and modifications are made for many exercises.

To find out how long a particular equipment modification takes, the training session may have to actually be performed. The rest periods may then have to be changed to account for the time needed for equipment modifications. Although it may be desirable to have 1-min rest periods in a particular training session, organizational problems such as equipment fit may make this impossible. Exercise machines typically require more modifications than free-weight exercises because of their fixed movement patterns and positions. These organizational problems must be resolved as well as possible without sacrificing the children's safety or making the training session ineffective.

EQUIPMENT ADJUSTMENTS

The most important equipment consideration when training children is whether the resistance training equipment fits each child properly. With free weights, body-weight exercises, or partner-assisted exercises fit is typically not a concern. With resistance training machines, however, fit can be a very critical concern, because most resistance training machines are made to properly fit an adult male. Therefore, most prepubescents are not tall enough and have shorter arms and legs than needed to properly fit many resistance training machines. If the machine does not properly fit the child, correct technique and full range of motion of the exercise are impossible.

The most critical problem of an ill-fitting machine is the chance that a body part may slip off its point of contact, such as a foot or arm pad, resulting in injury to the child. Another common problem of poor fit is that the bench for a machine or free-weight exercise is too wide to allow free movement of the shoulder during the exercise. When an exercise is performed with inappropriate technique because of ill-fitting equipment, too much stress can be placed on the child's joints and musculature.

If a piece of equipment cannot be safely adapted to properly fit a child, that particular piece of equipment should not be used by that child. Simple alterations of some machines—such as additional seat pads (e.g., for a knee-extension machine) or raising a bench by blocking it up (e.g., for bench press)—allow a trainee who is shorter than the machine was designed for to safely use the machine. Remember, just adjusting a seat height is often not enough to make a machine fit a child. Although the seat height may be appropriate, the points of contact on the machine for the arms or legs may not be. Therefore, adjustments also need to be made to allow proper positioning of the arms and/or legs on the contact points of the machine. In addition, raising the seat height may make it impossible for the child's feet to reach the floor. In many exercises the feet need to be in contact with the floor to aid in balance. Therefore, raising the seat may also make it necessary to place blocks under the feet so that they can be used to aid in balance during the exercise.

Altering a piece of equipment to fit one child does not guarantee that the equipment will fit another child. Proper fit must be checked before the equipment is used by each child. Care must be taken to ensure that additional padding or blocks do not slide during the exercise, which could result in injury. Sliding can be avoided in some alterations by attaching rubber mats to the top and bottom of blocks and to the back of additional pads.

APPROPRIATE RESISTANCE INCREASES

Another potential problem when prepubescents use certain resistance machines is that the resistance increments are too large to allow a smooth progression in resistance as the child becomes stronger. Many machines' weight stacks increase in increments of 10 lb to 20 lb (4.5 kg to 9.1 kg). If a child can bench press 30 lb (13.6 kg), a weight stack increment of 10 lb (4.5 kg) represents a 33% increase in resistance, which is too large an increase for a safe and smooth progression in resistance. This problem can be remedied on some machines by purchasing weights, usually 2.5 lb (1.1 kg) and 5 lb (2.3 kg), that are specially designed to be easily added and removed from the weight stack of the machine.

On some machines the starting resistance will be too great for a child to perform even one repetition. In this case the child will have to perform free-weight, body-weight, or partner-resisted exercises until he or she is strong enough to perform the desired number of repetitions using the machine. For example, if a child cannot perform leg presses on a machine because the starting resistance is too great, the child could perform body-weight squats and then squats holding light dumbbells in each hand until he or she is strong enough to perform leg presses at the starting resistance on the machine.

SUMMARY

Resistance training of children has gained acceptance and popularity primarily because strength gains can occur, bone development may be enhanced, and injuries might be prevented in other sports and activities with developmentally appropriate training programs. When designing a program, consider the developmental and physical differences among children, exercise tolerance, and safety issues so that acute and chronic injuries are minimized and the benefits to the participating children are maximized.

SELECTED READINGS

Bar-Or, O. 1989. Trainability of the prepubescent child. *Physician and Sportsmedicine* 17:65-82.

Blimkie, C.J.R. 1989. Age- and sex-associated variation in strength during childhood: Anthropometric, morphologic, neurologic, biomechanical, endocrinologic, genetic and physical activity correlates. In *Perspectives in exercise science and sports medicine.* Vol. 2, *Youth exercise and sport,* eds. C. Gisolfi and D. Lamb, 99-163. Indianapolis: Benchmark Press.

Blimkie, C.J.R. 1993. Resistance training during preadolescence. *Sports Medicine* 15:389-407.

Docherty, D.; Wenger, H.A.; and Collis, M.L. 1987. The effects of resistance training on aerobic and anaerobic power of young boys. *Medicine and Science in Sports and Exercise* 19:389-92.

Duda, M. 1986. Prepubescent strength training gains support. *Physician and Sportsmedicine* 14:157-61.

Freedson, P.S.; Ward, A.; and Rippe, J.M. 1990. Resistance training for youth. *Advances in Sports Medicine and Fitness* 3:57-65.

Fukunaga, T.; Funato, K.; and Ikegawa, S. 1992. The effects of resistance training on muscle area and strength in prepubescent age. *Annals of Physiology and Anthropology* 11:357-64.

Kraemer, W.J., and Fleck, S.J. 1993. *Strength training for young athletes.* Champaign, IL: Human Kinetics.

Martens, R. 1987. *Joy and sadness in children's sports.* Champaign, IL: Human Kinetics.

Moskwa, C.A., and Nicholas, J.A. 1989. Musculoskeletal risk factors in the young athlete. *Physician and Sportsmedicine* 17:49-59.

Ramsay, J.A.; Blimkie, C.J.R.; Smith, K.; Garner, S.; MacDougall, J.D.; and Sale, D.G. 1990. Strength training effects in prepubescent boys. *Medicine and Science in Sports and Exercise* 22:605-14.

Rotrella, R.J., and Bunker, L.K. 1987. *Parenting your superstar.* Champaign, IL: Leisure Press.

Rowland, T.W. 1989. Oxygen uptake and endurance fitness in children: A developmental perspective. *Pediatric Exercise Science* 1:313-28.

Weltman, A. 1989. Weight training in prepubertal children. Physiologic benefits and potential damage. In *Advances in pediatric sport sciences,* vol. 3, ed. O. Bar-Or, 101-30. Champaign, IL: Human Kinetics.

CHAPTER 11

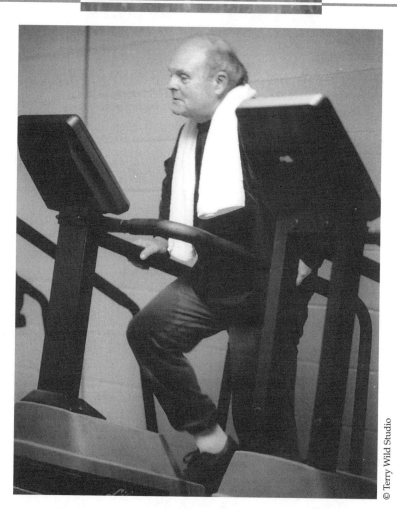

© Terry Wild Studio

Resistance Training for Seniors

It has been established over the past 10 years that seniors can benefit from participation in a resistance training program. In fact, Fiatarone and co-workers (1990) demonstrated that even individuals over the age of 90 can make strength gains over an 8-wk training period. This finding generated great attention. Improvements in strength and functional ability (e.g., improved mobility) can enhance the quality of life even of individuals with chronic illness. At the other end of the spectrum, seniors can demonstrate substantial strength. For example, a 180-lb (82-kg), 79-yr-old master power lifter squat-lifted 242 lb (110 kg). Strength training is one way that the age-related declines in strength and muscle mass can be diminished, which in turn results in improved quality of life.

AGE-RELATED LOSS OF MUSCULAR STRENGTH AND POWER

Strength is an important factor for functional abilities. Muscle weakness can advance until an elderly person cannot do common activities of daily living, such as household tasks, getting out of a chair, sweeping the floor, or taking out the trash. Reduced functional ability may result in nursing home placement. It is important to maintain strength as we age, because it is vital to health, functional abilities, and independent living.

Under normal conditions strength performances appear to peak between the ages of 20 and 30 yr, after which strength remains relatively stable or slightly decreases over the next 20 yr (Häkkinen, Kallinen, and Komi 1994). In the sixth decade of life a more dramatic decrease occurs in both men and women, although this decrease may be more dramatic in women. Cross-sectional studies may seriously underestimate the magnitude of strength loss with age (Bassey and Harries 1993). In fact, Bassey and Harries's (1993) cross-sectional data show a 2% loss of grip strength per year in elderly people. The loss of hand grip strength followed longitudinally over a 4-yr period, however, was 3% per year for men and nearly 5% for women.

Figure 11.1 depicts a general theoretical aging curve for muscle strength in trained and untrained people. The magnitude of strength decreases is related to gender and individual muscles, however.

Long-term involvement with strength training appears to offset the magnitude of strength loss and to enhance the actual absolute strength capabilities of an individual, but declines do occur even in competitive weight lifters (Kraemer and Koziris 1994; Meltzer 1994). The loss of strength in the lower extremities has also been shown to be greater than that of the upper extremities (Häkkinen, Kallinen, and Komi 1994). It appears that muscle strength losses are most dramatic after the age of 70 yr. For example, knee extensor strength of a group of healthy 80-yr-old men and women studied in the Copenhagen City Heart Study (Danneskoild-Samsoe et al. 1984) was found to be 30% lower than a previous population study (Aniansson and Gustavsson 1981) of 70-yr-old men and women. Cross-sectional as well as longitudinal data indicate that muscle strength declines by approximately 15% per decade in the sixth and seventh decades and about 30% thereafter (Danneskoild-Samsoe et al. 1984; Harries and Bassey 1990; Larsson 1978; Murray et al. 1985).

In addition to the loss in muscle strength, the muscle's ability to exert force rapidly (power development) appears to diminish with age. The ability of muscles to produce force rapidly is vital and may serve as a protective mechanism when falling. Falls in the elderly have been shown to be one of the top causes of injury, may lead to death, and are a major public health problem (Wolinsky and Fitzgerald 1994). Muscle power and its trainability in seniors has not received a great deal of study but may be even more important than strength for

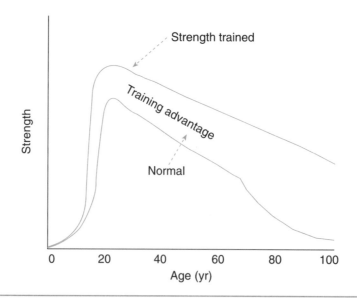

Fig. 11.1   A theoretical aging curve for muscle strength. The magnitude of change will vary for different muscle groups and by gender.

TABLE 11.1
Overview of Correlations Between Leg Extensor Power and Functional Performances

	Men	Women	Both genders
Chair-rising speed	0.45	0.83*	0.65*
Stair-climbing speed	0.76*	0.85*	0.81*
Walking speed	0.58*	0.93*	0.80*
Stair-climbing power	0.91*	0.86*	0.88*

* $p < .05$

Adapted, by permission, from E.J. Bassey et al., 1992, "Leg extensor power and functional performance in men and women," *Clinical Science* 82:321-27.

the functional abilities of the individual, as many everyday activities (walking, climbing stairs, lifting objects) require rapid force development or a certain degree of power to perform. In a study by Bassey and colleagues (1992) on elderly men (88.5 ±6 yr) and women (86.5±6 years) leg extensor power was significantly correlated with chair-rising speed, stair-climbing speed and power, and walking speed (table 11.1). Correlations between power and functional ability were greater in women than in men. For both genders, however, the data indicate that power is important for the performance of daily activities, and if power decreases, so does the ability to perform daily activities.

In examining the force-time curve characteristics of younger and older men and women, Häkkinen and Häkkinen (1991) suggested that the ability to produce force early (0 to 200 ms) in the force-time curve may be compromised by the aging process. The time needed to produce maximal isometric force was significantly longer in the older (70 yr) women than in middle-aged (50 yr) and younger (30 yr) women. The ability to rapidly produce force may decrease even more than maximal strength, especially at older ages. It has been estimated from cross-sectional studies that lower-limb power capabilities may be lost at a rate of 3.5% per year from the ages of 65 to 84 yr (A. Young and Skelton 1994). Conversely, peak anaerobic power in master endurance and power athletes expressed in watts per kilogram of body mass decreases linearly as a function of age at a rate of about 1% a year. This means that a 75-yr-old has only 50% of the anaerobic power of a 20-yr-old (Grassi et al. 1991).

In 1980 Bosco and Komi identified that aging (from 18 to 73 yr) resulted in reduced vertical jump

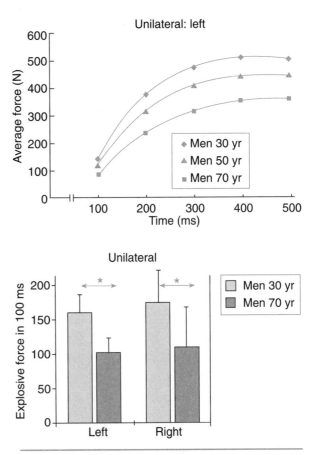

Fig. 11.2 Unilateral force development curves. * = significant differences between the two groups. Courtesy of Dr. Keijo Häkkinen from the University of Jyväskylä.

Adapted, with permission, from K. Häkkinen, U.M. Pastinen, R. Karsikas, and V. Linnamo, 1995, "Neuromuscular performance in voluntary bilateral and unilateral contraction and during electrical stimulation in men at different ages," *European Journal of Applied Physiology* 70:518-27; and from K. Häkkinen, W.J. Kraemer, and R. Newton, in press, "Muscle activation and force production during bilateral and unilateral concentric and isometric contractions of the knee extensors in men and women at different ages," *Electromyographic Clinical Neurophysiology*.

heights. Testing with stretch-shortening cycle jumps (e.g., drop jumps from various heights) showed even greater decreases caused by aging in vertical jump ability. The underlying effects on the elastic contractile components in the muscle may be affected by age and may affect power performance.

Decreased power may be one of the primary contributing factors to a loss of functional abilities and of safety mechanisms related to the prevention of injury from falls in older adults. Improvement in muscular power appears to be a primary training goal in older populations. Figures 11.2 and 11.3 depict the difference in rate of force development between older and younger individuals in bilateral (two limbs working together) and unilat-

eral (single limb) strength. It is evident that the ability to produce force in a short period of time is dramatically reduced by age in both men and women.

MECHANISMS OF MUSCLE STRENGTH AND POWER REDUCTIONS WITH AGE

A number of factors could contribute to the loss of muscle strength and power with age. How these factors interact with each other and what exact mechanisms predominate under certain conditions or at certain ages remains speculative. Following

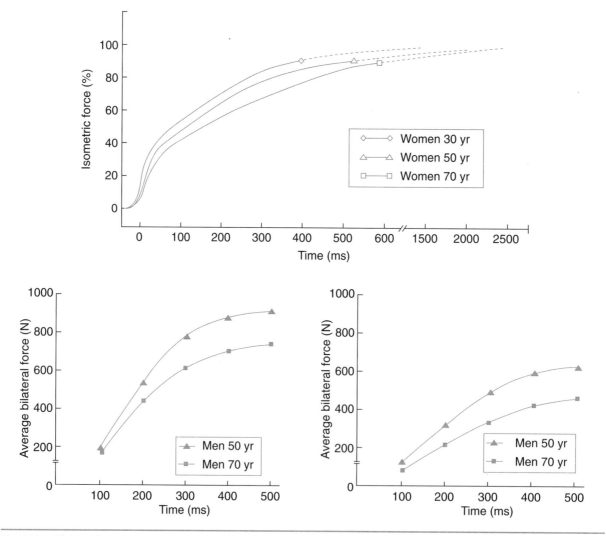

Fig. 11.3   Bilateral force development curves. Courtesy of Dr. Keijo Häkkinen from the University of Jyväskylä.

Adapted, by permission, from K. Häkkinen and A. Häkkinen, 1991, "Muscle cross-sectional area, force production and relaxation characteristics in women at different ages," *European Journal of Applied Physiology* 62:410-14; and from K. Häkkinen, W.J. Kraemer, M. Kallinen, V. Linnamo, U.M. Pastinen, and R. Newton, 1996, "Bilateral and unilateral neuromuscular function and muscle cross-sectional area in middle-aged and elderly men and women," *Journal of Gerontology and Biological Sciences* 51A:B21-B29.

are some of the primary factors associated with muscle weakness (Fiatarone and Evans 1993; Kraemer 1992a, 1992b):

- Senescent musculoskeletal changes
- Accumulation of chronic diseases
- Medications needed to treat diseases
- Nervous system changes
- Reductions in hormonal secretions
- Undernourishment
- Disuse atrophy

Senescent Musculoskeletal Changes

Decreased muscle mass has been suggested as the primary reason for the reduction in force production capabilities with age. This age-associated reduction in muscle mass has been termed sarcopenia (Evans and Campbell 1993). As one grows older, a general trend toward reduction in muscle mass is observed (Evans 1993; Evans and Campbell 1993; Frontera et al. 1991; Häkkinen and Häkkinen 1991; Häkkinen, Kallinen, and Komi 1994). It appears that

this effect on muscle mass is independent of muscle location (upper versus lower extremities) and function (extension versus flexion) (Frontera et al. 1991). A. Young, Stokes, and Crowe (1984) demonstrated that the quadriceps cross-sectional area of women in their 70s was 77% of that of women in their 20s. However, there is not only a decrease in cross-sectional muscle area, but also an increase of intramuscular fat, and such changes are most pronounced in women (Imamura et al. 1983).

It appears that the decline in muscle mass is caused by the reduction in the size of the individual muscle fibers, the loss of individual muscle fibers, or both (Frontera et al. 1988; Larsson 1982; Lexell et al. 1983). It also appears there is a preferential loss of Type II (fast-twitch) muscle fibers with aging. Figure 11.4 reviews the basic muscle fiber changes with aging. The number of muscle fibers in the midsection of the vastus lateralis of autopsy specimens is lower by about 23% in elderly men (age 70 to 73) than in young men (age 19 to 37) (Lexell et al. 1983). The decline is more marked in Type II muscle fibers, which fall from an average of 60% in sedentary young men to below 30% after the age of 80 (Larsson 1983). Thus, much of the

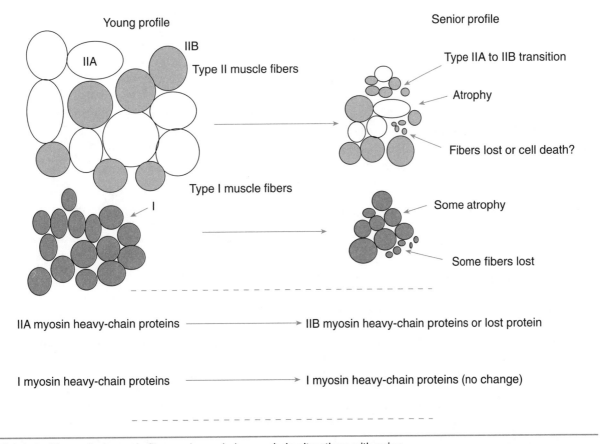

Fig. 11.4   Theoretical muscle fiber and myosin heavy-chain alterations with aging.

reduction in strength with aging is related to a selective atrophy of Type II muscle fibers.

In addition, the quality of protein may also be affected, because myosin heavy chains (MHC) make a shift to the slower type, which could affect the speed of myosin and actin crossbridge cycling during muscle actions (Sugiura et al. 1992). Furthermore, it has been known for some time that myosin ATPase activity decreases with aging (Syrovy and Gutmann 1970). The loss of Type II muscle fibers also means a loss of fast MHC proteins (Fry, Allemeier, and Staron 1994). Therefore, the loss of both quantity and quality of proteins in the contractile units of muscle provides a structural biochemical basis for the loss of muscle strength and power with age.

Nervous System Changes

The ability to activate muscle tissue is the primary determinant of whether or not muscle fibers are used in an activity and receive a training stimulus. In 1980 Moritani and DeVries examined 72-yr-old men before and after a strength training program consisting of two sets of 10 repetitions using 66% of 1 RM for elbow flexors, 3 d/wk for 8 wk. No significant changes were observed in muscle circumferences, but significant increases in the maximal integrated EMG were observed. This suggests that in older men neural factors were the primary mechanism mediating strength gains during an initial 8-wk period of strength training. Based on subsequent understanding of the time course of muscle fiber changes, it is not surprising that no hypertrophy was observed (Staron et al. 1994). Nevertheless, it appears that in older people, as in younger individuals, initial strength gains from training result from neural adaptations.

It is possible that each cell in the body has a minimum size, which is determined by genetic predisposition. When a cell shrinks below this size, cell death might occur. The loss of muscle fibers with aging may be a result of muscle cell death or of a denervation process caused by the loss of contact with the nerve (Häkkinen, Kallinen, and Komi 1994). Muscle fibers are lost with age, but some fibers undergo a reinnervation process with increased activity. Muscle fibers that are lost are subsequently replaced with fat or fibrous connective tissue. The loss of muscle fibers compromises the individual motor units' functional ability to produce force and affects basic metabolic functions of the entire muscle (such as reduced caloric expenditure caused by reduced muscle mass).

Aniansson, Grimby, and Hedberg (1992) suggested that in men between 76 and 80 yr of age who maintain physical activity, a compensatory hypertrophy of Type I and Type II muscle fibers is an adaptation for the loss of muscle fibers and motor units. Type I and II muscle fiber percentages do not change between the ages of 76 and 80 yr, but there is a significant reduction in the Type IIB fibers. This could be interpreted as a loss of muscle fibers or more likely as a transition of Type IIB to Type IIA muscle fibers caused by physical activity.

Using single-motor-unit EMG procedures, R.M. Nelson, Soderberg, and Urbscheit (1984) observed that large motor units were being used in older subjects (79 yr) where smaller motor units would typically be used in younger individuals. Later work by Doherty and colleagues (1993) indicates that the loss of motor units, even in healthy, active individuals, is a primary factor underlying age-associated reductions in strength. Using computerized EMG single-motor-unit analyses, it has been estimated that there is a 47% reduction in the number of motor units in older individuals (60 to 81 yr).

Questions about whether or not older individuals can activate their muscles maximally have been raised. Phillips and co-workers (1992) have reported twitch interpolation data that indicate that both old and young subjects could fully activate their muscles. Therefore, muscle weakness that occurs with aging is not caused by a failure in muscle activation. A.B. Brown, McCartney, and Sale (1990) also concluded that older individuals are able to fully activate their muscles, but activation for dynamic activities may differ from isometric muscle actions. The extent to which central voluntary neural drive decreases with increasing age is unclear.

It may be more probable that peripheral neuromuscular mechanisms (e.g., the neuromuscular junction) instead of decreased neural impulses are primarily responsible for the inability to activate muscle with aging if it does occur (Häkkinen, Kallinen, and Komi 1994).

Hormonal Changes

The endocrine system and its many hormones provide important regulatory signals for a variety of metabolic functions in the body. Of particular interest in resistance training are the anabolic hormones, such as testosterone, growth hormones, insulin, and growth factors, which help to stimulate development of the muscle and nerve tissues (Kraemer 1992a, 1992b). When an effective resistance exercise workout is performed, anabolic hormonal concentrations in serum increase above normal resting values during and after the workout (Kraemer, Gordon, et al; Kraemer et al. 1990, 1993), stimulating muscle remodeling and growth.

With age the endocrine system loses it ability to alter hormonal concentrations with exercise; reductions in resting concentrations of anabolic hormones are also observed with aging. Häkkinen and Pakarinen (1995) have demonstrated that for older men (70 yr) no changes take place in the circulating testosterone concentrations, whereas in younger (30 yr) and middle-aged men (50 yr) increases occur after a heavy resistance exercise protocol (i.e., five sets of 10 RM with 3-min rest between sets and exercises). This same pattern of change with aging was observed for growth hormone. Like men, older women also demonstrated a lack of growth hormone response to resistance training. Thus, testosterone and growth hormone responses to resistance exercise in older adults sup-

port the concept that the endocrine system is compromised with age (Chakravati and Collins 1976; Häkkinen and Pakarinen 1993; Hammond et al. 1974; Vermeulen, Rubens, and Verdonck 1972).

Ultimately this means that anabolic mechanisms related to tissue growth are affected by aging. Figure 11.5 reviews the hormonal changes to resistance exercise with aging. It is unclear whether or how a proper resistance training program can alter this change in the natural aging of the endocrine system. It might be that certain hormonal systems may be better maintained than others. In a case study of a 51-yr-old male competitive lifter, Fry and colleagues (Fry, Kraemer, et al. 1995) demonstrated that reductions in some hormonal responses to an exercise session took place despite over 35 yr of training. This older lifter had lower resting serum testosterone concentrations than young controls but a similar increase caused by response to exercise, whereas growth hormone did not change in response to resistance exercise. This study showed that despite long-term training the exercise-induced endocrine response was modified with age.

Nutritional Status

As individuals age, excess energy intake increases the fat stores. Positive energy balance and lack of activity are two of the major factors contributing to an increase in percent body fat and a decrease in percent muscle mass with aging. Meredith and co-workers (1992) supplemented the diet of a group of individuals with extra protein, carbohydrate, vitamins, minerals, and some fat, accounting for an additional 8 kcal and 0.33 g of protein per kilogram of ideal body mass per day. Another group did not receive the additional nutrients. A resistance training program was then undertaken for 12 wk. The supplemented-diet group showed a dramatic increase in muscle tissue, and changes in muscle size were proportional to caloric intake. Improved nutrition and better dietary management should enhance the effects of resistance training on muscle mass in older people. It appears that the need for adequate protein is vital for muscle hypertrophy in elderly people.

A resistance program for seniors should include exercise for all major muscle groups, so that many muscle fibers receive a stimulus for remodeling and hypertrophy. This means the muscle fibers will need additional protein. Without the needed protein and other nutrients, increases in lean body mass will be compromised. If a senior

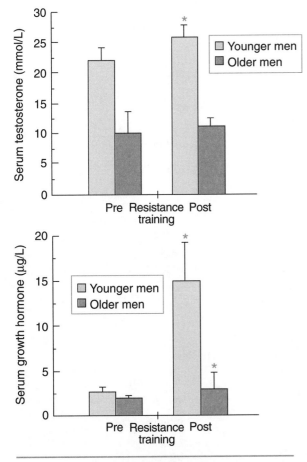

Fig. 11.5 Hormonal alterations with aging. * = significantly different from preexercise value. Data courtesy of Dr. William Kraemer's laboratory.

is undernourished, optimal adaptations to resistance training will not occur.

TRAINING ADAPTATIONS WITH AGE

A properly designed resistance training program can result in significant increases in muscle mass, muscle fiber hypertrophy, bone density, and strength-related performance improvements. At the present time, however, there is limited information concerning the long-term effect of resistance training on power output capabilities and endocrine function. Is it possible to actually produce improvements in the rate of force development and to shift the early portions of the force-time curve (0 to 200 ms) so more force can be produced quickly? It appears that it is theoretically possible, because improvements in neurological function indicating that force development can increase have been observed (A.B. Brown, McCartney, and Sale 1990; Moritani and DeVries 1980). No study has demonstrated that endocrine function can be restored with resistance exercise training. However, intensive investigation into these two areas of study is just starting to get underway. Table 11.2 reviews some of the adaptations with resistance exercise training in older people.

As a result of age-associated loss of muscle mass and strength, a great deal of attention has been focused on strategies for prevention or reversal of these losses. Resistance training has been demonstrated to be an effective means of increasing

TABLE 11.2
Basic Resistance Exercise Training Adaptations in Older Adults (60 yr and Older)

Experimental variable	Response
Muscle strength (1 RM)	Increased
Muscle power (30% of 1 RM)	No change*
Muscle fiber size	Increased (both types)
Isokinetic peak torque	
60°/s	Increased
240°/s	Increased, but less than 60°
Cross-sectional thigh muscle size	Increased
Regional bone mineral density	Increased
Total bone mineral density (men)	No change
Bone mineral density	No changes or increase
Pain levels	Decreased*
Intraabdominal fat	Decreased*
% fat	Decreased
Daily tasks	Improved
Gastrointestinal motility	Improved*
Flexibility	No change (unclear)*
Back strength	Increased
Peak oxygen consumption	Increased
Psychological factors	Positive effects
Neural factors	Enhanced*
Twitch half relaxation time	Increased*
Rate of force development	No change*

* Scientific data to make definite conclusions about training adaptations is limited.

strength and improving functional status in the elderly. Aniansson and Gustafsson (1981) demonstrated that a low-intensity resistance training regimen produced limited results, which led them to conclude that the elderly have a lower capacity to respond to strengthening exercises than younger people. Moritani and DeVries (1980) examined a higher-intensity training program in older men and concluded that the capacity for the elderly to increase strength is preserved. They also concluded that skeletal muscle has a reduced capacity for hypertrophy. They were unable to detect any evidence of muscle hypertrophy, however, but their methods were indirect, consisting of limb circumferences and skinfold determinations to estimate muscle size. Fiatarone and colleagues (1990) examined a group of very old (87- to 96-yr-old) men and women who trained the knee extensors for 8 wk. This study was the first to demonstrate that the capacity for muscle strength improvement is preserved even in the very old. This study also demonstrated a significant increase in muscle size using CAT scans.

Frontera and co-workers (1988) trained a group of sedentary older men (age 60 to 72 yr) using a high-intensity resistance training regimen (three sets of eight repetitions at 80% of 1 RM, 3 d/wk for 12 wk). The men demonstrated substantial strength gains (up to 200% increase in 1 RM), and computerized tomography and muscle biopsy analysis showed evidence of muscle hypertrophy. The capacity for high-intensity resistance training to increase muscle fiber size has also been demonstrated in older women. Charette and co-workers (1991) examined muscle biopsies taken before and after 12 wk of high-intensity resistance training and found an increase in Type II fiber area with no significant change in Type I area.

More recently Fiatarone and colleagues (1994) examined a larger group of very old, frail men and women and demonstrated that high-intensity resistance training (80% of 1 RM for 10 wk) is safe for this population and produced significant increases in strength but no significant increase in muscle size. It is important to note that the increase in strength was associated with an increase in gait speed, stair-climbing power, balance, and overall spontaneous activity.

Recent research efforts have focused on the effects of resistance training on muscle protein metabolism. W.W. Campbell and co-workers (1995) examined nitrogen balance before and after 12 wk of high-intensity resistance training (three sets of eight repetitions, 80% of 1 RM, upper- and lower-

body exercises) in a group of older men and women. They found that resistance training increases nitrogen retention. In addition, constant infusion of ^{13}Cleucine revealed that the training resulted in a significant increase in rate of whole-body protein synthesis.

In another study Yarasheski, Zachwieja, and Bier (1993) determined the rate of quadriceps muscle protein synthesis using the in vivo incorporation rate of intravenously infused ^{13}Cleucine into mixed-muscle protein in both young (24 yr) and older (63 to 66 yr) men and women before and at the end of 2 wk of resistance exercise training (2 to 4 sets of 4 to 10 repetitions at 60% to 90% of 1 RM, 5 d/wk). They observed that, although the older subjects had a lower rate of muscle protein synthesis before the training, both young and old subjects in the resistance exercise group experienced a significant increase in muscle protein synthesis. It is interesting to note that although growth hormone administration has been suggested as an anabolic agent (Rudman et al. 1990), when growth hormone administration is combined with resistance training, it does not cause any greater increase in muscle mass than training alone (Yarasheski et al. 1992). This finding indicates that the hormonal system in older individuals still functions to the extent needed to make some adaptations to resistance training.

While many resistance training studies have examined short-term adaptations in the elderly, only a few have examined strength and body composition changes during long training periods of 52 wk or greater. Morganti and co-workers (1995) examined 39 healthy women (59 ± 0.9 yr) who were randomly assigned to either a control group or a progressive resistance training group (three sets of eight repetitions, 80% of 1 RM, upper- and lower-body exercises) that trained twice weekly for 12 mo. Strength continued to improve with no evidence of plateauing during the 12 mo of the study. In the lat pull-down, knee extension, and leg press the greatest changes in strength were seen in the first 3 mo of the study. However, smaller but statistically significant increases were seen in the second 6 mo of the study.

Using a similar population of older women, Nelson and colleagues (1994) demonstrated that high-intensity resistance training had significant effects on bone health, with increases reported in femoral and lumbar spine density after 1 yr of training. In addition, the resistance training resulted in an improvement in balance, total level of physical activity, and muscle mass. Thus, resistance training has an effect on most of the major risk factors for an osteoporotic bone fracture.

It is clear that the capacity to adapt to increased levels of physical activity is preserved even in the very old. Regularly performed exercise has been demonstrated to result in a remarkable number of positive changes in elderly men and women. Because sarcopenia and weakness may be an almost universal characteristic of advancing age, strategies for preserving or increasing muscle mass in the elderly should be implemented. With increasing muscle strength, increased levels of spontaneous activity have been seen in both healthy, free-living older subjects and very old, frail men and women. Resistance training, in addition to its positive effects on bone density, energy metabolism, and functional status, may also be an important way to increase levels of physical activity in the elderly. Resistance training may be one of the most effective and least costly ways to preserve independent living in a wide segment of the population (Rogers and Evans 1993).

DEVELOPING A RESISTANCE TRAINING PROGRAM

The fundamental principles of resistance training program design are the same no matter what the trainees' ages. Because of variations in the functional capacity of many older individuals, the best program is individualized to meet the needs and medical concerns of each person. At present, periodized training has been used in only one training study for older adults (Newton et al. 1995), and more information on training variation is needed to optimize training for older adults.

It has been shown that higher-intensity resistance exercise (80% of 1 RM) can be tolerated and results in positive adaptations in the very old. Some data indicate that the intensity must be carefully applied so as not to initiate an overtraining syndrome in older adults (Hunter and Treuth 1995). It is quite possible that recovery from a training session takes longer, and the use of varied intensities in a periodized format may allow for more optimal adaptation. The resistance training programs used in most studies have been quite fundamental in design and have had positive results. Thus, in the early phases of training, advanced program design may not be required. Furthermore, many middle-aged and older adults may require an initial training period to get into shape before they can train at the level needed to make training ad-

aptations in the muscle later in a training program. A basic overview of programs that have been used for older adults is shown in table 11.3.

It is important to appreciate that the starting level of strength fitness in the frail elderly may be close to zero with a maximal force capability of only a couple of pounds. A progressive resistance training program may mean that an older individual may lift only 0.5 lb (0.2 kg) during a set. Thus, the resistance needed at the start of a program is minimal in many situations. Choosing the proper equipment to allow manipulations of such low resistance increments also calls for some care.

NEEDS ANALYSIS

The process for developing a strength training program for older adults has been outlined. It consists of pretesting and evaluation, setting individualized goals, designing a program, and developing evaluation methods. In older adults, resistance training should be part of a lifelong fitness lifestyle, so continual reevaluation of program goals and program design is necessary for optimal results and adherence. The American College of Sports Medicine (1995) has advised that people who start an exercise program be classified into one of three risk categories:

1. Apparently healthy individuals with no more than one coronary risk factor (e.g., hypertension, smoking)

2. Individuals who have signs or symptoms suggestive of possible cardiopulmonary or metabolic disease or with two or more major coronary risk factors

3. Individuals with known cardiac, pulmonary, or metabolic disease

Consultation with and consent of a physician are recommended in all cases, with additional functional exercise testing for class 3 recommended by the ACSM. If only a resistance training program is to be used in the fitness program, it is common to use a strength test or exercise protocol to evaluate individuals for symptoms specific to the exercise modality. One-RM strength testing and resistance exercise workouts using as much as 75% of 1 RM have been shown to result in fewer cardiopulmonary symptoms than graded treadmill exercise tests in cardiac patients with good left ventricular function (Faigenbaum et al. 1990). Resistance exercise that is not performed with a Valsalva maneuver is

> ### TABLE 11.3
> #### General Characteristics of Resistance Training Programs for Older Adults
>
> **Choice of exercise**
>
> The primary exercises focus on large muscle group exercises: 4-6 large muscle groups; 3-5 supplemental small muscle group exercises are usually added. Barbells, isokinetic machines, pneumatic machines, and stack plate machines have all been used.
>
> **Order of exercise**
>
> A warm-up is usually followed by exercising large muscle groups. This is followed by smaller muscle group exercise and cool-down activities.
>
> **Resistance used**
>
> The most common percentage that has been used is 80% of 1 RM for 8 repetitions. Studies have used varied resistances of 50%-85% of 1 RM; resistances rotated across days of 3-5 RM, 8-10 RM, and 6-8 RM or 6-8 repetitions with a resistance of 12-15 RM; half pyramid of 10 repetitions at 50% of 10 RM set 1, 75% of 10 RM set 2, and 100% of 10 RM set 3; and 8-12 RM.
>
> **Number of sets**
>
> Typically three sets are performed. Progression can go from one to three sets over training time. Tolerance of three sets has been shown by even the frail elderly.
>
> **Rest between sets and exercises**
>
> Typically 2-3 min have been used. Shorter rest periods have been associated with very light resistances where recovery is quicker.

considered a safe form of exercise but should be specifically evaluated in each individual case. The needs analysis and development of program goals should follow the steps outlined in chapter 5. The fundamental principles of training previously discussed in this text must be considered in the design and progression of a program for an older individual.

Evaluation of training progress should include strength testing (if possible on the equipment used in training), determination of body composition, functional abilities testing (e.g., walking, getting out of chair), measuring muscle size changes, nutritional assessment, and medical tracking of preexisting conditions.

Choice of Exercise

The choice of exercise varies when working with older adults in ways similar for any individual. At least one exercise for all the major muscle groups should be included in the program. The equipment used has to fit the individual, and the resistance used must accommodate the individual's functional capacity.

The progression of exercises throughout the program should activate as much of the skeletal muscle mass as possible so that adaptation can take place. Furthermore, use of only linear movements may not address some of the more common movement patterns in everyday life (e.g., twisting, turning).

On some machines even the minimal resistance is too great, and older adults can have difficulty producing the initial force to start the exercise movement. Also, the increments in resistance on some machines are too large, especially at the lighter resistances, to allow a smooth progression in resistance. Some modalities, such as isokinetics, pneumatics, or hydraulics, allow for easier initiation of the exercise movement and a smooth progression in the resistance used.

Programs have used all types of resistance tools, from free weights, food cans of different sizes, rubber tubing, or water-filled milk cartons. With any of these types of equipment, care must be taken that proper range of motion can be attained and that the individual can safely control the resistance throughout the full range of motion. Despite using the full range of motion in exercise training, older adults may need to supplement full range of motion resistance exercise training with specific flexibility exercise training (Hurley 1995).

Order of Exercise

Large–muscle group exercises are typically placed at the beginning of the workout. This reduces fatigue and allows for higher intensity or greater resistances in the large–muscle group exercises. Optimal stimulation of large muscle groups in the lower extremities (e.g., leg press, squat) and the upper body (e.g., bench press, seated rowing) should be a top priority in a program for older adults.

Rest Between Sets and Exercises

The rest between sets determines the metabolic demands of the resistance training workout. It can also produce a reduction in the resistance used if recovery is not sufficient before the next set or exercise is initiated. Because activation of muscle tissue depends on the resistance and the total amount of work performed, rest period lengths should be consistent with the program goals. Short rest periods can be used in circuit programs. The rest periods should be longer if heavier resistances are used and can be shortened as exercise tolerance is enhanced. The amount of rest is also dictated by the medical condition of the individual. For some older adults (e.g., those with type I diabetes) gains in strength are the major goal, so care must be taken not to create a metabolic stress by not properly controlling the length of rest between sets and exercises.

Number of Sets

The number of sets depends on the exercise volume desired. The volume of exercise that can be tolerated is initially low but increases as training continues. One-set programs are the simplest starting point. Single-set programs are typically used in the early phases of a program or when a person's exercise tolerance is low. According to the principle of progressive resistance training, the volume is increased by increasing the number of sets, so that the muscle starts to tolerate a higher volume of exercise. Usually programs for older adults do not involve more than three or four sets of a given exercise. If the muscle group needs more stimulation, another exercise for that muscle group can be added to the program. In addition, many programs for older adults use a warm-up set at a low per-

centage of the RM prior to performing a heavier set.

Resistance Used

The amount of resistance that can be tolerated by frail elderly adults in their 90s is at least 80% of 1 RM. The resistance needs to be carefully evaluated so that optimal increases occur. Hunter and Treuth (1995) found that training with lighter resistances (50% to 60% of 1 RM) results in greater increases in the 1 RM in older women than training with heavier resistances (70% to 80% of 1 RM). Program periodization appears to have potential in resistance training programs for older adults (Newton et al. 1995). But it is clear from the work done in the 1980s and early 1990s that older men and women can tolerate and positively adapt to heavy weight training programs (Fiatarone and Evans 1993).

Number of Repetitions

The resistance used and the number of repetitions performed affects the training adaptations in all populations, including the elderly. However, because of their high prevalence in older adults, cardiovascular problems and risks must also be carefully considered for safety reasons. A set performed to concentric failure results in higher blood pressures and heart rates than a set not performed to failure. In addition, performing sets to concentric failure using resistances in the range of 50% to 90% of 1 RM results in blood pressures that are higher than sets to failure below and above this range. The highest blood pressures and heart rates normally occur in the last few repetitions of a set. Therefore, for safety reasons it is recommended that older adults, especially those with cardiovascular problems or risks, do not perform sets to concentric failure, especially in the range of 50% to 90% of 1 RM. Performance of a Valsalva maneuver should also be discouraged in this population.

Designing a resistance program for older adults should follow the careful planning guidelines used for younger individuals. The program design, however, needs to consider health concerns of older adults such as cardiovascular problems and arthritis. Examples of total body workouts for older adults are described in table 11.4.

SUMMARY

We have discussed the positive and negative aspects of older adults' participation in resistance

TABLE 11.4
Example Resistance Training Programs for Seniors

Beginning home program

- For upper-body exercises, use soup cans or light resistance (2- to 5-lb [0.9- to 2.3-kg] hand dumbbells).
- Perform 1-3 sets of 8-10 repetitions.
- Take 1-2 min rest between sets and exercises.
- Concentrate on full range of motion movement and balance. A wall or solid chair can be used for help with balance in the beginning. Keep head up.
- Exercises: front shoulder raise, wall push-ups, standing single knee lifts, toe raises, arm curls, good-morning exercise, side bends, standing knee curls, single-arm shoulder press, 1/4 squat, single bent-over arm rows, side shoulder raise.

Program note: This is a light-resistance, calisthenic program to gain basic movement and range of motion abilities. Progression to heavier resistances, especially for the lower-body musculature, is vital for optimal progression.

Beginning program in the weight room

- Exercises: leg press, knee extensions, knee curls, calf raises, bench press, seated rows, upright rows, arm curls
- Order of exercises: large– to small–muscle group exercises
- Resistance used: 80% of 1 RM or 10-15 RM
- Number of sets: Start out with one and progress to three over a 12-wk program
- Rest between sets and exercises: 2-3 min or until recovered

Periodized program for weight room and long-term use

Use a 12-wk cycle (e.g., Mon., Wed., Fri.) followed by an active rest of 2 wk, and then repeat the cycle with appropriate variation in the program variables based on training goals and needs of the individual.

- Exercises: leg press/squats, knee extensions, knee curls, calf raises, bench press, seated rows, upright rows, arm curls
- Order of exercises: large– to small–muscle group exercises
- Resistance used: 8-10 RM (M), 3-5 RM (W), 12-15 RM (F)
- Number of sets: Start out with one and progress to three over the 12-wk cycle
- Rest between sets and exercises: 2-3 min (M), 3-4 min (W), 1-2 min (F)

training programs. The benefits to older adults are reported to be increased strength, endurance, muscle capacity, and flexibility; more energy; and improved self-image and confidence. The negative aspects include some pain or stiffness and other nonspecific problems. The positive and negative aspects of resistance training are therefore very similar to those in younger populations. Scientific investigations over the past 10 years have demonstrated that resistance training can be safely and successfully implemented in older populations. Even the frail and very sick elderly can benefit and improve their quality of life. Proper design and progression of a resistance training program for older adults is vital to optimal benefits from resistance exercise.

SELECTED READINGS

Brown, A.B.; McCartney, N.; and Sale, D.G. 1990. Positive adaptations to weight-lifting training in the elderly. *Journal of Applied Physiology* 69:1725-33.

Doherty, T.J.; Vandervoort, A.A.; Taylor, A.W.; and Brown, W.F. 1993. Effects of motor unit losses on strength in older men and women. *Journal of Applied Physiology* 74:868-74.

Evans, W.J., and Campbell, W.W. 1993. Sarcopenia and age-related changes in body composition and functional capacity. *Journal of Nutrition* 123:465-68.

Fiatarone, M.A.; O'Neill, E.F.; Ryan, N.D.; Clements, K.M.; Solares, G.R.; Nelson, M.E.; Roberts, S.B.; Kehayias, J.J.; Lipsitz, L.A.; and Evans, W.J. 1994. Exercise training and nutritional supplementation for physical frailty in very elderly people. *New England Journal of Medicine* 330:1769-75.

Frontera, W.R.; Meredith, C.N.; O'Reilly, K.P.; Knuttgen, H.G.; and Evans, W.J. 1988. Strength conditioning in older men: Skeletal muscle hypertrophy and improved function. *Journal of Applied Physiology* 64:1038-44.

Häkkinen, K.; Pastinen, U.M.; Karsikas, R.; and Linnamo, V. 1995. Neuromuscular performance in voluntary bilateral and unilateral contraction and during electrical stimulation in men at different ages. *European Journal of Applied Physiology* 70:518-27.

Hurley, B. 1995. Strength training in the elderly to enhance health status. *Medicine, Exercise, Nutrition and Health* 4:217-29.

Meredith, C.N.; Frontera, W.R.; O'Reilly, K.P.; and Evans, W.J. 1992. Body composition in elderly men: Effect of dietary modification during strength training. *Journal of the American Geriatric Society* 40:155-62.

Nelson, M.E.; Fiatarone, M.A.; Morganti, C.M.; Trice, I.; Greenberg, R.A.; and Evans, W.J. 1994. Effects of high-intensity strength training on multiple risk factors for osteoporotic fractures. *Journal of the American Medical Association* 272:1909-14.

Rogers, M.A., and Evans, W.J. 1993. Changes in skeletal muscle with aging: Effects of exercise training. In *Exercise and sport sciences reviews*, ed. J.O. Holloszy, vol. 21. Baltimore: Williams and Wilkins.

Young, A., and Skelton, D.A. 1994. Applied physiology of strength and power in old age. *International Journal of Sports Medicine* 15:149-51.

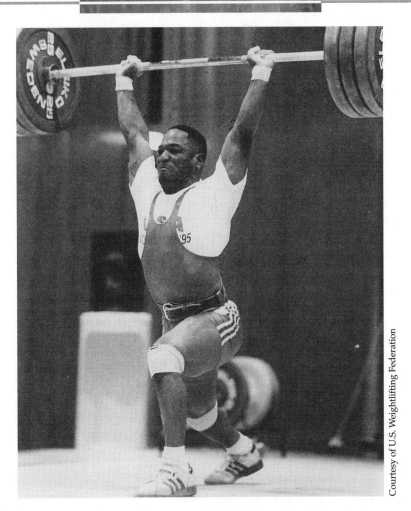

Courtesy of U.S. Weightlifting Federation

Resistance Training Sports

M any fitness training programs have their origin in competitive resistance sports. The folklore that surrounds resistance training originated from the resistance sports of body building, power lifting, and Olympic weight lifting. A great deal of empirical evidence about training has been generated by athletes in these sports (Kraemer and Koziris 1994). Consequently, when resistance training became popular, coaches, athletes, and fitness enthusiasts looked to athletes in resistance sports for help in designing exercise programs. It is important for coaches to understand the resistance training sports but also to realize that programs for those sports have very specific goals and needs.

Patterning a program after body building, power lifting, or Olympic weight lifting is appropriate if the trainee is interested in one of these sports. If the trainee is an athlete in another sport or is simply interested in basic muscular fitness, using a program for a resistance training sport may not be appropriate for that athlete's individual needs. Using

231

a resistance training sport program for other sports and fitness is a common mistake in resistance exercise prescription. A trainer who has a background in one of the resistance training sports must draw upon more than just his or her own competitive training experience to successfully develop programs for most people.

When examining published examples of competitive styles of training, it is important to realize that these training techniques are used by weight trainers with years of training experience. Some routines are too advanced for beginning and novice weight trainers. It is important to use the wealth of information available from the resistance training sports when designing a goal-specific training program. However, the goals of the resistance sports must be kept in mind when using their training concepts. The purpose of this chapter is to review the three resistance training sports and the general concepts used in the different training programs they employ.

OLYMPIC WEIGHT LIFTING

Weight lifting has been a part of the Olympic program for men since 1896. The first World Championship in weight lifting for women was held in 1987, and weight lifting is currently an Olympic demonstration sport for women.

Olympic weight-lifting competition is made up of two lifts: the snatch and the clean and jerk. Before 1972 a third lift called the standing press was also used in competition (Fair 1988). The objective in the snatch is to lift the barbell from the floor to an extended-arms overhead position in one continuous motion. The clean and jerk is actually two separate movements. The first (clean) is lifting the barbell in one continuous motion from the floor to a position resting on the front of the shoulders. The second (jerk) involves lifting the barbell to an extended-arms overhead position as shown in figure 12.1. The lifter must finish both lifts in an erect standing posture and have the barbell under control. As in power lifting, the goal is to total as much weight as possible in the competitive lifts. Each competitor is permitted three attempts for each of the competitive lifts. The competitor chooses his or her starting weight for each of the competitive lifts. After each attempt, whether successful or not, the lifter may choose to increase the weight on the bar for the next attempt. The nature of the competition makes the major training goal to increase maximal strength and power. Extensive reviews of

the training protocols used by various nations have been presented by Garhammer and Takano (1992). Totten and Javorek (1988) have detailed the United States Weightlifting Federation's approach to developmental training of weight lifters.

Acute Program Variables in Olympic Weight Lifting

The majority of exercises used in training are variations of the two competitive lifts. A major component of both competitive lifts is the pull. The object of the pull is to get the weight as high as possible off the floor before moving underneath it. The pull can be divided into two portions: from the floor to just above the knees and from just above the knees to as high as possible. Front and back squats also constitute a major portion of the training.

Choice of Exercise. The legs, shoulders, and entire back are the main muscle groups involved in the pulling movement. However, shoulder and arm strength are needed to get the weight overhead and hold it there. Because of the explosive nature of this sport and the need to balance the weight overhead, a large amount of training time must also be dedicated to perfecting technique of the two competitive lifts.

Order of Exercise. The order of exercise varies with the training period. For example, during the preparatory phase, squats and pulls might be performed early in a workout. In a competitive phase, squats and pulls would be performed later in a workout after performing full cleans and full snatches.

Training sessions normally include few single-joint or small–muscle group exercises. Many lifters perform abdominal and low-back exercises to strengthen the torso, because strength in this area is needed when supporting heavy weights overhead and during the pull of the competitive lifts. The abdominal exercises are also performed to help prevent low-back problems. These exercises are normally performed late in a training session.

Resistance. The goal of this sport is to lift the heaviest weight possible in the competitive lifts. To prepare the muscles to do this, heavy resistances (1 RM to 6 RM) must be used. Lighter resistances (8 RM to 10 RM), however, are used during preparatory training phases and for assistance exercises such as back extensions. The resistances used—especially for variations of the clean and snatch such as clean-and-snatch pulls, power cleans, and power snatches—are frequently calculated from the lifter's best clean, jerk, and snatch weights.

Number of Sets. The number of sets can vary considerably from training session to training session. Up to six sets of each exercise are typically performed per training session. However, some programs call for up to 12 sets of some exercises at various points in the training cycle.

Rest Periods. As in power lifting, the rest periods between sets and exercises are related to the resistances used. Rest periods are typically in the range of 3 to 4 min and can become longer when near 1-RM resistances are used. This allows sufficient recovery, so the exercises can be performed with good technique and heavy resistances.

Sample Olympic Lifting Program

Olympic lifters use periodized programs. Therefore, there is a great deal of variation in training sessions, depending on when in the training year a session occurs. Attention to technique during all exercises is necessary to develop the skill needed to lift the heaviest possible weight. In addition, most

exercises are performed in an explosive manner to develop the power needed to accelerate the weight during the pull phase of the competitive lifts.

Many lifters perform two training sessions per day to increase the total training volume and to maintain high training intensity (tables 12.1 and 12.2). Training is normally performed 4 to 6 d/wk. The notation used in the tables represents sets × repetitions at a percentage of 1 RM. For example, 3 × 2 at 60% means three sets of two repetitions each using 60% of 1 RM. A question mark means the weight varies, based on the individual lifter's strength.

POWER LIFTING

Although not an Olympic sport, power lifting has increased dramatically in popularity throughout the world over the past 20 years. Power lifting gained Amateur Athletic Union (AAU) acceptance only in the early 1960s. The first official U.S. National Power Lifting Championships for men were held in 1965. Based on memberships in national

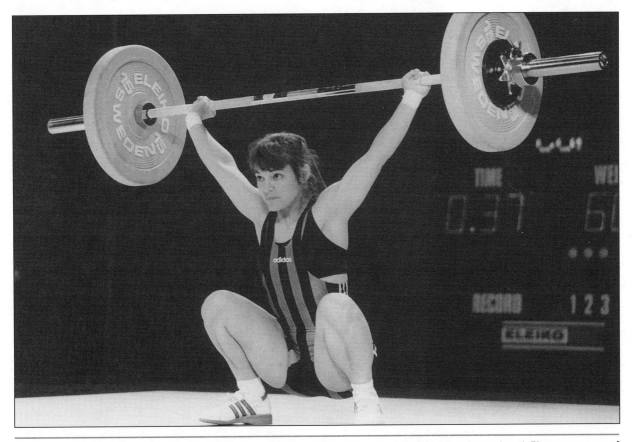

Fig. 12.1 An Olympic weight lifter in the bottom position of a snatch after catching the bar overhead. Photo courtesy of U.S. Weightlifting Federation.

TABLE 12.1
Sample Olympic Lifting Program: Preparatory Phase

Monday

A.M.

Overhead press 3 × 2 at 60%, 3 × 2 at 70%
Snatch 3 × 2 at 60%, 3 × 2 at 70%,
    2 × 2 at 80%
Back squat 3 × 3 at 60%, 4 × 2 at 70%,
    3 × 2 at 80%

P.M.

Hang-clean 3 × 3 at 60%, 3 × 2 at 70%,
    3 × 2 at 80%
Clean pull 2 × 4 at 70%, 2 × 4 at 80%,
    2 × 4 at 85%
Back extension 4 × 10 at ?

Tuesday

A.M.

Power clean 3 × 3 at 60%, 3 × 3 at 70%,
    3 × 2 at 80%
Power snatch 3 × 3 at 60%, 3 × 3 at 70%,
    2 × 2 at 80%
Jerk 3 × 3 at 70%, 2 × 2 at 80%
Romanian deadlift 5 × 5 at 80%

Wednesday

Rest

Thursday

A.M.

Back squat 2 × 5 at 70%, 2 × 5 at 80%,
    2 × 3 at 90%
Power clean 3 × 3 at 60%, 2 × 3 at 70%,
    2 × 2 at 80%
Jerk 2 × 3 at 70%, 2 × 3 at 80%,
    2 × 2 at 90%

P.M.

Hang snatch 3 × 3 at 65%, 2 × 3 at 75%,
    2 × 2 at 80%
Snatch pull 2 × 4 at 60%, 2 × 3 at 70%,
    2 × 3 at 80%
Romanian deadlift 5 × 5 at 80%

Friday

A.M.

Full snatch 3 × 3 at 65%, 3 × 3 at 75%,
    3 × 3 at 85%
Snatch pull 3 × 4 at 70%, 3 × 4 at 80%,
    3 × 3 at 90%
Hang-clean 3 × 3 at 60%, 3 × 3 at 70%,
    3 × 2 at 80%
Front squat 3 × 5 at 70%, 2 × 4 at 80%,
    2 × 3 at 90%

Saturday

A.M.

Overhead press 1 × 4 at 60%, 1 × 4 at 70%,
    2 × 3 at 80%
Clean 3 × 3 at 60%, 2 × 3 at 70%,
    2 × 3 at 80%
Back squat 2 × 5 at 60%, 2 × 5 at 70%,
    2 × 5 at 80%

P.M.

Hang-snatch 3 × 3 at 60%, 2 × 3 at 70%,
    2 × 2 at 75%
Snatch pull 3 × 4 at 70%, 2 × 4 at 80%,
    2 × 4 at 90%
Back extension 4 × 10 at ?

Sunday

Rest

TABLE 12.2
Sample Olympic Lifting Program: Competitive Phase

Monday

A.M.

Snatch 3 × 3 at 70%, 3 × 2 at 80%,
  2 × 2 at 90%
Clean and jerk 2 × 3 at 70%, 2 × 2 at 80%,
  2 × 2 at 90%, 2 × 1 at 100% (jerk only in
  last repetition in a set)
Jerk 1 × 2 at 70%, 1 × 2 at 80%,
  1 × 2 at 90%, 1 × 2 at 100%

P.M.

Front squat 3 × 2 at 70%, 3 × 2 at 90%,
  3 × 2 at 100%
Snatch pull 2 × 3 at 70%, 1 × 3 at 80%,
  1 × 3 at 90%, 1 × 3 at 100%
Back extension 3 × 10 at ?

Tuesday

A.M.

Power snatch 3 × 2 at 65%, 2 × 2 at 75%,
  2 × 2 at 85%
Power clean 3 × 2 at 65%, 2 × 2 at 75%,
  2 × 2 at 85%
Clean pull 3 × 2 at 80%, 2 × 2 at 90%,
  2 × 2 at 100%
Back squat 2 × 3 at 70%, 2 × 3 at 80%,
  2 × 3 at 90%
Overhead press 2 × 3 at 65%, 2 × 3 at 75%

Wednesday

Rest

Thursday

A.M.

Snatch 2 × 3 at 70%, 2 × 2 at 80%,
  1 × 2 at 90%
Clean and jerk 2 × 2 at 75%, 2 × 2 at 85%,
  1 × 2 at 90% (jerk only in last repetition in
  a set)
Jerk 1 × 2 at 75%, 1 × 2 at 85%,
  1 × 2 at 90%

P.M.

Front squat 1 × 3 at 70%, 2 × 2 at 80%,
  2 × 2 at 90%
Snatch pull 2 × 3 at 60%, 2 × 3 at 70%,
  2 × 3 at 80%
Back extension 3 × 10 at ?

Friday

Hang-clean 1 × 3 at 60%, 2 × 2 at 70%,
  2 × 2 at 80%, 1 × 2 at 90%
Clean and jerk 1 × 3 at 60%, 2 × 2 at 70%,
  2 × 2 at 80% (jerk only in last repetition
  in a set)
Clean pull 2 × 3 at 70%, 3 × 2 at 80%,
  3 × 2 at 90%
Back squat 3 × 2 at 70%, 3 × 2 at 80%,
  3 × 2 at 90%

sport organizations and competitions held world-wide, there are 10 times more power lifting competitors than Olympic weight lifting competitors. This rapid rise in power lifting's popularity can be attributed to the facts that the power lifts are easy to learn and are similar to those used in typical weight training programs and that heavy weights can be lifted in competition (Hatfield 1981; Hatfield and McLaughlin 1985).

Power lifting has flourished in North America

because the lifts used in power lifting were identified by American football coaches as "strength" lifts, and the competitive lifts were therefore endorsed for use in conditioning programs. This led to extensive participation in power lifting by athletes who had played high school or college American football (Pullo 1992).

The three lifts in power lifting are the squat, the bench press, and the deadlift. The objective in the squat is to descend from a standing position with the barbell across the shoulders to a position in which the thighs are parallel to the floor and then to return to the erect starting position as shown in figure 12.2. In the bench press the lifter lies supine on a bench, lowers the barbell from an extended-arms position to the chest, and then pushes the barbell back to the starting position. In the deadlift the barbell is lifted from the floor to thigh level, and the lifter ends in an erect standing position. Many different types of programs are used by competitive power lifters (Hatfield 1981; Kraemer and Koziris 1994; Todd 1978). However, in all cases the major training goal is to lift as much as possible for one repetition in the three competitive lifts.

Acute Program Variables in Power Lifting

Training for power lifting emphasizes practice of the three competitive lifts: the squat, bench press, and deadlift.

Choice of Exercise. Assistance exercises are chosen to develop the strength of the muscles that assist or stabilize prime movers or are prime movers for the competitive lifts. Assistance exercises might include flys, back extensions, and decline presses.

Order of Exercise. The usual progression is from the larger–muscle group exercises (the competitive lifts) to the smaller–muscle group exercises (assistance exercises). This progression helps to ensure that the practice of the competitive lifts is completed before fatigue of smaller muscle groups limits their performance. Only coaches' and athletes' anecdotal observations support the use of this common exercise order.

Resistance. Because the criterion of power lifting is 1-RM strength, almost all resistances used are heavy (i.e., 1 RM to 8 RM). Ten- and 12-RM resistances are used for warm-ups or during a high-volume, low-intensity period. Most power lifters avoid frequent training with 1-RM resistances. Although the reasons for this are highly

speculative and influenced by individual preferences, most lifters want to train as heavily as they can with other RM resistances (e.g., 2 RM to 6 RM) and hope to see an increase in the 1 RM after a period of training. Since progress in 1-RM strength in advanced lifters is slow and the absolute magnitudes of increase can be very small (e.g., 1 kg to 3 kg), many athletes do not want to face such slow progress day to day. In training, the use of a different resistance for each set is popular. For example, an ascending half pyramid involves lifting heavier and heavier resistances for each set (e.g., 8 RM, 6 RM, 4 RM, and 2 RM).

Number of Sets. The number of sets typically ranges from 3 to 10 for a primary exercise, followed by 3 or 4 sets of assistance exercises. Because sets will determine the volume of the workout, different numbers of sets are used to vary the volume of exercise over a training period.

Rest Periods. In power lifting, rest periods are relatively long (e.g., 2 to 7 min) and are related to the intensity of the previous sets; the heavier the resistance, the longer the rest period. This allows recovery between sets so the heaviest possible resistance for each set can be used.

Training Styles

In addition to pyramid programming, multiple sets, and periodized programs, many other program styles are used to train for power lifting, including

- forced repetition,
- eccentric (negative) training,
- functional isometrics, and
- periodization.

The periodization of training used by power lifters is very similar to that of Olympic weight lifters in that the year-long program includes a preparatory period, a competitive period, and a transition period. The major difference is that the amount of workout time that must be dedicated to skill practice of the lifts in power lifting is dramatically less.

During the preparatory period, emphasis is not placed on technique development, and the power lifter therefore can use heavier resistances earlier in the training period. As in training for Olympic weight lifting, the competitive period is dedicated to participation in power-lifting meets and the transition period has lower intensity and volume, which allows for rest and recovery. Because of the much heavier resistances used in training and competition, the transition period may be longer in the sport of power lifting than in Olympic weight lifting. A typical power-lifting cycle is shown in table 12.3, table 12.4 gives a typical week's training program schedule, and table 12.5 shows a sample power-lifting program for 8 wk of training leading up to competition.

TABLE 12.3
Typical Power-Lifting Cycle

Time	Load	Frequency of training
4 wk	10 RM	3-4 d/wk
4 wk	6 RM	4 d/wk
4 wk	3 RM	5 d/wk
4 wk	2-3 RM	6 d/wk

POWER PRODUCTION: WEIGHT LIFTING VERSUS POWER LIFTING

The Olympic lifts have been extensively analyzed, and the total power output of the snatch is similar to that of the clean phase of the clean and jerk (Garhammer 1980, 1981b, 1989; Häkkinen, Alén, and Komi 1984). The power output of a lift depends on which portion of the lifting movement is analyzed. The clean portion includes two pull phases: from the floor to the knees and from the knees until the bar reaches maximal upward velocity. The jerk portion consists of moving the bar from the finished clean position to the overhead position. For example, a 125-kg man attempting a 260.5-kg clean-and-jerk-lift can produce average power of 4191 W for the entire pull, 6981 W in the second pull, and 4570 W during the jerk (Garhammer 1993). Typically, the power output of the jerk is similar to that of the top pull of the snatch and of the clean (Garhammer 1981a, 1982-83, 1985, 1991a, 1991b).

A 100-kg power lifter deadlifting or squat-lifting 375 kg would produce 1274 W, considerably less than the power output of the clean or snatch (Garhammer 1993). Other studies confirm this difference (Garhammer and McLaughlin 1980). A 75-kg power lifter bench-pressing 200 kg would produce 343 W, or 4.6 W per kilogram of body

TABLE 12.4
Sample Power-Lifting Program

Monday

Bench press: 10, 8, 6, 4, 2, 2 (a pyramid program), or periodization cycle of RM loads as in table 12.3 over each 4-wk time period
Assistance exercises
    Incline press: 8, 8, 8
    Press behind neck: 8, 8, 8
    Triceps extension: 8, 8, 8
    Biceps curl: 10, 10, 10

Sit-up (bent leg) with load: 2 × 20
Crunch: 10, 10, 10
Calf raise: 10, 10, 10

Tuesday

Squat: 10, 8, 6, 4, 2, 2 (pyramid program), or periodization cycle of RM loads as in table 12.3 over each 4-wk time period
Assistance exercises
    Lat pull-down: 8, 8, 8
    Seated row: 8, 8, 8
    T-bar row: 8, 8, 8
    Upright row: 10, 10, 10
    Knee extension: 10, 10, 10
    Knee curl: 10, 10, 10

Thursday

Bench press (close-grip): 6 × 8 (light day)
Assistance exercises
    Incline bench: 8, 8, 8
    Press behind neck: 8, 8, 8
    Triceps extension: 8, 8, 8
    Biceps curl: 10, 10, 10

Sit-up (bent leg): 20, 20, 20
Hanging knee-up: 10, 10, 10
Calf raise: 10, 10, 10

Friday

Deadlift: 10, 8, 6, 4, 2, 2 (pyramid program), or periodization cycle of RM loads as in table 12.3 over each 4-wk time period
Squats: 6 sets of 8
Assistance exercises
    Lat pull-down: 8, 8, 8
    Seated row: 8, 8, 8
    T-bar row: 8, 8, 8
    Knee extension (doubles): 6, 6, 6, 6
    Knee curl: 10, 10, 10

Wednesday is a day of complete rest and Saturday and Sunday are days of active rest.

All repetitions are RM resistances (e.g., 8 = 8 RM) unless otherwise noted. Warm-up and stretching exercises (not listed) are performed before and after each workout.

TABLE 12.5
Typical 8-wk Cycle for Contest Preparation for Trained Power Lifters

Week	Monday	Tuesday	Wednesday	Thursday	Friday	Saturday
1	Bench, assistance 75%-80% × 5 × 8-10	Squat and deadlift, assistance 75%-80% × 5 × 8-10	Bench, assistance 75%-80% × 5 × 8-10	Squat and deadlift, assistance 75%-80% × 5 × 8-10	Bench, assistance 75%-80% × 5 × 8-10	Squat and deadlift, assistance 75%-80% × 5 × 8-10
2	Same as week 1, but cut assistance work to three sets of eight, and add the competitive lifts for two sets of five at 85%-90% 1 RM.					
3	Same as week 2, except drop to 2 × 8 for assistance exercises, and increase to 3 × 5 × 85%-90% for the competitive lifts.					
4	Bench, assistance 85% × 2 × 6-8 Bench 90%-95% × 3 × 2-3	Squat and deadlift, assistance 85% × 2 × 6-8 90%-95% × 3 × 2-3	Bench, assistance 85% × 5 × 3-5	Squat and deadlift, assistance 85% × 5 × 3-5	Bench, assistance 85% × 5 × 2-5	Squat and deadlift, assistance 85% × 5 × 3-5
5	Same as week 4. Use 3 × 3-5 for assistance work on Wednesday through Saturday, and add the competitive styles for 3 × 3 on Friday and Saturday.					
6	Bench, competitive style 85% × 2 × 5 90% × 3 × 3	Squat and deadlift, assistance to 90% × 5 × 5	Bench, assistance to 90% × 5 × 5	Rest	Bench, competitive style 85% × 2 × 5 95% × 3 × 3	Squat and deadlift, competitive style 90% × 2 × 5 95% × 3 × 3
7	Bench, competitive style 90% × 2 × 5 95% × 3 × 3 98% × 2 × 2	Squat and deadlift, competitive style 90% × 2 × 5 95% × 3 × 3 98% × 2 × 2	Rest	Competitive bench same as Monday	Competitive squat and deadlift same as Tuesday	Rest
8	Bench, competitive style 90% × 2 × 5 95% × 3 × 3 98% × 2 × 2	Squat and deadlift, competitive style to 80% for 3 or 4 single reps only	Rest	Squat, bench, and deadlift to 70% for 3 or 4 single reps only	Rest	Contest (each lift): 95% × 1 98% × 1 100% × 1

Notation used is percentage of 1 RM × number of sets × repetition range; assistance = assistance exercise for that competitive lift; competitive = higher RM weight emphasizing correct technique.

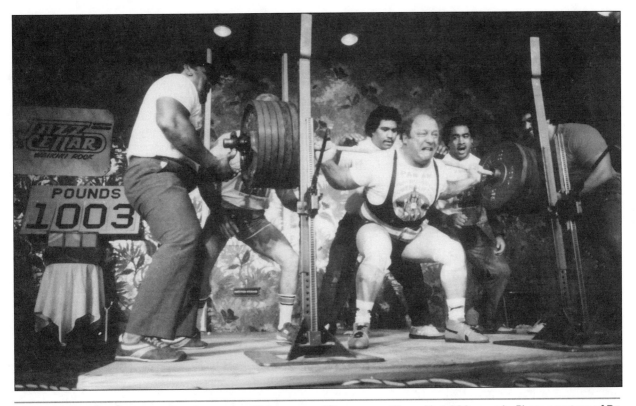

Fig. 12.2 Dr. Fred Hatfield performing a squat lift in a power lifting competition with 1,003 pounds. Photo courtesy of Dr. Fred Hatfield, Clearwater, FL.

weight. It is interesting to note that the sport called "power lifting" really does not have a high-power component but rather a high-force component.

BODY BUILDING

The sport of body building gained great popularity in the 1970s. Today there are many amateur and professional body-building competitions for men, women, and couples. Body builders have specific programs designed to address the needs for balanced muscular size, symmetry, and definition. Body builders also spend a great deal of time developing their posing ability and specific posing routines for competition. In a body-building competition each contestant is judged on the three characteristics of balanced muscularity in different compulsory poses (flexed and unflexed) and a free posing routine. Body builders must also pay attention to cosmetic appearance (e.g., tanned body, hair cut), which helps to enhance their competitiveness. Dietary habits that minimize body fat also play a large role in final preparations for the contest. Ultimately superior muscularity and mass, symmetry, harmony among different body parts, muscle den-

sity, and visible separation of muscles lead to success (Tesch 1992b).

As with any sport, body building has a wide range of training styles. There are, however, several basic components to all body-building programs. Body building is one of the more metabolically strenuous resistance training sports, as it is common opinion that body builders have to "punish themselves" in order to see progress (Tesch 1992b). Whether this is true or not, some of the highest blood lactate concentrations (over 20 mmol/L) have been observed with body-building workouts (Kraemer et al. 1987).

Acute Program Variables in Body Building

Body-building workouts, in general, contain more exercises than those of the other resistance training sports. This stems from the belief that working a particular muscle at different angles and with several exercises will lead to optimal gains in muscle size. The use of many different exercise angles is also thought to contribute to the symmetrical appearance of the hypertrophied muscle.

Choice of Exercise. The body builder selects exercises that will develop and balance the body's appearance. In body building one goal is balance; one part of the body should not overshadow others. Beginners frequently concentrate on upper-body musculature, letting their lower body lag behind. This asymmetrical development scores poorly in competition. More-advanced body builders must use exercises that emphasize less-developed or weak parts of their physiques.

Order of Exercise. Generally a body builder progresses from large–muscle group to small–muscle group exercises. The order of exercises for a given body part is believed to be more important than the order in which body parts are exercised. Many programs use a split routine: Only certain body parts (e.g., back and chest) are exercised during a particular workout. This allows for a large training volume for a single body part in a workout. Body builders use many systems of resistance training, but the most common is super setting (discussed in chapter 6). The order of exercise becomes more important if super sets are performed in a workout.

Resistance. The resistances used by body builders typically range from 8 RM to 12 RM. Because the sport does not require the athlete to exhibit superior maximal strength, there is no real need to train with exceptionally heavy resistances. Many exercises prohibit the use of heavy weights because of the angles used, poor mechanical advantage, and the small relative size of some of the muscle groups exercised. The resistance used (8 RM to 12 RM) appears to be important in the performance of large training volumes (load $\times$ repetitions $\times$ sets) in body-building workouts. This high-volume stress may be a primary stimulus for the hypertrophy observed in these athletes.

Number of Sets. It is most common for body builders to use multiple sets of an exercise. Sometimes as many as 10 to 15 sets of a particular exercise are performed, but usually 3 to 6 sets are used. A particular muscle is stressed using several exercises.

Rest Periods. Probably the most distinctive feature of a body-building workout, besides the high exercise volume, is the short length of rest periods. Rests between sets and exercises are rarely longer than 90 s and sometimes less than 30 s. This variable appears to be important in promoting the muscular definition and vascularity observed in body builders. It may also be a vital factor in helping body builders to maintain a high metabolic intensity, which along with diet may

contribute to the low body fat observed in these athletes.

Figure 12.3 demonstrates one of the various poses and the high level of body development exhibited by these athletes in competition. Table 12.6 describes a typical body-building workout. The basic features of this workout are common to all types of body-building programs. This workout is primarily for an off-season program. As the body builder approaches competition, adjustment must be made in sets, repetitions, length of rest periods, and number of days to exercise certain muscle groups. Diet and posing must be considered in the total training program, so adjustments will be essential.

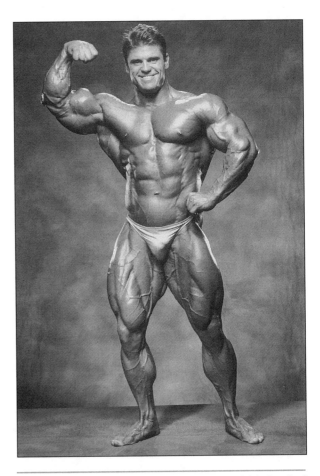

Fig. 12.3 Various poses demonstrate the high level of body development exhibited by body builders in competition. Photo courtesy of Dr. Fred Hatfield, Clearwater, FL.

Training Styles

The program in table 12.6 is an example of one possible set of workouts. By manipulating the acute variables, there are many other workout possibilities.

TABLE 12.6
Sample Body-Building Workout

Monday

6:00 A.M. (Back, heavy)

Warm-up
2 × 12 Wide-grip lat pulls to chest

Lat pulls (wide-grip)
2 × 10 to chest
2 × 10 behind neck

Low cable pulls
3 × 10-8-6 (heavy)

Close-grip pull-downs
3 × 10-8-6 (heavy)

Straight-leg deadlifts
2 × 12-10 (medium to heavy)

Hyperextensions
2 × 25

Tuesday

6:00 A.M. (Shoulders)

Warm-up
2 × 12 Dumbbell or machine lateral raises
1 × 10 Shoulder press (fronts)

Dumbbell laterals
3 × 10-8-8 (heavy)

Seated press (behind or in front of neck)
3 × 10-8-6 (heavy)

Dumbbell posterior pulls
3 × 10-8-8

Upright row
2 × 10

Shrugs
2 × 12-10

Neck machine
2 × 12

Wednesday

10:00 A.M. (Legs)

Warm-up
2 × 12 Knee extensions

Knee extensions
3 × 12-10-10 (heavy)

Front squats
3 × 10-8-8 (heavy)

Leg press
3 × 10-8-8 (heavy)

Double-leg curl
3 × 10-8-8 (heavy)

Single-leg curl
3 × 10-8-8 (medium)

10:00 A.M. (Chest, heavy)

Warm-up
2 × 12 Dumbbell laterals
1 × 10 Incline bench
1 × 10 Flat bench (135 lb [61.2 kg])
1 × 10 Flat bench (medium weight)

Bench press
3 × 10-8-8 (heavy)

Semi-incline
3 × 8

Incline press (bar or dumbbell)
3 × 8

Dumbbell fly
2 × 8

10:00 A.M. (Arms)

Warm-up
2 × 10 Curls
2 × 10 Triceps extension
1 × 8 Dips

Preacher curls (low cable)
3 × 10-8-6 (heavy)

Triceps extensions
3 × 12-10-8 (heavy)

Straight bar curl (E-Z curls)
3 × 8 (heavy) } Super set

Close-grip press
3 × 10-8-6 (heavy)

Concentration curls
2 × 8 } Super set

Flat-back triceps extensions
2 × 10

(continued)

TABLE 12.6
(continued)

Thursday

6:00 A.M. (Back)

Warm-up
Same as Monday

Low cables (standard or reverse grip)
2 × 12-10 (slide second set, i.e., do 10, drop
  the pin 4 or 5 plates, and do 2 × 12-10-8
  to 10 more)

Lat pulls (wide-grip)
2 × 12-10 Pull to front (slide second set)
2 × 12-10 Pull to back of neck (slide second
  set)

Close-grip high pull-downs
2 × 12-10 (slide second set)

Prone leg raises
2 × 20 (Use 10-lb [4.5-kg] dumbbell)

Hyperextensions
2 × 20

Friday

6:00 A.M. (Shoulders)

Warm-up
Same as Tuesday

Dumbbell or machine lateral raises
2 × 12-10 (slide second set, i.e., dumbbell = 35
  lb [15.9 kg] × 8; 20 lb [9.1 kg] × 8)

Front press
2 × 10

Cable posterior pulls
2 × 12-10 (slide second set 10-8-8)

Upright row (low cable)
2 × 12-10-10 (drop the weight once, i.e., 8
  plates for 10, 4 plates for 10)

Shrugs
1 × 12-10-10 (drop the resistance twice)

Neck
1 × 12-10-10 (front and back) (slide same as
  above)

Saturday

10:00 A.M. (Legs)

Warm-up
Same as Wednesday

Knee extensions
3 × 12-10

Hack squats
3 × 12-10-10

Knee press
2 × 12

Single-knee curl
2 × 12-10

Double-knee curl
3 × 12-10-8 (forced reps on last set to failure)

10:00 A.M. (Chest)

Warm-up
Same as Monday

Incline press (bar or dumbbell)
3 × 12-10-8

Semi-incline (dumbbell)
3 × 12-10-10 (heavy)

Flat bench
2 × 10 (slide second set, i.e., 1 × 10 at 255 lb
  [115.7 kg], slide 50 lb [22.7 kg], 1 × 8 to 10
  lb [4.5 kg] at 205 lb, no rest)

Dumbbell flys
2 × 10

10:00 A.M. (Arms)

Warm-up
Same as Tuesday

Dumbbell concentration curl
3 × 10

Triceps extension
3 × 12-10-10

*Spider curls (arms raised laterally to shoulder
  height and curled in from that position)*
3 × 10-8-8

Dips (with weight)
3 × 10

Preacher curls
2 × 10-8

Reverse-grip push-downs
2 × 12-10

TABLE 12.6
(continued)

Monday-Friday

P.M.

Calves
1. Calf raises using leg press   Pick two movements.
2. Calf raises
3. Seated calf raises   Do 3 × 12.
4. Donkeys (calf raises)   Do 3 × 12.

Tuesday-Thursday

P.M.

Abdominals
1. Incline hip flexor   Start out with one general exercise (i.e., include sit-ups) and as you
2. Incline sit-ups   fatigue, isolate exercise to the part of the abdomen on which you
3. Incline leg raises   want to concentrate. As you become more fit, add other exercises
4. Rope crunches   to your abdominal routine.
5. Weight semi-crunch
6. Crunches
7. V-ups

Note. The beginning of the week is heavy (80% of 1 RM or greater), concentrated exercise. The second time through, the exercise is medium to moderately heavy, with higher reps (8-10 RM and 12-15 RM).

The workouts must take into account the competition schedule. The primary systems of training used by body builders include

- super setting,
- burn sets,
- multiple sets,
- agonist/antagonist orders,
- trisets,
- cheat systems,
- isolated exercises,
- exhaustion sets, and
- super pump systems.

ANABOLIC DRUG USE

A detailed discussion of anabolic drugs is beyond the scope of this book, but excellent books and reviews have been published (NSCA 1993; Yesalis 1993). Anabolic drug use to enhance muscle size and strength has been for almost 50 years, and is still, a part of weight lifting, power lifting, and body building. Experimentation with anabolic drugs in Olympic weight lifting can be traced back at least as far as 1954 to the World Weight Lifting Championships, where the U.S. team physician was reportedly told by his Soviet counterpart that the Soviets were taking testosterone (Yesalis 1993). Since that time further experimentation with anabolic drugs has continued.

In 1958 Ciba Pharmaceutical Company released Dianabol (methandrostenolone), a synthetic testosterone, and experimentation continued. Reports about the efficacy of the drug spread by word of mouth through the lifting communities. By the 1964 Olympics anabolic-androgenic steroids were being used by almost all athletes in the strength sports. It has been estimated that over 88% of elite power lifters use anabolic steroids (Yesalis 1993). The potential health hazards from use of these drugs is not dramatic enough to discourage their use by many athletes. New federal laws have made anabolic steroids illegal to possess or distribute in the United States. More comprehensive drug testing programs, especially for Olympic-related competitions, and bans from future competitions on positive testing indicate that efforts are being made by sport governing bodies to discourage anabolic drug use.

In body building, attempts have been made to limit drug use, and drug-free and natural bodybuilding contests have taken place over the past 10 years. Nevertheless, fans of elite body building like the larger and larger body sizes of competitors, and this limits the desire of certain organizations to take a harder stand against anabolic drugs. Drugs often allow short-cuts in training techniques and programming, resulting in less concern about the training program and more emphasis on pharmacology.

Drug testing became a routine part of Olympic sports in the 1980s. The international governing body for power lifting does not finance a drug testing program comparable to the Olympic program. Limited attempts at drug testing (i.e., random testing) have been made in body building but not at the national or international level. This has resulted in a split in the power-lifting and body-building governance structures to include drug-free power-lifting associations (e.g., American Drug Free Power Lifting Association) and natural body-building competitions. Although the new drug-free and natural associations philosophically support the promotion of "clean" competitions, limited funding has been available to support any type of extensive random drug testing to verify the drug-free status of the competitors.

With the increased availability of additional growth-promoting drugs (e.g., growth hormone), concern about anabolic drug use in Olympic weight lifting, power lifting, body building, and strength and power sports in general does and will continue to exist. Through drug use some men and women attempt to go beyond their genetic limitations in order to achieve high levels of competitive excellence. Yet no study has ever demonstrated that an individual with less than optimal genetics can achieve superior results from drug use. Too often competitors with little or no chance to compete at the highest levels abuse anabolic drugs in the hope of negating genetic predisposition.

SUMMARY

As with any program, the design of programs for resistance sports should address the needs and goals of the activity for which it is designed. Good programs for the resistance training sports are designed to meet the goals of the individual sport. Therefore, these programs do not meet the needs and goals of many recreational weight trainers or athletes in other sports. However, information concerning program design when the program goal is to increase 1-RM strength or power and muscle size can be obtained by examining programs for these sports. This information can then be used when designing portions of a weight training program where the goals correspond to those of a resistance training sport.

SELECTED READINGS

Garhammer, J. 1991. A comparison of maximal power outputs between elite male and female weightlifters in competition. *International Journal of Sport and Biomechanics* 7:3-11.

Garhammer, J. 1993. A review of power output studies of Olympic and power lifting: Methodology, performance prediction, and evaluation tests. *Journal of Strength and Conditioning Research* 7:76-89.

Garhammer, J., and Takano, B. 1992. Training for weightlifting. *Strength and power in sports* 5:357-81.

Hatfield, F.C., and McLaughlin, T.M. 1985. Powerlifting. In *Encyclopedia of physical education, fitness, and sports*, ed. T.K. Cureton, vol. 4, 587-93. Reston, VA: AAHPERD.

Kraemer, W.J., and Koziris, L.P. 1994. Olympic weightlifting and power lifting. In *Physiology and nutrition for competitive sport*, eds. D.R. Lamb, H.G. Knuttgen, and R. Murray, 1-54. Carmel, IN: Cooper.

Tesch, P.A. 1992. Training for bodybuilding. In *Strength and power in sport*, ed. P.V. Komi, 370-80. Oxford: Blackwell Scientific.

Yesalis, C.E. 1993. *Anabolic steroids in sport and exercise*. Champaign, IL: Human Kinetics.

References

Abe, T.; Kawakami, Y.; Ikegawa, S.; Kanehisa, H.; and Fukunaga, T. 1992. Isometric and isokinetic knee joint performance in Japanese alpine ski racers. *Journal of Sports Medicine and Physical Fitness* 31:353-57.

Adams, G.R.; Hather, B.M.; Baldwin, K.M.; and Dudley, G.A. 1993. Skeletal muscle myosin heavy chain composition and resistance training. *Journal of Applied Physiology* 74:911-15.

Adams, J.E. 1965. Injuries to the throwing arm: A study of traumatic changes in the elbow of boy baseball players. *California Medicine* 102:127-32.

Adams, K.; O'Shea, J.P.; O'Shea, K.L.; and Climstein, M. 1992. The effect of six weeks of squat, plyometric and squat-plyometric training on power production. *Journal of Applied Sport Science Research* 6:36-41.

Alén, M.; Pakarinen, A.; Häkkinen, K.; and Komi, P.V. 1988. Responses of serum androgenic-anabolic and catabolic hormones to prolonged strength training. *International Journal of Sports Medicine* 9:229-33.

Allen, T.E.; Byrd, R.J.; and Smith, D.P. 1976. Hemodynamic consequences of circuit weight training. *Research Quarterly* 47:299-307.

Allsen, P.E.; Parsons, P.; and Bryce, G.R. 1977. Effect of menstrual cycle on maximum oxygen uptake. *Physician and Sportsmedicine* 5:53-55.

Alway, S.E. 1994. Characteristics of the elbow flexors in women bodybuilders using androgenic-anabolic steroids. *Journal of Strength and Conditioning Research.* 8:161-69.

Alway, S.E.; Grumbt, W.H.; Gonyea, W.J.; and Stray-Gundersen, J. 1989. Contrasts in muscle and myofibers of elite male and female bodybuilders. *Journal of Applied Physiology* 67:24-31.

Alway, S.E.; MacDougall, J.D.; and Sale, D.G. 1989. Contractile adaptations in the human triceps surae after isometric exercise. *Journal of Applied Physiology* 66:2725-32.

Alway, S.E.; Sale, D.G.; and MacDougall, J.D. 1990. Twitch contractile adaptations are not dependent on the intensity of isometric exercise in the human triceps surae. *European Journal of Applied Physiology* 60:346-52.

Alway, S.E.; Stray-Gundersen, J.; Grumbt, W.H.; and Gonyea, W.J. 1990. Muscle cross-sectional area and torque in resistance-trained subjects. *European Journal of Applied Physiology* 60:86-90.

Alway, S.E.; Winchester, P.K.; Davis, M.E.; and Gonyea. W.J. 1989. Regionalized adaptations and muscle fiber proliferation in stretch-induced enlargement. *Journal of Applied Physiology* 66:771-81.

American College of Sports Medicine. 1990. The recommended quantity and quality of exercise for developing and maintaining cardiorespiratory muscular fitness in healthy adults. *Medicine and Science in Sports and Exercise* 22:265-74.

American College of Sports Medicine. 1991. *Guidelines for exercise testing and prescription.* 4th ed. Philadelphia: Lea and Febiger.

American College of Sports Medicine. 1995. *ACSM's guidelines for exercise testing and prescription.* 5th ed. Baltimore, MD: Williams and Wilkins.

Amusa, L.O., and Obajuluwa, V.A. 1986. Static versus dynamic training programs for muscular strength using the knee-extensors in healthy young men. *Journal of Orthopaedic and Sports Physical Therapy* 8:243-47.

Anderson, T., and Kearney, J.T. 1982. Muscular strength and absolute and relative endurance. *Research Quarterly for Exercise and Sport* 53:1-7.

Aniansson, A.; Grimby, G.; and Hedberg, M. 1992. Compensatory muscle fiber hypertrophy in elderly men. *Journal of Applied Physiology* 73:812-16.

Aniansson, A., and Gustafsson, E. 1981. Physical training in elderly men with specific reference to quadriceps muscle strength and morphology. *Clinical Physiology* 1:87-98.

Antonio, J., and Gonyea, W.J. 1994. Muscle fiber splitting in stretch-enlarged avian muscle. *Medicine and Science in Sports and Exercise* 26:970-77.

Ariel, G. 1977. Barbell vs. dynamic variable resistance. *U.S. Sports Association News* 1:7.

Atha, J. 1981. Strengthening muscle. *Exercise and Sport Science Reviews* 9:1-73.

Baker, D.; Wilson, G.; and Carlyon, R. 1994. Periodization: The effect on strength of manipulating volume and intensity. *Journal of Strength and Conditioning Research* 8:235-42.

Barham, J.N. 1960. A comparison of the effectiveness of isometric and isotonic exercise when performed at different frequencies per week. PhD diss., Louisiana State University.

Barker, M.; Wyatt, T.J.; Johnson, R.L.; Stone, M.H.; O'Bryant, H.S.; Poe, C.; and Kent, M. 1993. Performance factors, psychological assessment, physical characteristics, and football playing ability. *Journal of Strength and Conditioning Research* 7:224-33.

Barnett, L.S. 1985. Little league shoulder syndrome: Proximal humeral epiphyseolysis in adolescent baseball pitchers. *Journal of Bone and Joint Surgery* 7A:495-96.

Bartholomeu, S.A. 1985. Plyometrics and vertical jump training. Master's thesis, University of North Carolina, Chapel Hill.

Bass, A.; Mackova, E.; and Vitek, V. 1973. Activity of some enzymes of energy supplying metabolism in rat soleus after tenotomy of synergistic muscles and in contralateral control muscle. *Physiologica Bohemoslovaca* 22:613-21.

Bassey, E.J.; Fiatarone, M.A.; O'Neill, E.F.; Kelly, M.; Evans, W.J.; and Lipsitz, L.A. 1992. Leg extensor power and functional performance in very old men and women. *Clinical Science* 82:321-27.

Bassey, E.J., and Harries, U.J. 1993. Normal values for handgrip strength in 920 men and women aged over 65 years, and longitudinal changes over 4 years in 620 survivors. *Clinical Science* 84:331-37.

Bauer, T.; Thayer, R.E.; and Baras, G. 1990. Comparison of training modalities for power development in the lower extremity. *Journal of Applied Sport Science Research* 4:115-21.

Baumgartner, T., and Wood, S. 1984. Development of shoulder-girdle strength-endurance in elementary children. *Research Quarterly for Exercise and Sport* 55:169-71.

Beedle, B.; Jessee, C.; and Stone, M.H. 1991. Flexibility characteristics among athletes who weight train. *Journal of Applied Sport Science Research* 5:150-54.

Behm, D.G., and Sale, D.G. 1993. Intended rather than actual movement velocity determines velocity-specific training response. *Journal of Applied Physiology* 74:359-68.

Belanger, A., and McComas, A.J. 1981. Extent of motor unit activation during effort. *Journal of Applied Physiology* 51:1131-35.

Bell, G.J.; Petersen, S.R.; Maclean, I.; Reid, D.C.; and Quinney, H.A. 1992. Effect of high velocity resistance training on peak torque, cross sectional area and myofibrillar ATPase activity. *Journal of Sports Medicine and Physical Fitness* 32:10-17.

Bell, G.J.; Petersen, S.R.; Wessel, J.; Bagnall, K.; and Quinney, H.A. 1991a. Adaptations to endurance and low velocity resistance training performed in a sequence. *Canadian Journal of Sport Science* 16:186-92.

Bell, G.J.; Petersen, S.R.; Wessel, J.; Bagnall, K.; and Quinney, H.A. 1991b. Physiological adaptations to concurrent endurance training and low velocity resistance training. *International Journal of Sports Medicine* 12:384-90.

Bell, G.J.; Snydmiller, G.D.; Neary, J.P.; and Quinney, H.A. 1989. The effect of high and low velocity resistance training on anaerobic power output in cyclists. *Journal of Human Movement Studies* 16:173-81.

Bell, G.J.; Syrotuik, D.G.; Attwood, K.; and Quinney, H.A. 1993. Maintenance of strength gains while performing endurance training in oarswomen. *Journal of Applied Physiology* 18:104-15.

Bender, J., and Kaplan, H. 1963. The multiple angle testing method for the evaluation of muscle strength. *Journal of Bone and Joint Surgery* 45A:135-40.

Berger, R.A. 1962a. Comparison of static and dynamic strength increases. *Research Quarterly* 33:329-33.

Berger, R.A. 1962b. Effect of varied weight training programs on strength. *Research Quarterly* 33:168-81.

Berger, R.A. 1962c. Optimum repetitions for the development of strength. *Research Quarterly* 33:334-38.

Berger, R.A. 1963a. Comparative effects of three weight training programs. *Research Quarterly* 34:396-98.

Berger, R.A. 1963b. Comparison between static training and various dynamic training programs. *Research Quarterly* 34:131-35.

Berger, R.A. 1963c. Effects of dynamic and static training on vertical jump ability. *Research Quarterly* 34:419-24.

Berger, R.A. 1965. Application of research findings in progressive resistance exercise to physical therapy. *Journal of the Association of Physical and Mental Rehabilitation* 19:200-203.

Berger, R.A., and Hardage, B. 1967. Effect of maximum loads for each of ten repetitions on strength improvement. *Research Quarterly* 38:715-18.

Blair, S.N.; Kohl, H.W.; Paffenbarger, R.S.; Clark, D.G.; Cooper, K.H.; and Gibbons, L.W. 1989. Physical fitness and all-cause mortality: A prospective study of healthy men and women. *Journal of the American Medical Association* 262:2395-2401.

Blattner, S.E., and Noble, L. 1979. Relative effects of isokinetic and plyometric training on vertical jumping performance. *Research Quarterly* 50:583-88.

Blessing, D.; Stone, M.; Byrd, R.; Wilson, D.; Rozenek, R.; Pushparani, D.; and Liper, H. 1987. Blood lipid and hormonal changes from jogging and weight training of middle-aged men. *Journal of Applied Sport Science Research* 1:25-29.

Blimkie, C.J.R. 1989. Age- and sex-associated variation in strength during childhood: Anthropometric, morphologic, neurologic, biomechanical, endocrinologic, genetic and physical activity correlates. In *Perspectives in exercise science and sports medicine*. Vol. 2, *Youth exercise and sport*, eds. C. Gisolfi and D. Lamb, 99-163. Indianapolis: Benchmark Press.

Blimkie, C.J.R. 1993. Resistance training during preadolescence. *Sports Medicine* 15:389-407.

Blimkie, C.J.R.; Ramsay, J.; Sale, D.; MacDougall, D.; Smith, K.; and Garner, S. 1989. Effects of 10 weeks resistance training on strength development in pre-pubertal boys. In *Children and exercise XIII*, eds. S. Oseid and K.-H. Carlsen, 183-97. Champaign, IL: Human Kinetics.

Blomqvist, C.G., and Saltin, B. 1983. Cardiovascular adaptations to physical training. *Annual Review of Physiology* 45:169-89.

Bobbert, M.F. 1990. Drop jumping as a training method for jumping ability. *Sports Medicine* 9:7-22.

Bonde-Petersen, F. 1960. Muscle training by static, concentric and eccentric contractions. *Acta Physiologica Scandinavica* 48:406-16.

Bonde-Petersen, F., and Knuttgen, H.G. 1971. Effect of training with eccentric muscle contractions on human skeletal muscle metabolites. *Acta Physiologica Scandinavica* 80:16A-17A.

Borges, O., and Essen-Gustavsson, B. 1989. Enzyme activities in Type I and II muscle fibres of human skeletal muscle in relation to age and torque development. *Acta Physiologica Scandinavica* 136:29-36.

Bosco, C., and Komi, P.V. 1980. Influence of aging on the mechanical behavior of leg extensor muscles. *European Journal of Applied Physiology* 45:209-19.

Bosco, C.; Montanari, G.; Ribacchi, R.; Giovenali, P.; Latteri, F.; Iachelli, G.; Faina, M.; Colli, R.; Dal Monte, A.; La Rosa, M.; Cortili, G.; and Saibene, F. 1987. Relationship between the efficiency of muscular work during jumping and the energetics of running. *European Journal of Applied Physiology* 56:138-43.

Bosco, C., and Pittera, C. 1982. Zur trainings Wirkung neuentwickeher Sprungubungen auf die Explosivkraft. *Leistungssport* 12:36-39.

Bosco, C.; Tarkka, I.; and Komi, P.V. 1982. Effects of elastic energy and myoelectrical potentiation of triceps surae during stretch-shortening cycle exercises. *Sports Medicine* 3:137-40.

Boyer, B.T. 1990. A comparison of the effects of three strength training programs on women. *Journal of Applied Sport Science Research* 4: 88-94.

Braith, R.W.; Graves, J.E.; Leggett, S.H.; and Pollock, M.L. 1993. Effect of training on the relationship between maximal and submaximal strength. *Medicine and Science in Sports and Exercise* 25:132-38.

Brazell-Roberts, J.V., and Thomas, L.E. 1989. Effects of weight training frequency on the self-concept of college females. *Journal of Applied Sports Science Research* 3:40-43.

Bricourt, V.A.; Germain, P.S.; Serrurier, B.D.; and Guezennec, C.Y. 1994. Changes in testosterone muscle receptors: Effects of an androgen treatment on physically trained rats. *Cellular and Molecular Biology* 40:291-94.

Brooks, G.A.; Butterfield, G.E.; Wolfe, R.R.; Groves, B.M.; Mazzeo, R.S.; Sutton, J.R.; Wolfel, E.E.; and Reeves, J.T. 1991. Decreased reliance on lactate during exercise after acclimatization to 4,300 m. *Journal of Applied Physiology* 71:333-41.

Brooks, G.A., and Fahey, T.D. 1984. *Exercise physiology: Human bioenergetics and its applications*. New York: Wiley.

Brooks-Gunn, J., and Rubb, D.N. 1983. The experience of menarche from a developmental perspective. In *Girls at puberty: Biological and psychosocial perspectives*, eds. J. Brooks-Gunn and A.C. Peterson, 155-77. New York: Plenum Press.

Brose, D.E., and Hanson, D.L. 1967. Effects of overload training on velocity and accuracy of throwing. *Research Quarterly* 38:528-33.

Brown, A.B.; McCartney, N.; and Sale, D.G. 1990. Positive adaptations to weight-lifting training in the elderly. *Journal of Applied Physiology* 69:1725-33.

Brown, B.S.; Gorman, D.R.; DiBrezzom, R.; and Fort, I. 1988. Anaerobic power changes following short term, task specific, dynamic and static overload training. *Journal of Applied Sport Science Research* 2:35-38.

Brown, C.H., and Wilmore, J.H. 1974. The effects of maximal resistance training on the strength and body composition of women athletes. *Medicine and Science in Sports* 6:174-77.

Brown, E.; Lillegard, W.; Henderson, R.; Wilson, D.; Lewis, E.; Hough, D.; and Stringer, K. 1992. Efficacy and safety of strength training with free weights in prepubescents to early postpubescents (Abstract). *Medicine and Science in Sports and Exercise* 24:S82.

Burke, J.; Thayer, R.; and Belcamino, M. 1994. Comparison of effects of two interval-training programmes on lactate and ventilatory thresholds. *British Journal of Sports Medicine* 28:18-21.

Caiozzo, V.J.; Laird, T.; Chow, K.; Prietto, C.A.; and McMaster, W.C. 1983. The use of precontractions to enhance the in-vivo force velocity relationship. *Medicine and Science in Sports and Exercise* 14:162.

Caiozzo, V.J.; Perrine, J.J.; and Edgerton, V.R. 1981. Training-induced alterations of the in vivo force-velocity relationship of human muscle. *Journal of Applied Physiology: Respiratory, Environmental and Exercise Physiology* 51:750-54.

Callister, R.; Shealy, M.J.; Fleck, S.J.; and Dudley, G.A. 1988. Performance adaptations to sprint, endurance and both modes of training. *Journal of Applied Physiology* 2:46-51.

Cameron, K.R.; Wark, J.D.; and Telford, R.D. 1992. Stress fractures and bone loss—the skeletal cost of intense athleticism? *Excel* 8:39-55.

Campbell, D.E. 1967. Maintenance of strength during a season of sports participation. *American Corrective Therapy Journal* 21:193-95.

Campbell, R.C. 1962. Effects of supplemental weight training on the physical fitness of athletic squads. *Research Quarterly* 33:343-48.

Campbell, W.W.; Crim, M.C.; Young, V.R.; Joseph, L.J.; and Evans, W.J. 1995. Effects of resistance training and dietary protein intake on protein metabolism in older adults. *American Journal of Applied Physiology* 268:E1143-53.

Cann, C.E.; Martin, M.C.; Genant, H.K.; and Jaffe, R. 1984. Decreased spinal mineral content in amenorrheic female. *Journal of the American Medical Association* 251:626-29.

Cannon, R., and Cafarelli, E. 1987. Neuromuscular adaptations to training. *Journal of Applied Physiology* 63:2396-2402.

Capen, E.K. 1950. The effect of systematic weight training on power, strength and endurance. *Research Quarterly* 21:83-93.

Capen, E.K.; Bright, J.A.; and Line, P.Q. 1961. The effects of weight training on strength, power, muscular endurance and anthropometric measurements on a select group of college women. *Journal of the Association for Physical and Mental Rehabilitation* 15:169-73.

Carolyn, B., and Cafarelli, E. 1992. Adaptations in coactivation after isometric resistance training. *Journal of Applied Physiology* 73:911-17.

Carpinelli, R.N., and Gutin, B. 1991. Effects of miometric and pliometric muscle actions on delayed muscle soreness. *Journal of Applied Sport Science* 5:66-70.

Chakravati, S.; Forecast, J.D.; Newton, J.R.; Oram, D.H.; Studd, J.W.; and Collins, W. 1976. Hormonal profiles after menopause. *British Medical Journal* 2:784-87.

Chang, D.E.; Buschbacker, L.P.; and Edlich, R.F. 1988. Limited mobility in power lifters. *American Journal of Sports Medicine* 16:280-84.

Charette, S.L.; McEvoy, L.; Pyka, G.; Snow-Harter, C.; Guido, D.; Wiswell, R.A.; and Marcus, R. 1991. Muscle hypertrophy response to resistance training in older women. *Journal of Applied Physiology* 70:1912-16.

Chromiak, J.A., and Mulvaney, D.R. 1990. A review: The effects of combined strength and endurance training on strength development. *Journal of Applied Sport Science Research* 4:55-60.

Chu, E. 1950. The effect of systematic weight training on athletic power. *Research Quarterly* 21:188-94.

Ciriello, V.M.; Holden, W.C.; and Evans, W.J. 1983. The effects of two isokinetic training regimens on muscle strength and fiber composition. In *Biochemistry of exercise*, eds. H.G. Knuttgen, J.A. Vogel, and S. Poortmans, 787-93. Champaign, IL: Human Kinetics.

Clarke, D.H. 1973. Adaptations in strength and muscular endurance resulting from exercise. *Exercise and Sport Science Reviews* 1:73-102.

Clarke, D.H. 1986. Sex differences in strength and fatigability. *Research Quarterly* 57:144-49.

Clarke, D.H.; Vaccaro, P.; and Andersen, N. 1984. Physiologic alterations in 7- to 9-year-old boys following a season of competitive wrestling. *Research Quarterly for Exercise and Sport* 55:318-22.

Clarkson, P.M.; Nosaka, K.; and Braun, B. 1992. Muscle function after exercise-induced muscle damage and rapid adaptation. *Medicine and Science in Sports and Exercise* 24:512-20.

Clarkson, P.M., and Tremblay, I. 1988. Exercise-induced muscle damage, repair and adaptation in humans *Journal of Applied Physiology*. 65:1-6.

Clutch, D.; Wilton, C.; McGown, C.; and Bryce, G.R. 1983. The effect of depth jumps and weight training on leg strength and vertical jump. *Research Quarterly* 54:5-10.

Colan, S.; Sanders, S.P.; McPherson, D.; and Borrow, K.M. 1985. Left ventricular function in elite athletes with physiologic cardiac hypertrophy. *Journal of the American College of Cardiology* 6:545-49.

Coleman, A.E. 1977. Nautilus vs. universal gym strength training in adult males. *American Corrective Therapy Journal* 31:103-7.

Colliander, E.B., and Tesch, P. 1988. Blood pressure in resistance-trained athletes. *Canadian Journal of Sport Science* 13:31-34.

Colliander, E.B., and Tesch, P.A. 1989. Bilateral eccentric and concentric torque of quadriceps and hamstring in females and males. *European Journal of Applied Physiology* 59:227-32.

Colliander, E.B., and Tesch, P.A. 1990a. Effects of eccentric and concentric muscle actions in resistance training. *Acta Physiologica Scandinavica* 140:31-39.

Colliander, E.B., and Tesch, P.A. 1990b. Responses to eccentric and concentric resistance training in females and males. *Acta Physiologica Scandinavica* 141:149-56.

Conale, S.T., and Belding, R.H. 1980. Osteochondral lesions of the talus. *Journal of Bone and Joint Surgery* 62A:97-102.

Conroy, B.P.; Kraemer, W.J.; Maresh, C.M.; and Dalsky, G.P. 1992. Adaptive responses of bone to physical activity. *Medicine, Exercise, Nutrition, and Health* 1:64-74.

Conroy, B.P.; Kraemer, W.J.; Maresh, C.M.; Dalsky, G.P.; Fleck, S.J.; Stone, M.H.; Miller, P.; and Fry, A.C. 1993. Bone mineral density in elite junior weightlifters. *Medicine and Science in Sports and Exercise* 25:1103-9.

Cornelius, W.L. 1985. Flexibility: The effective way. *National Strength and Conditioning Association Journal* 7:62-64.

Cornelius, W.L.; Ebrahim, K.; Watson, J.; and Hill, D.W. 1992. The effects of cold application and modified PNF stretching techniques on hip joint flexibility in college males. *Research Quarterly for Exercise and Sport* 63:311-14.

Costill, D.L.; Coyle, E.F.; Fink, W.F.; Lesmes, G.R.; and Witzmann, F.A. 1979. Adaptations in skeletal muscle following strength training. *Journal of Applied Physiology: Respiratory, Environmental and Exercise Physiology* 46:96-99.

Cote, C.; Simoneau, J.-A.; Lagasse, P.; Boulay, M.; Thibault, M.-C.; Marcotte, M.; and Bouchard, C. 1988. Isokinetic strength training protocols: Do they induce skeletal muscle fiber hypertrophy? *Archives of Physical Medicine and Rehabilitation* 69:281-85.

Coyle, E.F.; Feiring, D.C.; Rotkis, T.C.; Cote, R.W.; Roby, F.B.; Lee, W.; and Wilmore, J.H. 1981. Specificity of power improvements through slow and fast isokinetic training. *Journal of Applied Physiology: Respiratory, Environmental and Exercise Physiology* 51:1437-42.

Crist, D.M.; Peake, G.T.; Egan, P.A.; and Waters, D.L. 1988. Body composition response to exogenous GH during training in highly conditioned adults. *Journal of Applied Physiology* 65:579-84.

Cureton, K.J.; Collins, M.A.; Hill, D.W.; and McElhannon, F.M. 1988. Muscle hypertrophy in men and women. *Medicine and Science in Sports and Exercise* 20:338-44.

Dale, E.; Gerlach, D.; and Wilhite, A. 1979. Menstrual dysfunction in distance runners. *Obstetrics and Gynecology* 54:47-53.

Dalsky, G.P.; Stocke, K.S.; Ehasani, A.A.; Slatopolsky, E.; Lee, W.C.; and Birge, S.J. 1988. Weight-bearing exercise training and lumbar bone mineral content in post menopausal female. *Annals of Internal Medicine* 108:824-28.

Dalton, S.E. 1992. Overuse injuries in adolescent athletes. *Sports Medicine* 13 (1): 58-70.

Danneskoild-Samsoe, B.; Kofod, V.; Munter, J.; Grimby, G.; and Schnohr, P. 1984. Muscle strength and functional capacity in 77-81 year old men and women. *European Journal of Applied Physiology* 52:123-35.

Darden, E. 1973. Weight training systems in the U.S.A. *Journal of Physical Education* 44:72-80.

Davies, A.H. 1977. Chronic effects of isokinetic and allokinetic training on muscle force, endurance, and muscular hypertrophy. *Dissertation Abstracts International* 38:153A.

Davies, B.N.; Greenwood, E.J.; and Jones, S.R. 1988. Gender differences in the relationship of performance in the handgrip and standing long jump tests to lean limb volume in young adults. *European Journal of Applied Physiology* 58:315-20.

Davies, C.T.M., and Young, K. 1983. Effects of training at 30 and 100% maximal isometric force on the contractile properties of the triceps surae of man. *Journal of Physiology* 36:22-23.

Davies, J.; Parker, D.F.; Rutherford, O.M.; and Jones, D.A. 1988. Changes in strength and cross sectional area of the elbow flexors as a result of isometric strength training. *European Journal of Applied Physiology* 57:667-70.

Davies, R. 1966. A molecular theory of muscle contraction: Calcium dependent contractions with hydrogen bond formation plus ATP-dependent extensions of part of the myosin-actin cross-bridges. *Nature* 199:1068-74.

Dawood, M.Y. 1983. Dysmenorrhea. *Clinical Obstetrics and Gynecology* 26:719-27.

De Cree, C.; Vermeulen, A.; and Ostyn, M. 1991. Are high-performance young women athletes doomed to become low-performance old wives? A reconsideration of the increased risk of osteoporosis in amenorrheic women. *Journal of Sports Medicine and Physical Fitness* 31:108-14.

DeKoning, F.L.; Binkhorst, R.A.; Vissers, A.C.A.; and Vos, J.A. 1982. Influence of static strength training on the force-velocity relationship of the arm flexors. *International Journal of Sports Medicine* 3:25-28.

Deligiannis, A.; Zahopoulou, E.; and Mandroukas, K. 1988. Echocardiographic study of cardiac dimensions and function in weight lifters and body builders. *International Journal of Sports Cardiology* 5:24-32.

DeLorme, T.L.; Ferris, B.G.; and Gallagher, J.R. 1952. Effect of progressive exercise on muscular contraction time. *Archives of Physical Medicine* 33:86-97.

DeLorme, T.L., and Watkins, A.L. 1948. Techniques of progressive resistance exercise. *Archives of Physical Medicine* 29:263-73.

DeLuca, C.J.; LeFever, R.S.; McCue, M.P.; and Xenakis, A.P. 1982. Behavior of human motor units in different muscles during linearly varying contractions. *Journal of Physiology* 329:113-28.

DeRenne, C.; Ho, K.; and Blitzblau, A. 1990. Effects of weighted implement training on throwing velocity. *Journal of Sport Science Research* 4:16-19.

Deschenes, M.R.; Maresh, C.M.; Armstrong, L.E.; Covault, J.M.; Kraemer, W.J.; and Crivello, J.F. 1994. Endurance and resistance exercise induce muscle fiber type specific responses in androgen binding capacity. *Journal of Steroid Biochemistry and Molecular Biology* 50:175-79.

Deschenes, M.R.; Maresh, C.M.; Crivello, J.F.; Armstrong, L.E.; Kraemer, W.J.; and Covault, J. 1993. The effects of exercise training of different intensities on neuromuscular junction morphology. *Journal of Neurocytology* 22:603-15.

Deschenes, M.R.; Maresh, C.M.; and Kraemer, W.J. 1994. The neuromuscular junction: Structure, function, and its role in the excitation of muscle. *Journal of Strength and Conditioning Research* 8:103-9.

Desmedt, J.E. 1981. The size principle of motoneuron recruitment in ballistic or ramp-voluntary contractions in man. In *Progress in clinical neurophysiology*. Vol. 9, *Motor unit types, recruitment and plasticity in health and disease*, ed. J.E. Desmedt, 250-304. Basel: Karger.

Desmedt, J.E., and Godaux, E. 1977. Ballistic contractions in man: Characteristic recruitment pattern of single motor units of the tibialis muscle. *Journal of Physiology* 264:673-94.

DeSouza, M.J., and Metzger, D.A. 1991. Reproductive dysfunction in amenorrheic athletes and anorexic patients: A review. *Medicine and Science in Sports and Exercise* 23:995-1007.

DeVries, H.A. 1980. *Physiology of exercise for physical education and athletics*. Dubuque, IA: Brown.

Dibrizzo, R.; Fort, I.L.; and Brown, B. 1988. Dynamic strength and work variations during three stages of the menstrual cycle. *Journal of Orthopaedic and Sports Physical Therapy* 10:110-16.

DiPrampero, P.E., and Margaria, R. 1978. Relationship between O_2 consumption, high energy phosphates and the kinetics of the O_2 debt in exercise. *Pflugers Archives* 304:11-19.

Doherty, T.J.; Vandervoort, A.A.; Taylor, A.W.; and Brown, W.F. 1993. Effects of motor unit losses on strength in older men and women. *Journal of Applied Physiology* 7:868-74.

Dohm, G.L.; Williams, R.T.; Kasperek, G.J.; and Van, R.J. 1982. Increased excretion of urea and N tanmethylhistidine by rats and humans after a bout of exercise. *Journal of Applied Physiology* 52:458-66.

Donnelly, A.E.; Clarkson, P.M.; and Maughan, R.J. 1992. Exercise-induced muscle damage: Effects of light exercise on damaged muscle. *European Journal of Applied Physiology* 64:350-53.

Doolittle, R.L., and Engebretsen, J. 1972. Performance variations during the menstrual cycle. *Journal of Sports Medicine and Physical Fitness* 12:54-58.

Drinkwater, B.L. 1984. Women and exercise: Physiological aspects. In *Exercise and sport science reviews*, ed. R.L. Terjung, 21-52. Lexington, KY: MAL Callamore Press.

Duchateau, J., and Hainaut, K. 1984. Isometric or dynamic training: Differential effects on mechanical properties of a human muscle. *Journal of Applied Physiology* 56:296-301.

Dudley, G.A., and Djamil, R. 1985. Incompatibility of endurance and strength training modes of exercise. *Journal of Applied Physiology* 59:1446-51.

Dudley, G.A., and Fleck, S.J. 1987. Strength and endurance training: Are they mutually exclusive? *Sports Medicine* 4:79-85.

Dudley, G.A., and Harris, R.T. 1992. Use of electrical stimulation in strength and power training. In *Strength and power in sport*, ed. P.V. Komi, 329-37. Oxford: Blackwell Scientific.

Dudley, G.A.; Harris, R.T.; Duvoisin, M.R.; Hather, B.M.; and Buchanan, P. 1990. Effect of voluntary vs. artificial activation on the relationship of muscle torque to speed. *Journal of Applied Physiology* 69:2215-21.

Dudley, G.A.; Tesch, P.A.; Miller, B.J.; and Buchanan, P. 1991. Importance of eccentric actions in performance adaptations to resistance training. *Aviation, Space, and Environmental Medicine* 62:543-50.

Ebbling, C.B., and Clarkson, P.M. 1990. Muscle adaptation

prior to recovery following eccentric exercise. *European Journal of Applied Physiology* 60:26-31.

Edgerton, V.R. 1978. Mammalian muscle fiber types and their adaptability. *American Zoologist* 18:113-25.

Edwards, R.H.T.; Hill, D.K.; and McDonnell, M.N. 1972. Monothermal and intramuscular pressure measurements during isometric contractions of the human quadriceps muscle. *Journal of Physiology* 224:58-59.

Effron, M.B. 1989. Effects of resistance training on left ventricular function. *Medicine and Science in Sports and Exercise* 21:694-97.

Ellenbecker, T.S.; Davies, G.J.; and Rowinski, M.J. 1988. Concentric versus eccentric isokinetic strengthening of the rotator cuff. *American Journal of Sports Medicine* 16:64-69.

Elliot, D.L., and Goldberg, L. 1983. Weight lifting and amenorrhea. *Journal of the American Medical Association* 249:354.

Elliot, D.L.; Goldberg, L.; Kuehl, K.S.; and Katlin, D.H. 1987. Characteristics of anabolic-androgenic steroid-free, competitive male and female body builders. *Physician in Sportsmedicine* 15:169-79.

Elliott, B.C.; Wilson, G.J.; and Kerr, G.K. 1989. A biomechanical analysis of the sticking region in the bench press. *Medicine and Science in Sports and Exercise* 21:450-62.

Essen, B.; Jansson, E.; Henriksson, J.; Taylor, A.W.; and Saltin, B. 1975. Metabolic characteristics of fiber types in human skeletal muscle. *Acta Physiologica Scandinavica* 95:153-65.

Etnyre, B.R., and Lee, E.J. 1987. Comments on proprioceptive neuromuscular facilitation. *Research Quarterly for Exercise and Sport* 58:184-88.

Etnyre, B.R., and Lee, E.J. 1988. Chronic and acute flexibility of men and women using three different stretching techniques. *Research Quarterly for Exercise and Sport* 59:222-28.

Evans, W.J. 1993. Sarcopenia: The age-related loss in skeletal muscle mass. In *Musculoskeletal soft-tissue aging: Impact on mobility*, eds. J.A. Buckwalter, V.M. Goldberg, and S.L.Y. Woo, 217-29. Rosemont, IL: American Academy of Orthopedic Surgeons.

Evans, W.J., and Campbell, W.W. 1993. Sarcopenia and age-related changes in body composition and functional capacity. *Journal of Nutrition* 123:465-68.

Ewing, J.L.; Wolfe, D.R.; Rogers, M.A.; Amundson, M.L.; and Stull, G.A. 1990. Effects of velocity of isokinetic training on strength, power, and quadriceps muscle fibre characteristics. *European Journal of Applied Physiology* 61:159-62.

Exner, G.U.; Staudte, H.W.; and Pette, D. 1973. Isometric training of rats: Effects upon fast and slow muscle and modification by an anabolic hormone in female rats. *Pflugers Archives* 345:1-4.

Fahey, T.D.; Akka, L.; and Rolph, R. 1975. Body composition and $\dot{V}O_2$max of exceptional weight trained athletes. *Journal of Applied Physiology* 39:559-61.

Fahey, T.D., and Brown, C.H. 1973. The effects of anabolic steroid on the strength, body composition and endurance of college males when accompanied by a weight training program. *Medicine and Science in Sports* 5:272-76.

Fahey, T.D.; DelValle-Zuris, A.; Oehlsen, G.; Trieb, M.; and Seymour, J. 1979. Pubertal stage differences in hormonal and hematological responses to maximal exercise in males. *Journal of Applied Physiology* 46:823-27.

Fahey, T.D.; Rolph, R.; Moungmee, P.; Nagel, J.; and Mortara, S. 1976. Serum testosterone, body composition and strength of young adults. *Medicine and Science in Sports* 8:31-34.

Faigenbaum, A.D. 1993. Strength training: A guide for teachers and coaches. *National Strength and Conditioning Association Journal* 15:20-29.

Faigenbaum, A.D.; Skrinar, G.S.; Cesare, W.F.; Kraemer, W.J.; and Thomas, H.E. 1990. Physiologic and symptomatic responses of cardiac patients to resistance exercise. *Archives of Physical Medicine and Rehabilitation* 71:395-98.

Faigenbaum, A.D.; Zaichowsky, L.; Westcott, W.; Micheli, L.; and Fehlandt, A. 1993. The effects of twice a week strength training program on children. *Pediatric Exercise Science* 5:339-46.

Fair, J.D. 1988. Olympic weightlifting and the introduction of steroids: A statistical analysis of world championship results 1948-1972. *International Journal of History of Sport* 5:96-114.

Falkel, J.E.; Fleck, S.J.; and Murray, T.F. 1992. Comparison of central hemodynamics between powerlifters and body builders during resistance exercise. *Journal of Applied Sport Science Research* 6:24-35.

Falkel, J.E.; Sawka, M.N.; Levine, L.; and Pandolf, K.B. 1985. Upper to lower body muscular strength and endurance ratios for women and men. *Ergonomics* 28:1661-70.

Fardy, P.S. 1977. Training for aerobic power. In *Toward an understanding of human performance*, ed. E.J. Burke, 10-14. Ithaca, NY: Movement Press.

Fardy, P.S.; Maresh, C.M.; Abbott, R.; and Kristiansen, T. 1976. An assessment of the influence of habitual physical activity, prior sport participation, smoking habits and aging upon indices of cardiovascular fitness: Preliminary report of a cross-section and retrospective study. *Journal of Sports Medicine and Physical Fitness* 16:77-90.

Farley, C.T.; Blickhan, R.; Saito, J.; and Taylor, C.R. 1991. Hopping frequency in humans: A test of how springs set stride frequency in bouncing gaits. *Journal of Applied Physiology* 71:2127-32.

Faulkner, J.A.; Claflin, D.R.; and McCully, K.K. 1986. Power output of fast and slow fibers from human skeletal muscles. In *Human muscle power*, eds. N.L. Jones, N. McCartney, and A.J. McComas, 88. Champaign, IL: Human Kinetics.

Fiatarone, M.A., and Evans, W.J. 1993. The etiology and reversibility of muscle function in the aged. *Journal of Gerontology* 48:77-83.

Fiatarone, M.A.; Marks, E.C.; Ryan, N.D.; Meredith, C.N.; Lipsitz, L.A.; and Evans, W.J. 1990. High-intensity strength training in nonagenarians. Effects on skeletal muscle. *Journal of the American Medical Association* 263:3029-34.

Fiatarone, M.A.; O'Neill, E.F.; Ryan, N.D.; Clements, K.M.; Solares, G.R.; Nelson, M.E.; Roberts, S.B.; Kehayias, J.J.; Lipsitz, L.A.; and Evans, W.J. 1994. Exercise training and nutritional supplementation for physical frailty in very elderly people. *New England Journal of Medicine* 330:1769-75.

Fleck, S.J. 1979. Varying frequency and intensity of isokinetic strength training. *Dissertation Abstracts International* 39:2126A.

Fleck, S.J. 1988. Cardiovascular adaptations to resistance training. *Medicine and Science in Sports and Exercise* 20:S146-51.

Fleck, S.J. 1992. Cardiovascular response to strength training. In *Strength and power in sport*, ed. P.V. Komi, 305-15. Oxford: Blackwell Scientific.

Fleck, S.J.; Case, S.; Puhl, J.; and Van Handle, P. 1985. Physical and physiological characteristics of elite women volleyball players. *Canadian Journal of Applied Sport Sciences* 10:122-26.

Fleck, S.J., and Dean, L.S. 1985. Influence of weight training experience on blood pressure response to exercise. *Medicine and Science in Sport and Exercise* 17:185.

Fleck, S.J., and Dean, L.S. 1987. Previous resistance-training experience and the pressor response during resistance exercise. *Journal of Applied Physiology* 63:116-20.

Fleck, S.J.; Falkel, J.; Harman, E.; Kraemer, W.J.; Frykman, P.; Maresh, C.M.; Goetz, K.L.; Campbell, D.; Rosenstein, M.; and Rosenstein, R. 1989. Cardiovascular responses during resistance training (Abstract). *Medicine and Science in Sports and Exercise* 21:S114.

Fleck, S.J.; Henke, C.; and Wilson, W. 1989. Cardiac MRI of elite junior Olympic weight lifters. *International Journal of Sports Medicine* 10:329-33.

Fleck, S.J., and Schutt, R.C. 1985. Types of strength training. *Clinics in Sports Medicine* 4:150-69.

Fogelholm, M.; Kaprio, J.; and Sarna, S. 1994. Healthy lifestyles of former Finnish world class athletes. *Medicine and Science in Sports and Exercise* 26:224-29.

Ford, H.T.; Puckett, J.R.; Drummond, J.P.; Sawyer, K.; Gantt, K.; and Fussell, C. 1983. Effects of three combinations of plyometric and weight training programs on selected physical fitness test items. *Perceptual and Motor Skills* 56:919-22.

Fox, E.L. 1979. *Sports physiology*. Philadelphia: Saunders.

Fox, E.L., and Mathews, D.K. 1981. *The physiological basis of physical education and athletics*. Philadelphia: Saunders.

Freedson, P.S.; Micheuic, P.M.; Loucks, A.B.; and Birandola, R.M. 1983. Physique, body composition, and psychological characteristics of competitive female body builders. *Physician and Sportsmedicine* 11:85-93.

Freedson, P.S.; Ward, A.; and Rippe, J.M. 1990. Resistance training for youth. *Advances in Sports Medicine and Fitness* 3:57-65.

Frick, M.H.; Elovainio, R.O.; and Somer, T. 1967. The mechanism of bradycardia evoked by physical training. *Cardiology* 51:46-54.

Frisch, R.E., and McArthur, J.W. 1974. Menstrual cycles: Fatness as a determinant of minimum weight and height necessary for their maintenance or onset. *Science* 185:949-51.

Froelicher, V.F. 1983. *Exercise testing and training*. New York: LeJacq.

Frontera, W.R.; Hughes, V.A.; Lutz, K.J.; and Evans, W.J. 1991. A cross-sectional study of muscle strength and mass in 45- to 78-year-old men and women. *Journal of Applied Physiology* 71:644-50.

Frontera, W.R.; Meredith, C.N.; O'Reilly, K.P.; Knuttgen, H.G.; and Evans, W.J. 1988. Strength conditioning in older men: Skeletal muscle hypertrophy and improved function. *Journal of Applied Physiology* 64:1038-44.

Fry, A.C.; Allemeier, C.A.; and Staron, R.S. 1994. Correlation between percentage fiber type area and myosin heavy chain content in human skeletal muscle. *European Journal of Applied Physiology* 68:246-51.

Fry, A.C., and Kraemer, W.J. 1991. Physical performance characteristics of American collegiate football players. *Journal of Applied Sport Science Research* 5:126-38.

Fry, A.C.; Kraemer, W.J.; Stone, M.H.; Fleck, S.J.; Kearney, J.T.; Triplett, N.T.; and Gordon, S.E. 1995. Acute endocrine responses with long-term weightlifting in a 51-year old male weightlifter (Abstract). *Journal of Strength and Conditioning Research* 9:193.

Fry, A.C.; Kraemer, W.J.; van Borselen, F.; Lynch, J.M.; Marsit, J.L.; Roy, E.P.; Triplett, N.T.; and Knuttgen, H.G. 1994. Performance decrements with high-intensity resistance exercise overtraining. *Medicine and Science in Sports and Exercise* 26:1165-73.

Fry, A.C.; Powell, D.R.; and Kraemer, W.J. 1992. Validity of isokinetic and isometric testing modalities for assessing short-term resistance exercise strength gains. *Journal of Sport Rehabilitation* 1:275-83.

Fry, A.C.; Stone, M.H.; Thrush, J.T.; and Fleck, S.J. 1995. Precompetition training sessions enhance competitive performance of high anxiety junior weightlifters. *Journal of Strength and Conditioning Research* 9:37-42.

Fukunaga, T.; Funato, K.; and Ikegawa, S. 1992. The effects of resistance training on muscle area and strength in prepubescent age. *Annals of Physiology and Anthropology* 11:357-64.

Funato, K.; Fukunaga, T.; Asami, T.; and Ikeda, S. 1987. Strength training for prepubescent boys and girls. In *Proceedings of the Department of Sports Science*, pp. 9-19. University of Tokyo.

Gajda, B. 1965. The new revolutionary phase or sequence system of training. *Iron Man* 26:14-17.

Gardner, G. 1963. Specificity of strength changes of the exercised and nonexercised limb following isometric training. *Research Quarterly* 34:98-101.

Garfinkel, S., and Cafarelli, E. 1992. Relative changes in maximal force, EMG, and muscle cross-sectional area after isometric training. *Medicine and Science in Sports and Exercise* 24:1220-27.

Garhammer, J. 1980. Power production by Olympic weightlifters. *Medicine and Science in Sports and Exercise* 12:54-60.

Garhammer, J. 1981a. Biomechanical characteristics of the 1978 world weightlifting champions. In *Biomechanics*, vol. VII-B, 300-304. Baltimore: University Park Press.

Garhammer, J. 1981b. Equipment for the development of athletic strength and power. *National Strength and Conditioning Association Journal* 3:24-26.

Garhammer, J. 1982-83. Elite weightlifting project biomechanics reports. Submitted to the Sports Medicine Division, U.S. Olympic Committee, and the U.S. Weightlifting Federation. December 1982, November 1983.

Garhammer, J. 1985. Biomechanical profiles of Olympic weightlifters. *International Journal of Sport and Biomechanics* 1:122-30.

Garhammer, J. 1989. Weight lifting and training. In *Biomechanics of sport*, ed. C.L. Vaughan, 169-211. Boca Raton, FL: CRC Press.

Garhammer, J. 1991a. A comparison of maximal power outputs between elite male and female weightlifters in competition. *International Journal of Sport and Biomechanics* 7:3-11.

Garhammer, J. 1991b. Maximal human power output capacity and its determination for male and female athletes. In *Proceedings of the XIII International Congress on Biomechanics*, December 9-13, 1991, *Book of Abstracts*, pp. 67-68. Perth: University of Western Australia.

Garhammer, J. 1993. A review of power output studies of Olympic and powerlifting: Methodology, performance prediction, and evaluation tests. *Journal of Strength and Conditioning Research* 7:76-89.

Garhammer, J., and McLaughlin, T. 1980. Power output as a function of load variation in Olympic and power lifting. *Journal of Biomechanics* 3:198.

Garhammer, J., and Takano, B. 1992. Training for weightlifting. *Strength and Power in Sports* 5:357-81.

Gasser, G.A., and Brooks, G.A. 1979. Metabolism and lactate after prolonged exercise to exhaustion. *Medicine and Science in Sports* 11:76.

Gettman, L.R., and Ayres, J.J. 1978. Aerobic changes through 10 weeks of slow and fast speed isokinetic training. *Medicine and Science in Sports* 10:47.

Gettman, L.R.; Ayres, J.J.; Pollock, M.L.; Durstine, J.C.; and Grantham, W. 1979. Physiological effects on adult men of circuit strength training and jogging. *Archives of Physical Medicine and Rehabilitation* 60:115-20.

Gettman, L.R.; Ayres, J.J.; Pollock, M.L.; and Jackson, A. 1978. The effect of circuit weight training on strength, cardiorespiratory function and body composition of adult men. *Medicine and Science in Sports* 10:171-76.

Gettman, L.R.; Culter, L.A.; and Strathman, T. 1980. Physiological changes after 20 weeks of isotonic vs. isokinetic circuit training. *Journal of Sports Medicine and Physical Fitness* 20:265-74.

Gettman, L.R., and Pollock, M.L. 1981. Circuit weight training: A critical review of its physiological benefits. *Physician and Sportsmedicine* 9:44-60.

Gilliam, G.M. 1981. Effects of frequency of weight training on muscle strength enhancement. *Journal of Sports Medicine* 21:432-36.

Gladden, L.B., and Colacino, D. 1978. Characteristics of volleyball players and success in a national tournament. *Journal of Sports Medicine and Physical Fitness* 18:57-64.

Goldberg, L.; Elliot, D.L.; and Kuehl, K.S. 1988. Cardiovascular changes at rest and during mixed static and dynamic exercise after weight training. *Journal of Applied Sport Science Research* 2:42-45.

Goldberg, L.; Elliot, D.L.; and Kuehl, K.S. 1994. A comparison of the cardiovascular effects of running and weight training. *Journal of Strength and Conditioning Research* 8:219-24.

Golden, C.L., and Dudley, G.A. 1992. Strength after bouts of eccentric or concentric actions. *Medicine and Science in Sports and Exercise* 24:926-33.

Goldspink, G. 1992. Cellular and molecular aspects of adaptation in skeletal muscle. In *Strength and power in sport*, ed. P.V. Komi, 211-29. Oxford: Blackwell Scientific.

Gollhofer, A. 1987. Innervation characteristics of m. gastrocnemius during landing on different surfaces. In *Biomechanics XB*, ed. B. Jonsson, 701-6. Champaign, IL: Human Kinetics.

Gollnick, P.D.; Timson, B.F.; Moore, R.L.; and Riedy, M. 1981. Muscular enlargement and number of fibers in skeletal muscles of rats. *Journal of Applied Physiology: Respiratory, Environmental and Exercise Physiology* 50:936-43.

Gonyea, W.J. 1980. Role of exercise in inducing increases in skeletal muscle fiber number. *Journal of Applied Physiology: Respiratory, Environmental and Exercise Physiology* 48:421-26.

Gonyea, W.J., and Sale, D. 1982. Physiology of weight-lifting exercise. *Archives of Physical Medicine and Rehabilitation* 63:235-37.

Gonyea, W.J.; Sale, D.; Gonyea, F.; and Mikesky, A. 1986. Exercise induced increases in muscle fiber number. *European Journal of Applied Physiology.* 55:137-41.

Gordon, A.M.; Huxley, A.F.; and Julian, F.J. 1966. The variation in isometric tension with sarcomere length in vertebrate muscle fibers. *Journal of Physiology* 184:170-92.

Gordon, S.E.; Kraemer, W.J.; and Pedro, J.G. 1991. Increased acid-base buffering capacity via dietary supplementation: Anaerobic exercise implications. *Journal of Applied Nutrition* 43:40-48.

Gordon, S.E.; Kraemer, W.J.; Vos, N.H.; Lynch, J.M.; and Knuttgen, H.G. 1994. Effect of acid base balance on the growth hormone response to acute, high-intensity cycle exercise. *Journal of Applied Physiology* 76:821-29.

Grassi, B.; Cerretelli, P.; Narici, M.V.; and Marconi, C. 1991. Peak anaerobic power in master athletes. *European Journal of Applied Physiology* 62:394-99.

Graves, J.E., and James, R.J. 1990. Concurrent augmented feedback and isometric force generation during familiar and unfamiliar muscle movements. *Research Quarterly for Exercise and Sport* 61:75-79.

Graves, J.E.; Pollock, M.L.; Jones, A.E.; Colvin, A.B.; and Leggett, S.H. 1989. Specificity of limited range of motion variable resistance training. *Medicine and Science in Sports and Exercise* 21:84-89.

Graves, J.E.; Pollock, M.L.; Leggett, S.H.; Braith, R.W.; Carpenter, D.M.; and Bishop, L.E. 1988. Effect of reduced frequency on muscular strength. *International Journal of Sports Medicine* 9:316-19.

Gray, D.P., and Dale, E. 1984. Variables associated with secondary amenorrhea in women runners. *Journal of Sports Sciences* 1:55-67.

Green, H.J. 1986. Muscle power: Fibre type recruitment, metabolism and fatigue. In *Human muscle power*, eds. N.L. Jones, N. McCartney, and A.J. McComas, 65-79. Champaign, IL: Human Kinetics.

Grimby, G.; Bjorntorp, P.; Fahlen, M.; Hoskins, T.A.; Hook, O.; Oxhof, H.; and Saltin, B. 1973. Metabolic effects of isometric training. *Scandinavian Journal of Clinical Laboratory Investigation* 31:301-5.

Grimby, L., and Hannerz, J. 1977. Firing rate and recruitment order of toe extensor motor units in different modes of voluntary contraction. *Journal of Physiology* (London) 264:867-79.

Grimby, L.; Hannerz, J.; and Hedman, B. 1981. The fatigue and voluntary discharge properties of single motor units in man. *Journal of Physiology* 36:545-54.

Grumbs, V.L.; Seagal, D.; Halligan, J.B.; and Lower, G. 1982. Bilateral radius and ulnar fractures in adolescent weight lifters. *American Journal of Sports Medicine* 10:375-79.

Haggmark, T.; Jansson, E.; and Eriksson, E. 1982. Fiber type area and metabolic potential of the thigh muscle in man after knee surgery and immobilization. *International Journal of Sports Medicine* 2:12-17.

Haggmark, T.; Jansson, E.; and Svane, B. 1978. Cross-sectional area of the thigh muscle in man measured by computed tomography. *Scandinavian Journal of Clinical and Laboratory Investigation* 38:354-60.

Häkkinen, K. 1985. Factors affecting trainability of muscular strength during short term and prolonged training. *National Strength and Conditioning Association Journal* 7:32-37.

Häkkinen, K. 1989. Neuromuscular and hormonal adaptations during strength and power training. *Journal of Sports Medicine* 29:9-26.

Häkkinen, K. 1992. Neuromuscular responses in male and female athletes to two successive strength training sessions in one day. *Journal of Sports Medicine and Physical Fitness* 32:234-42.

Häkkinen, K. 1993a. Changes in physical fitness profile in female basketball players during the competitive season including explosive type strength training. *Journal of Sports Medicine and Physical Fitness* 33:19-26.

Häkkinen, K. 1993b. Neuromuscular fatigue during heavy resistance loading in men at different ages. In *Proceedings of the XIV International Congress of Biomechanics*, Vol. I, Paris, July 4-8, 1993, pp. 538-39.

Häkkinen, K.; Alén, M.; and Komi, P.V. 1984. Neuromuscular, anaerobic, and aerobic performance of elite power athletes. *European Journal of Applied Physiology* 53:97-105.

Häkkinen, K.; Alén, M.; and Komi, P.V. 1985. Changes in isometric force- and relaxation-time, electromyographic and muscle fibre characteristics of human skeletal muscle during strength training and detraining. *Acta Physiologica Scandinavica* 125:573-85.

Häkkinen, K., and Häkkinen, A. 1991. Muscle cross-sectional area, force production and relaxation characteristics in women at different ages. *European Journal of Applied Physiology* 62:410-14.

Häkkinen, K., and Komi, P.V. 1981. Effect of different combined concentric and eccentric muscle work on maximal strength development. *Journal of Human Movement Studies* 7:33-44.

Häkkinen, K., and Komi, P.V. 1983. Changes in neuromuscular performance in voluntary and reflex contraction during strength training in man. *International Journal of Sports Medicine* 4:282-88.

Häkkinen, K., and Komi, P.V. 1985a. Changes in electrical and mechanical behavior of leg extensor muscles during heavy resistance strength training. *Scandinavian Journal of Sports Science* 7:55-64.

Häkkinen, K., and Komi, P.V. 1985b. The effect of explosive type strength training on electromyographic and force production characteristics of leg extensor muscles during concentric and various stretch-shortening cycle exercises. *Scandinavian Journal of Sports Science* 7:65-76.

Häkkinen, K., and Komi, P.V. 1986. Effects of fatigue and recovery on electromyographic and isometric force- and relaxation-time characteristics of human skeletal muscle. *European Journal of Applied Physiology* 55:588-96.

Häkkinen, K.; Komi, P.V.; and Alén, M. 1985. Effect of explosive type strength training on isometric force- and relaxation-time, electromyographic and muscle fiber characteristics of leg extensor muscles. *Acta Physiologica Scandinavica* 125:587-600.

Häkkinen, K.; Komi, P.V.; and Tesch, P.A. 1981. Effect of combined concentric and eccentric strength training and detraining on force-time, muscle fiber and metabolic characteristics of leg extensor muscles. *Scandinavian Journal of Sports Science* 3 (2): 50-58.

Häkkinen, K.; Kraemer, W.J.; Kallinen, M.; Linnamo, V.; Pastinen, U.M.; and Newton, R.U. 1996. Bilateral and unilateral neuromuscular function and muscle cross-sectional area in middle-aged and elderly men and women. *Journal of Gerontology and Biological Sciences* 51A:B21-B29.

Häkkinen, K.; Kraemer, W.J.; and Newton, R.U. In press. Muscle activation and force production during bilateral and unilateral concentric and isometric contractions of the knee extensors in men and women at different ages. *Electromyography and Clinical Neurophysiology*.

Häkkinen, K., and Pakarinen, A. 1991. Serum hormones in male strength athletes during intensive short term strength training. *European Journal of Applied Physiology* 63:194-99.

Häkkinen, K., and Pakarinen, A. 1993. Muscle strength and serum testosterone, cortisol and SHBG concentrations in middle-aged and elderly men and women. *Acta Physiologica Scandinavica* 148:199-207.

Häkkinen, K., and Pakarinen, A. 1995. Acute hormonal responses to heavy resistance exercise in men and women at different ages. *International Journal of Sports Medicine* 16:507-13.

Häkkinen, K.; Pakarinen, A.; Alén, M.; Kauhanen, H.; and Komi, P.V. 1987. Relationships between training volume, physical performance capacity, and serum hormone concentration during prolonged training in elite weight lifters. *International Journal of Sports Medicine* 8:61-65.

Häkkinen, K.; Pakarinen, A.; Alén, M.; Kauhanen, H.; and Komi, P.V. 1988a. Daily hormonal and neuromuscular responses to intensive strength training in 1 week. *International Journal of Sports Medicine* 9:422-28.

Häkkinen, K.; Pakarinen, A.; Alén, M.; Kauhanen, H.; and Komi, P.V. 1988b. Neuromuscular and hormonal adaptations in athletes to strength training in two years. *Journal of Applied Physiology* 65:2406-12.

Häkkinen, K.; Pakarinen, A.; Alén, M.; Kauhanen, H.; and Komi, P.V. 1988c. Neuromuscular and hormonal responses in elite athletes to two successive strength training sessions in one day. *European Journal of Applied Physiology* 57:133-39.

Häkkinen, K.; Pakarinen, A.; Alén, M.; and Komi, P.V. 1985. Serum hormones during prolonged training of neuromuscular performance. *European Journal of Applied Physiology* 53:287-93.

Häkkinen, K.; Pakarinen, A.; Komi, P.V.; Ryushi, T.; and Kauhanen, H. 1989. Neuromuscular adaptations and hormone balance in strength athletes, physically active males, and females during intensive strength training. In *Proceedings of the XII International Congress of Biomechanics*, no. 8, eds. R.J. Gregor, R.F. Zernicke, and W.C. Whiting, 889-94. Champaign, IL: Human Kinetics.

Häkkinen, K.; Pakarinen, A.; Kyrolainen, H.; Cheng, S.; Kim, D.H.; and Komi, P.V. 1990. Neuromuscular adaptations and serum hormones in females during prolonged training. *International Journal of Sports Medicine* 11:91-98.

Häkkinen, K.; Pastinen, U.M.; Karsikas, R.; and Linnamo, V. 1995. Neuromuscular performance in voluntary bilateral and unilateral contraction and during electrical stimulation in men at different ages. *European Journal of Applied Physiology* 70:518-27.

Hamill, B.P. 1994. Relative safety of weightlifting and weight training. *Journal of Strength and Conditioning Research* 8:53-57.

Hammond, G.L.; Kontturi, M.; Vihko, P.; and Vihko, R. 1974. Serum steroids in normal males and patients with prostatic diseases. *Clinical Endocrinology* 9:113-21.

Harman, E. 1983. Resistive torque analysis of 5 Nautilus exercise machines. *Medicine and Science in Sports and Exercise* 15:113.

Harman, E.A.; Rosenstein, R.; Frykman, P.; and Nigro, G. 1989. Effect of a belt on intra-abdominal pressure during weight lifting. *Medicine and Science in Sports and Exercise* 21:186-90.

Harries, U.J., and Bassey, E.J. 1990. Torque-velocity relationships for the knee extensors in women in their 3rd and 7th decades. *European Journal of Applied Physiology* 60:87-190.

Harr Romeny, B.M.; Denier Van Der Gon, J.J.; and Gielen, C.C. 1982. Changes in recruitment order of motor units in the human biceps muscle. *Experimental Neurology* 78:360-68.

Hatfield, F.C. 1981. *Powerlifting: A scientific approach.* Chicago: Contemporary Books.

Hatfield, F.C., and Krotee, M.L. 1978. *Personalized weight training for fitness and athletics from theory to practice.* Dubuque, IA: Kendall/Hunt.

Hatfield, F.C., and McLaughlin, T.M. 1985. Powerlifting. In *Encyclopedia of physical education, fitness, and sports,* ed. T.K. Cureton, vol. 4, 587-93. Reston, VA: AAHPERD.

Hather, B.M.; Mason, C.E.; and Dudley, G.A. 1991. Histochemical demonstration of skeletal muscle fiber types and capillaries on the same transverse section. *Clinical Physiology* (Oxford) 11:127-34.

Hather, B.M.; Tesch, P.A.; Buchanan, P.; and Dudley, G.A. 1992. Influence of eccentric actions on skeletal muscle adaptations to resistance training. *Acta Physiologica Scandinavica* 143:177-85.

Hatta, H.; Atomi, Y.; Yamamoto, Y.; Shinohara, S.; and Yamada, S. 1989. Incorporation of blood lactate and glucose into tissues in rats after short-term strenuous exercise. *International Journal of Sports Medicine* 10:272-78.

Hayward, V.H.; Johannes Ellis, S.M.; and Romer, J.F. 1986. Gender differences in strength. *Research Quarterly for Exercise and Sport* 57:154-59.

Hejna, W.F.; Rosenberg, A.; Buturusis, D.J.; and Krieger, A. 1982. The prevention of sports injuries in high school students through strength training. *National Strength and Conditioning Association Journal* 4:28-31.

Henderson, J.M. 1970. The effects of weight loadings and repetitions, frequency of exercise and knowledge of theoretical principles of weight training on changes in muscular strength. *Dissertation Abstracts International* 31A:3320.

Henneman, E.; Somjen, G.; and Carpenter, D.O. 1985. Functional significance of cell size in apinal motoneurons. *Journal of Neurophysiology* 28:560-80.

Hennessy, L.C., and Watson, A.W.S. 1994. The interference effects of training for strength and endurance simultaneously. *Journal of Strength and Conditioning Research* 8:12-19.

Henriksson-Larsen, K. 1985. Distribution, number and size of different types of fibres in whole cross-sections of female m. tibialis anterior. An enzyme histochemical study. *Acta Physiologica Scandinavica* 123:229-35.

Hensinger, R.N. 1982. Back pain and vertebral changes simulating Scheuermann's disease. *Orthopaedic Transactions* 6:1.

Hermansen, L.; Machlum, S.; Pruett, E.R.; Vaage, O.; Waldrum, H.; and Wessel-Aas, T. 1976. Lactate removal at rest and during exercise. In *Metabolic adaptation to prolonged physical exercise,* eds. H. Howard and J.R. Pootsmans, 101-5. Basel: Birhauser Verlag.

Hetherington, M.R. 1976. Effect of isometric training on the elbow flexion force torque of grade five boys. *Research Quarterly for Exercise and Sport* 47:41-47.

Hetrick, G.A., and Wilmore, J.H. 1979. Androgen levels and muscle hypertrophy during an eight week weight training program for men/women. *Medicine and Science in Sports* 11:102.

Hettinger, R. 1961. *Physiology of strength.* Springfield, IL: Charles C Thomas.

Hettinger, R., and Muller, E. 1953. Muskelleistung und Muskeltraining. *Arbeits Physiologie* 15:111-26.

Hickson, R.C. 1980. Interference of strength development by simultaneously training for strength and endurance. *European Journal of Applied Physiology* 45:255-69.

Hildebrandt, W.; Schutze, H.; and Stegemann, J. 1992. Cardiovascular limitations of active recovery from strenuous exercise. *European Journal of Applied Physiology and Occupational Physiology* 64:250-57.

Ho, K.W.; Roy, R.R.; Tweedle, C.D.; Heusner, W.W.; Van Huss, W.D.; and Carrow, R. 1980. Skeletal muscle fiber splitting with weight-lifting exercise in rats. *American Journal of Anatomy* 157:433-40.

Hoeger, W.W.K.; Barette, S.L.; Hale, D.F.; and Hopkins, D.R. 1987. Relationship between repetitions and selected percentages of one repetition maximum. *Journal of Applied Sport Science Research* 1:11-13.

Hoeger, W.W.K.; Hopkins, D.R.; Barette, S.L.; and Hale, D.F. 1990. Relationship between repetitions and selected percentages of one repetition maximum: A comparison between untrained and trained males and females. *Journal of Applied Sport Science Research* 4:47-54.

Hoffman, J.R.; Fry, A.C.; Howard, R.; Maresh, C.M.; and Kraemer, W.J. 1991. Strength, speed, and endurance changes during the course of a Division I basketball season. *Journal of Applied Sport Science Research* 5:144-49.

Hoffman, J.R.; Kraemer, W.J.; Fry, A.C.; Deschenes, M.; and Kemp, M. 1990. The effects of self-selection for frequency of training in a winter conditioning program for football. *Journal of Applied Sport Science Research* 4:76-82.

Hoffman, T.; Stauffer, R.W.; and Jackson, A.S. 1979. Sex difference in strength. *American Journal of Sports Medicine* 7:265-67.

Hogan, M.C.; Gladden, L.B.; Kurdak, S.S.; and Poole, D.C. 1995 Increased [lactate] in working dog muscle reduces tension development independent of pH. *Medicine and Science in Sports and Exercise* 27:371-77.

Holmdahl, D.C., and Ingelmark, R.E. 1948. Der bau des Gelenknorpels unterverschiedenen funktionellen Verhaltnissen. *Acta Anatomica* 6:113-16.

Hortobágyi, T.; Houmard, J.A.; Stevenson, J.R.; Fraser, D.D.; Johns, R.A.; and Israel, R.G. 1993. The effects of detraining on power athletes. *Medicine and Science in Sports and Exercise* 25:929-35.

Hortobágyi, T.; Katch, F.I.; and LaChance, P.F. 1991. Effects of simultaneous training for strength and endurance on upper and lower body strength and running performance. *Journal of Sports Medicine and Physical Fitness* 31:20-30.

Horvath, B. 1959. What's new in muscles? *Muscle Sculpture* 2:39-44.

Housh, D.J.; Housh, T.J.; Johnson, G.O.; and Chu, W.-K. 1992. Hypertrophic response to unilateral concentric isokinetic training. *Journal of Applied Physiology* 73:65-70.

Houston, M.E.; Froese, E.A.; Valeriote, S.P.; Green, H.J.; and Ramey, D.A. 1983. Muscle performance, morphology and metabolic capacity during strength train-ing and detraining: A one leg model. *European Journal of Applied Physiology and Occupational Physiology* 51:25-35.

Houston, M.E.; Norman, R.W.; and Froese, E.A. 1988. Mechanical measures during maximal velocity knee extension exercise and their relation to fibre composition of the human vastus lateralis muscle. *European Journal of Applied Physiology* 58:1-7.

Howald, H. 1982. Training-induced morphological and functional changes in skeletal muscle. *International Journal of Sports Medicine* 3:1-12.

Hudson, J. 1978. Physical parameters used for female exclusion from law enforcement and athletics. In *Women and sport: From myth to reality*, ed. G.A. Ogleby, 19-57. Philadelphia: Lea and Febiger.

Hultman, E.; Bergstrom, J.; and Anderson, N.M. 1967. Breakdown and resynthesis of phosphorylcreatine and adenosine triphosphate in connection with muscular work in man. *Scandinavian Journal of Clinical Laboratory Investigation* 19:56-66.

Hunter, G.; Demment, R.; and Miller, D. 1987. Development of strength and maximum oxygen uptake during simultaneous training for strength and endurance. *Journal of Sports Medicine and Physical Fitness* 27:269-75.

Hunter, G.R. 1985. Changes in body composition, body build and performance associated with different weight training frequencies in males and females. *National Strength and Conditioning Association Journal* 7:26-28.

Hunter, G.R.; McGuirk, J.; Mitrano, N.; Pearman, P.; Thomas, B.; and Arrington, R. 1989. The effects of a weight training belt on blood pressure during exercise. *Journal of Applied Sport Science Research* 3:13-18.

Hunter, G.R., and Treuth, M.S. 1995. Relative training intensity and increases in strength in older women. *Journal of Strength and Conditioning Research* 9:188-91.

Hurley, B. 1995. Strength training in the elderly to enhance health status. *Medicine, Exercise, Nutrition and Health* 4:217-29.

Hurley, B.F. 1989. Effects of resistance training on lipoprotein-lipid profiles: A comparison to aerobic exercise training. *Medicine and Science in Sports and Exercise* 21:689-93.

Hurley, B.F.; Hagberg, J.M.; Seals, D.R.; Ehasani, A.A.; Goldberg, A.P.; and Holloszy, J.O. 1987. Glucose tolerance and lipid-lipoprotein levels in middle-aged powerlifters. *Clinical Physiology* 7:11-19.

Hurley, B.F.; Seals, D.R.; Ehasani, A.A.; Cartier, L.J.; Dalsky, G.P.; Hagberg, J.M.; and Holloszy, J.O. 1984. Effects of high-intensity strength training on cardiovascular function. *Medicine and Science in Sports and Exercise* 16:483-88.

Hurley, B.F.; Seals, D.R.; Hagberg, J.M.; Goldberg, A.C.; Ostrove, S.M.; Holloszy, J.O.; Wiest, W.G.; and Goldberg, A.P. 1984. High density lipoprotein cholesterol in body builders vs. power lifters. *Journal of the American Medical Association* 252:507-13.

Hutton, R.S. 1992. Neuromuscular basis of stretching exercises. In *Strength and power in sport*, ed. P.V. Komi, 29-38. Oxford: Blackwell Scientific.

Hutton, R.S., and Atwater, S.W. 1992. Acute and chronic adaptations of muscle proprioceptors in response to increased use. *Sports Medicine* 14:406-21.

Huxley, H. 1969. The mechanism of muscular contraction. *Science* 164:1356-66.

Ikai, M., and Fukunaga, T. 1968. Calculation of muscle strength per unit cross-sectional area of human muscle by means of ultrasonic measurements. *International Zeitschrift fur Angewandte Physiologie* 26:26-32.

Ikai, M., and Fukunaga, T. 1970. A study on training effect on strength per unit cross-sectional area of muscle by means of ultrasonic measurement. *European Journal of Applied Physiology* 28:173-80.

Ikai, M., and Steinhaus, A.H. 1961. Some factors modifying the expression of human strength. *Journal of Applied Physiology* 16:157-63.

Imamura, K.; Ashida, H.; Ishikawa, T.; and Fujii, M. 1983. Human major psoas muscle and sacrospinalis muscle in relation to age: A study by computed tomography. *Journal of Gerontology* 38:678-81.

Ingelmark, B.E., and Elsholm, R. 1948. A study on variations in the thickness of the articular cartilage in association with rest and periodical load. *Uppsala Lakaretorenings Foxhandlingar* 53:61-64.

Ingjer, F. 1969. Effects of endurance training on muscle fiber ATP-ase activity, capillary supply and mitochondrial content in man. *Journal of Physiology* 294:419-32.

Ishida, K.; Moritani, T.; and Itoh, K. 1990. Changes in voluntary and electrically induced contractions during strength training and detraining. *European Journal of Applied Physiology* 60:244-48.

Jackson, A.; Jackson, T.; Hnatek, J.; and West, J. 1985. Strength development: Using functional isometrics in an isotonic strength training program. *Research Quarterly for Exercise and Sport* 56:234-37.

Jacobson, P.C.; Bever, W.; Brubb, S.A.; Taft, T.N.; and Talmage, R.V. 1984. Bone density in female college athletes and older athletic females. *Journal of Orthopaedic Research* 2:328-32.

Jenkins, W.L.; Thackaberry, M.; and Killian, C. 1984. Speed-specific isokinetic training. *Journal of Orthopaedic and Sports Physical Therapy* 6:181-83.

Jensen, C., and Fisher, G. 1979. *Scientific basis of athletic conditioning.* Philadelphia: Lea and Febiger.

Johnson, B.L.; Adamczy, K.J.W.; Tennoe, K.O.; and Stromme, S.B. 1976. A comparison of concentric and eccentric muscle training. *Medicine and Science in Sports* 8:35-38.

Johnson, J.H.; Colodny, S.; and Jackson, D. 1990. Human torque capability versus machine resistive torque for four eagle resistance machines. *Journal of Applied Sport Science Research* 4:83-87.

Jones, A. 1973. The best kind of exercise. *Ironman* 32:36-38.

Jones, D.A., and Rutherford, O.M. 1987. Human muscle strength training: The effects of three different regimes and the nature of the resultant changes. *Journal of Physiology* 391:1-11.

Kamen, G.; Kroll, W.; and Zigon, S.T. 1984. Exercise effects upon reflex time components in weight lifters and distance runners. *Medicine and Science in Sports and Exercise* 13:198-204.

Kanakis, C., and Hickson, C. 1980. Left ventricular responses to a program of lower-limb strength training. *Chest* 78:618-21.

Kanehisa, H., and Miyashita, M. 1983a. Effect of isometric and isokinetic muscle training on static strength and dynamic power. *European Journal of Applied Physiology* 50:365-71.

Kanehisa, H., and Miyashita, M. 1983b. Specificity of velocity in strength training. *European Journal of Applied Physiology* 52:104-6.

Kaneko, M.; Fuchimoto, T.; Toji, H.; and Suei, K. 1983. Training effect of different loads on the force-velocity relationship and mechanical power output in human muscle. *Scandinavian Journal of Sports Science* 5:50-55.

Karlsson, J.; Bonde-Petersen, F.; Henriksson, J.; and Knuttgen, H.G. 1975. Effects of previous exercise with arms or legs on metabolism and performance in exhaustive exercise. *Journal of Applied Physiology* 38:208-11.

Katch, U.L.; Katch, F.I.; Moffatt, R.; and Gittleson, M. 1980. Muscular development and lean body weight in body builders and weight lifters. *Medicine and Science in Sports and Exercise* 12:340-44.

Kauhanen, H., and Häkkinen, K. 1989. Short term effects of voluminous heavy resistance training and recovery on the snatch technique in weightlifting. In *Proceedings of the XII International Congress of Biomechanics*, eds. R.J. Gregor, R.F. Zernicke, and W.C. Whitting. Abstracts, 31.

Keul, J.; Haralambie, G.; Bruder, M.; and Gottstein, H.J. 1978. The effect of weight lifting exercise on heart rate and metabolism in experienced lifters. *Medicine and Science in Sports and Exercise* 10:13-15.

Kitai, T.A., and Sale, D.G. 1989. Specificity of joint angle in isometric training. *European Journal of Applied Physiology* 58:744-48.

Knapik, J.J.; Mawdsley, R.H.; and Ramos, M.U. 1983. Angular specificity and test mode specificity of isometric and isokinetic strength training. *Journal of Orthopedic Sports Physical Therapy* 5:58-65.

Knuttgen, H.G., and Kraemer, W.J. 1987. Terminology and measurement in exercise performance. *Journal of Applied Sport Science Research* 1:1-10.

Kokkonen, J.; Bangerter, B.; Roundy, E.; and Nelson, A. 1988. Improved performance through digit strength gains. *Research Quarterly for Exercise and Sport* 59:57-63.

Komi, P.V. 1973. Measurement of the force-velocity relationship in human muscle under concentric and eccentric contractions. *Medicine and Sport* 8:224-29.

Komi, P.V. 1979. Neuromuscular performance: Factors influencing force and speed production. *Scandinavian Journal of Sports Sciences* 1:2-15.

Komi, P.V., and Buskirk, E.R. 1972. Effect of eccentric and concentric muscle conditioning on tension and electrical activity of human muscle. *Ergonomics* 15:417-34.

Komi, P.V., and Häkkinen, K. 1988. Strength and power. In *The Olympic book of sports medicine*, eds. A. Dirix, H.G. Knuttgen, and K. Tittel, 183. Boston: Blackwell Scientific.

Komi, P.V.; Kaneko, M.; and Aura, O. 1987. EMG activity of the leg extensor muscles with special reference to mechanical efficiency in concentric and eccentric exercise. *International Journal of Sports Medicine* 8:22-29.

Komi, P.V., and Karlsson, J. 1978. Skeletal muscle fiber types, enzymes activities and physical performance in young males and females. *Acta Physiologica Scandinavica* 103:210-18.

Komi, P.V.; Karlsson, J.; Tesch, P.; Suominen, H.; and Heikkinen, E. 1982. Effects of heavy resistance and explosive-type strength training methods and mechanical, functional and metabolic aspects of performance. In *Exercise and sports biology*, ed. P.V. Komi, 99-102. International Series on Sports Sciences, vol. 12. Champaign, IL: Human Kinetics.

Koutedakis, Y.; Boreham, C.; Kabitsis, C.; and Sharp, N.C.C. 1992. Seasonal deterioration of selected physiological variables in elite male skiers. *International Journal of Sports Medicine* 13:548-51.

Kowalchuk, J.M.; Heigenhauser, F.J.F.; Lininger, M.I.; Obminski, G.; Sutton, J.R.; and Jones, N.L. 1988. Role of lungs and inactive muscle in acid-base control after maximal exercise. *Journal of Applied Physiology* 65:2090-96.

Kraemer, W.J. 1983a. Detraining the "bulked up" athlete: Prospects for lifetime health and fitness. *National Strength and Conditioning Association Journal* 5:10-12.

Kraemer, W.J. 1983b. Exercise prescription in weight training: Manipulating program variables. *National Strength and Conditioning Association Journal* 5:58-59.

Kraemer, W.J. 1983c. Exercise prescription in weight training: A needs analysis. *National Strength and Conditioning Association Journal* 5:64-65.

Kraemer, W.J. 1988. Endocrine responses to resistance exercise. *Medicine and Science in Sports and Exercise* 20 (suppl.): S152-57.

Kraemer, W.J. 1992a. Endocrine responses and adaptations to strength training. In *Strength and power in sport*, ed. P.V. Komi, 291-304. Oxford: Blackwell Scientific.

Kraemer, W.J. 1992b. Hormonal mechanisms related to the expression of muscular strength and power. In *Strength and power in sport*, ed. P.V. Komi, 64-76. Oxford: Blackwell Scientific.

Kraemer, W.J. 1992c. Involvement of eccentric muscle action may optimize adaptations to resistance training. *Sports Science Exchange* 4:230-38. (Gatorade Sports Science Institute, Chicago).

Kraemer, W.J. 1994. Neuroendocrine responses to resistance exercise. In *Essentials of strength and conditioning*, ed. T.R. Baechle, 86-107. Champaign, IL: Human Kinetics.

Kraemer, W.J. In press. A series of studies: The physiological basis for strength training in American football: Fact over philosophy. *Journal of Strength and Conditioning Research*.

Kraemer, W.J.; Deschenes, M.R.; and Fleck, S.J. 1988. Physiological adaptations to resistance training implications for athletic conditioning. *Sports Medicine* 6:246-56.

Kraemer, W.J., and Fleck, S.J. 1993. *Strength training for young athletes*. Champaign IL: Human Kinetics.

Kraemer, W.J.; Fleck, S.J.; and Deschenes, M. 1988. A review: Factors in exercise prescription of resistance training. *National Strength and Conditioning Association Journal* 10:36-41.

Kraemer, W.J.; Fleck, S.J.; Dziados, J.E.; Harman, E.A.; Marchitelli, L.J.; Gordon, S.E.; Mello, R.; Frykman, P.N.; Koziris, L.P., and Triplett, N.T. 1993. Changes in hormonal concentrations following different heavy resistance exercise protocols in women. *Journal of Applied Physiology* 75:594-604.

Kraemer, W.J., and Fry, A.C. 1995. Strength testing: Development and evaluation of methodology. In *Physiological assessment of human fitness*, eds. P. Maud and C. Foster. Champaign, IL: Human Kinetics.

Kraemer, W.J.; Fry, A.C.; Frykman, P.N.; Conroy, B.; and Hoffman, J. 1989. Resistance training and youth. *Pediatric Exercise Science* 1:336-50.

Kraemer, W.J.; Fry, A.C.; Warren, B.J.; Stone, M.H.; Fleck, S.J.; Kearney, J.T.; Conroy, B.P.; Maresh, C.M.; Weseman, C.A.; Triplett, N.T.; and Gordon, S.E. 1992. Acute hormonal responses in elite junior weightlifters. *International Journal of Sports Medicine* 13:103-9.

Kraemer, W.J.; Gordon, S.E.; Fleck, S.J.; Marchitelli, L.J.; Mello, R.; Dziados, J.E.; Friedl, K.; Harman, E.; Maresh, C.; and Fry, A.C. 1991. Endogenous anabolic hormonal and growth factor responses to heavy resistance exercise in males and females. *International Journal of Sports Medicine* 12:228-35.

Kraemer, W.J., and Koziris, L.P. 1992. Muscle strength training: Techniques and considerations. *Physical Therapy Practice* 2:54-68.

Kraemer, W.J., and Koziris, L.P. 1994. Olympic weightlifting and power lifting. In *Physiology and nutrition for competitive sport*, eds. D.R. Lamb, H.G. Knuttgen, and R. Murray, 1-54. Carmel, IN: Cooper.

Kraemer, W.J.; Marchitelli, L.; McCurry, D.; Mello, R.; Dziados, J.E.; Harman, E.; Frykman, P.; Gordon, S.E.; and Fleck, S.J. 1990. Hormonal and growth factor responses to heavy resistance exercise. *Journal of Applied Physiology* 69:1442-50.

Kraemer, W.J.; Noble, B.J.; Clark, M.J.; and Culver, B.W. 1987. Physiologic responses to heavy-resistance exercise with very short rest periods. *International Journal of Sports Medicine* 8:247-52.

Kraemer, W.J.; Patton, J.; Gordon, S.E.; Harman, E.A.; Deschenes, M.R.; Reynolds, K.; Newton, R.U.; Triplett, N.T.; and Dziados, J.E. 1995. Compatibility of high intensity strength and endurance training on hormonal and skeletal muscle adaptations. *Journal of Applied Physiology* 78 (3):976-89.

Kraemer, W.J.; Patton, J.F.; Knuttgen, H.G.; Hannan, C.J.; Kittler, T.; Gordon, S.; Dziados, J.E.; Fry, A.C.; Frykman, P.N.; and Harman, E.A. 1991. The effects of high intensity cycle exercise on sympatho-adrenal medullary response patterns. *Journal of Applied Physiology* 70:8-14.

Kraemer, W.J.; Patton, J.F.; Knuttgen, H.G.; Marchitelli, L.J.; Cruthirds, C.; Damokosh, A.; Harman, E.; Frykman, P.; and Dziados, J.E. 1989. Hypothalamic pituitary-adrenal responses to short duration high-intensity cycle exercise. *Journal of Applied Physiology* 66:161-66.

Kraemer, W.J.; Vogel, J.A.; Patton, J.F.; Dziados, J.E.; and Reynolds, K.L. 1987. *The effects of various physical training programs on short duration high intensity load bearing performance and the Army physical fitness test.* USARIEM Technical Report, 30/87 August.

Kusintz, I., and Kenney, C. 1958. Effects of progressive weight training on health and physical fitness of adolescent boys. *Research Quarterly* 29:295-301.

Lacerte, M.; deLateur, B.J.; Alquist, A.D.; and Questad, K.A. 1992. Concentric versus combined concentric-eccentric isokinetic training programs: Effect on peak torque of human quadriceps femoris muscle. *Archives of Physical Medicine and Rehabilitation* 73:1059-62.

Lamb, D.R. 1978. *Physiology of exercise: Response and adaptations.* New York: Macmillan.

Lander, J.E.; Bates, B.T.; Sawhill, J.A.; and Hamill, J.A. 1985. Comparison between free-weight and isokinetic bench pressing. *Medicine and Science in Sports and Exercise* 17:344-53.

Lander, J.E.; Hundley, J.R.; and Simonton, R.L. 1992. The effectiveness of weight-belts during multiple repetitions of the squat exercise. *Medicine and Science in Sports and Exercise* 24:603-9.

Lander, J.E.; Simonton, R.; and Giacobbe, J. 1990. The effectiveness of weight-belts during the squat exercise. *Medicine and Science in Sports and Exercise* 22:117-26.

Larsson, L. 1978. Morphological and functional characteristics of the aging skeletal muscle in man. *Acta Physiological Scandinavica* 457 (suppl.): 1-36.

Larsson, L. 1982. Physical training effects on muscle morphology in sedentary males at different ages. *Medicine and Science in Sports and Exercise* 14:203-6.

Larsson, L. 1983. Histochemical characteristics of human skeletal muscle during aging. *Acta Physiologica Scandinavica* 117:469-71.

Laubach, L.L. 1976. Comparative muscular strength of men and women: A review of the literature. *Aviation, Space and Environmental Medicine* 47:534-42.

Laurent, D.; Reutenauer, H.; Payen, J.F.; Favre-Javin, A.; Eterradossi, J.; Lekas, J.F.; and Rossi, A. 1992. Muscle bioenergetics in skiers: Studies using NMR. *International Journal of Sports Medicine* 13(Suppl.1):S150-52.

Laurent, G.J.; Sparrow, M.P.; Bates, P.C.; and Millward, D.J. 1978. Collagen content and turnover in cardiac and skeletal muscles of the adult fowl and the changes during stretch-induced growth. *Biochemistry Journal* 176:419-27.

Laycoe, R.R., and Marteniuk, R.G. 1971. Leaning and tension as factors in strength gains produced by static and eccentric training. *Research Quarterly* 42:299-305.

Lee, A.; Craig, B.W.; Lucas, J.; Pohlman, R.; and Stelling, H. 1990. The effect of endurance training, weight training and a combination of endurance and weight training upon the blood lipid profile of young male subjects. *Journal of Applied Sport Science Research* 4:68-75.

Legwold, G. 1982. Does lifting weights harm a prepubescent athlete? *Physician and Sportsmedicine* 10:141-44.

Leighton, J. 1955. Instrument and technique for measurement of range of joint motion. *Archives of Physical Medicine and Rehabilitation* 36:571-78.

Leighton, J. 1957a. Flexibility characteristics of four specialized skill groups of college athletes. *Archives of Physical Medicine and Rehabilitation* 38:24-28.

Leighton, J. 1957b. Flexibility characteristics of three specialized skill groups of champion athletes. *Archives of Physical Medicine and Rehabilitation* 38:580-83.

Leighton, J.R.; Holmes, D.; Benson, J.; Wooten, B.; and Schmerer, R. 1967. A study of the effectiveness of ten different methods of progressive resistance exercise on the development of strength, flexibility, girth, and body weight. *Journal of the Association of Physical and Mental Rehabilitation* 21:78-81.

Lemon, P.W., and Mullin, J.P. 1980. Effect of initial muscle glycogen levels on protein catabolism during exercise. *Journal of Applied Physiology: Respiratory, Environmental and Exercise Physiology* 48:624-29.

Lesmes, G.R.; Costill, D.L.; Coyle, E.F.; and Fink, W.J. 1978. Muscle strength and power changes during maximal isokinetic training. *Medicine and Science in Sports* 4:266-69.

Lewis, S.; Nygaard, E.; Sanchez, J.; Egelbald, H.; and Saltin, B. 1984. Static contraction of the quadriceps muscle in man: Cardiovascular control and responses to one-legged strength training. *Acta Physiologica Scandinavica* 122:341-53.

Lexell, J.; Henriksson-Larsen, K.; Winblad, B.; and Sjostrom, M. 1983. Distribution of different fiber types in human skeletal muscles: Effects of aging studied in whole muscle cross section. *Muscle and Nerve* 6:588-95.

Lieber, R.L., and Friden, J. 1993. Muscle damage is not a function of muscle force but active muscle strain. *Journal of Applied Physiology* 74:520-26.

Lieber, R.L.; Woodburn, T.M.; and Friden, J. 1991. Muscle damage induced by eccentric contractions of 25% strain. *Journal of Applied Physiology* 70:2498-2507.

Liederman, E. 1925. *Secrets of strength.* New York: Earle Liederman.

Lind, A.R., and Petrofsky, J.S. 1978. Isometric tension from rotary stimulation of fast and slow cat muscles. *Muscle and Nerve* 1:213-18.

Lindh, M. 1979. Increase of muscle strength from isometric quadriceps exercises at different knee angles. *Scandinavian Journal of Rehabilitation Medicine* 11:33-36.

Lipscomb, A.B. 1975. Baseball pitching in growing athletes. *Journal of Sports Medicine* 3:25-34.

Liu, H.; Liu, P.; and Qin, X. 1987. *Investigation of menstrual cycle in female weightlifters.* Beijing: Department of Exercise Physiology, National Institute of Sports Science.

Loucks, A.B., and Horvath, S.M. 1985. Athletic amenorrhea: A review. *Medicine and Science in Sports and Exercise* 17:56-72.

Lusiani, L.; Ronsisvalle, G.; Bonanome, A.; Castellani, V.; Macchia, C.; and Payan, A. 1986. Echocardiographic evaluation of the dimensions and systolic properties of the left ventricle in freshman athletes during physical training. *European Heart Journal* 7:196-203.

Luthi, J.M.; Howald, H.; Claassen, H.; Rosler, K.; Vock, P.; and Hoppler, H. 1986. Structural changes in skeletal muscle tissue with heavy-resistance exercise. *International Journal of Sports Medicine* 7:123-27.

MacDougall, J.D. 1992. Hypertrophy or hyperplasia. In *Strength and power in sport*, ed. P.V. Komi, 230-38. Oxford: Blackwell Scientific.

MacDougall, J.D.; Sale, D.G.; Alway, S.E.; and Sutton, J.R. 1984. Muscle fiber number in biceps brachii in body builders and control subjects. *Journal of Applied Physiology: Respiratory, Environmental and Exercise Physiology* 57:1399-1403.

MacDougall, J.D.; Sale, D.G.; Elder, G.C.B.; and Sutton, J.R. 1982. Muscle ultrastructural characteristics of elite power lifters and body builders. *European Journal of Applied Physiology* 48:117-26.

MacDougall, J.D.; Sale, D.G.; Moroz, J.R.; Elder, G.C.B.; Sutton, J.R.; and Howard, H. 1979. Mitochondrial volume density in human skeletal muscle following heavy resistance training. *Medicine and Science in Sports and Exercise* 11:164-66.

MacDougall, J.D.; Tuxen, D.; Sale, D.G.; Moroz, J.R.; and Sutton, J.R. 1985. Arterial blood pressure response to heavy resistance exercise. *Journal of Applied Physiology* 58:785-90.

MacDougall, J.D.; Ward, G.R.; Sale, D.G.; and Sutton, J.R. 1977. Biochemical adaptation of human skeletal muscle to heavy resistance training and immobilization. *Journal of Applied Physiology* 43:700-703.

Madsen, N., and McLaughlin, T. 1984. Kinematic factors influencing performance and injury risk in the bench press exercise. *Medicine and Science in Sports and Exercise* 16:429-37.

Manning, R.J.; Graves, J.E.; Carpenter, D.M.; Leggett, S.H.; and Pollock, M.L. 1990. Constant vs. variable resistance knee extension training. *Medicine and Science in Sports and Exercise* 22:397-401.

Mannion, A.F.; Jakeman, P.M.; and Willan, P.L.T. 1992. Effect of isokinetic training of the knee extensors on isokinetic strength and peak power output during cycling. *European Journal of Applied Physiology* 65:370-75.

Marcinik, E.J.; Potts, J.; Schlabach, G.; Will, S.; Dawson, P.; and Hurley, B.F. 1991. Effects of strength training on lactate threshold and endurance performance. *Medicine and Science in Sports and Exercise* 23:739-43.

Maresh, C.M.; Abraham, A.; DeSouza, M.J.; Deschenes, M.R.; Kraemer, W.J.; Armstrong, L.E.; Maguire, M.S.; Gabaree, C.L.; and Hoffman, J.R. 1992. Oxygen consumption following exercise of moderate intensity and duration. *European Journal of Applied Physiology* 65:421-26.

Maresh, C.M.; Allison, T.G.; Noble, B.J.; Drash, A.; and Kraemer, W.J. 1989. Substrate and endocrine responses to race-intensity exercise following a marathon run. *International Journal of Sports Medicine* 10:101-6.

Markiewitz, A.D., and Andrish, J.T. 1992. Hand and wrist injuries in the preadolescent athlete. *Clinics in Sports Medicine* 11:203-25.

Massey, B.H., and Chaudet, N.L. 1956. Effects of heavy resistance exercise on range of joint movement in young male adults. *Research Quarterly* 27:41-51.

Masterson, G.L., and Brown, S.P. 1993. Effects of weighted rope jump training on power performance tests in col-

legians. *Journal of Strength and Conditioning Research* 7:108-14.

Matveyev, L. 1981. *Fundamentals of sports training*. Moscow: Progress.

Maud, P.J., and Shultz, B.B. 1986. Gender comparisons in anaerobic power and anaerobic capacity tests. *British Journal of Sports Medicine* 20:51-54.

Maughan, R.J.; Harmon, M.; Leiper, J.B.; Sale, D.; and Delman, A. 1986. Endurance capacity of untrained males and females in isometric and dynamic muscular contractions. *European Journal of Applied Physiology* 55:395-400.

Mayhew, J.L., and Gross, P.M. 1974. Body composition changes in young women with high intensity weight training. *Research Quarterly* 45:433-40.

Mayhew, J.L., and Salm, P.C. 1990. Gender differences in anaerobic power tests. *European Journal of Applied Physiology* 60:133-38.

McCarthy, J.P.; Agre, J.C.; Graf, B.K.; Poziniak, M.A.; and Vailas, A.C. 1995. Compatibility of adaptive responses with combining strength and endurance training. *Medicine and Science in Sports and Exercise* 27:429-36.

McCartney, N.; McKelvie, R.S.; Martin, J.; Sale, D.G.; and MacDougall, J.D. 1993. Weight-training-induced attenuation of the circulatory response of older males to weight lifting. *Journal of Applied Physiology* 74:1056-60.

McDonagh, M.J.N., and Davies, C.T.M. 1984. Adaptive responses of mammalian skeletal muscle to exercise with high loads. *European Journal of Applied Physiology* 52:139-55.

McDonagh, M.J.N.; Hayward, C.M.; and Davies, C.T.M. 1983. Isometric training in human elbow flexor muscles. *Journal of Bone and Joint Surgery* 65:355-58.

McGee, D.; Jessee, T.C.; Stone, M.H.; and Blessing, D. 1992. Leg and hip endurance adaptations to three weight-training programs. *Journal of Applied Sports Science Research* 6:92-95.

McGovern, M. 1984. Effects of circuit weight training on the physical fitness of prepubescent children. *Dissertation Abstracts International* 45:452A-53A.

McLaughlin, T.M.; Dillman, C.J.; and Lardner, T.J. 1977. A kinematic model of performance of the parallel squat. *Medicine and Science in Sports* 9:128-33.

McLoughlin, P.; McCaffrey, N.; and Moynihan, J.B. 1991. Gentle exercise with a previously inactive muscle group hastens the decline of blood lactate concentration after strenuous exercise. *European Journal of Applied Physiology* 62:274-78.

McMorris, R.O., and Elkins, E.C. 1954. A study of production and evaluation of muscular hypertrophy. *Archives of Physical Medicine and Rehabilitation* 35:420-26.

Meltzer, D.E. 1994. Age dependence of Olympic weightlifting ability. *Medicine and Science in Sports and Exercise* 26:1053-67.

Meredith, C.N.; Frontera, W.R.; O'Reilly, K.P.; and Evans, W.J. 1992. Body composition in elderly men: Effect of dietary modification during strength training. *Journal of the American Geriatric Society* 40:155-62.

Mero, A. 1988. Blood lactate production and recovery from

anaerobic exercise in trained and untrained boys. *European Journal of Applied Physiology* 57:660-66.

Meyer, R.A., and Terjung, R.L. 1979. Differences in ammonia and adenylate metabolism in contracting fast and slow muscle. *American Journal of Physiology* 237:C11-C18.

Meyers, C.R. 1967. Effect of two isometric routines on strength, size and endurance in exercised and non-exercised arms. *Research Quarterly* 38:430-40.

Micheli, L.J. 1983. Overuse injuries in children's sports: The growth factor. *Orthopedic Clinics of North America* 14:337-60.

Miles, D.S.; Owens, J.J.; Golden, J.C.; and Gothsall, R.W. 1987. Central and peripheral hemodynamics during maximal leg extension exercise. *European Journal of Applied Physiology* 56:12-17.

Miller, A.E.J.; MacDougall, J.D.; Tarnopolsky, M.A.; and Sale, D.G. 1992. Gender differences in strength and muscle fiber characteristics. *European Journal Applied Physiology* 66:254-62.

Miller, B.P. 1982. The effects of plyometric training on the vertical jump performance of adult female subjects. *British Journal of Sports Medicine* 16:113-15.

Milner-Brown, H.S.; Stein, R.B.; and Yemin, R. 1973. The orderly recruitment of human motor units during voluntary contractions. *Journal of Physiology* 230:359-70.

Misner, S.E.; Broileau, R.A.; Massey, B.H.; and Mayhew, J. 1974. Alterations in the body composition of adult men during selected physical training. *Journal of the American Geriatrics Society* 22:33-38.

Moffroid, M.; Whipple, R.; Hofkosh, J.; Lowman, E.; and Thistle, H. 1969. A study of isokinetic exercise. *Physical Therapy* 49:735-47.

Moffroid, M.T., and Whipple, R.H. 1970. Specificity of speed of exercise. *Physical Therapy* 50:1693-99.

Moore, M.A., and Hutton, R.S. 1980. Electromyographic investigation of muscle stretching techniques. *Medicine and Science in Sports and Exercise* 12:322-29.

Morehouse, C. 1967. Development and maintenance of isometric strength of subjects with diverse initial strengths. *Research Quarterly* 38:449-56.

Morgan, D.W.; Cruise, R.J.; Girardian B.W.; Lutz-Schneider, V.; Morgan, D.H.; and Qi, W.M. 1986. HDL-C concentrations in weight-trained, endurance-trained, and sedentary females. *Physician in Sportsmedicine* 14:166-81.

Morganroth, J.; Maron, B.J.; Henry, W.L.; and Epstein, J.E. 1975. Comparative left ventricular dimensions in trained athletes. *Annals of Internal Medicine* 82:521-24.

Morganti, C.M.; Nelson, M.E.; Fiatarone, M.A.; Dallal, G.E.; Economos, C.D.; Crawford, B.M.; and Evans, W.J. 1995. Strength improvements with 1 yr of progressive resistance training in older women. *Medicine and Science in Sports and Exercise* 27:906-12.

Moritani, T. 1992. Time course of adaptations during strength and power training. In *Strength and power in sport,* ed. P.V. Komi, 266-78. Oxford: Blackwell.

Moritani, T., and DeVries, H.A. 1979. Neural factors versus hypertrophy in the time course of muscle strength gain. *American Journal of Physical Medicine* 82:521-24.

Moritani, T., and DeVries, H.A. 1980. Potential for gross hypertrophy in older men. *Journal of Gerontology* 35:672-82.

Morrow, J.R., and Hosler, W.W. 1981. Strength comparisons in untrained men and trained women athletes. *Medicine and Science in Sports and Exercise* 13:194-98.

Morrow, J.R.; Jackson, A.S.; Hosler, W.W.; and Kachurick, J.K. 1979. The importance of strength, speed and body size for team success in women's intercollegiate volleyball. *Research Quarterly* 50:429-37.

Moskwa, C.A., and Nicholas, J.A. 1989. Musculoskeletal risk factors in the young athlete. *Physician and Sportsmedicine* 17 (11): 49-59.

Murray, J., and Weber, A. 1974. The cooperative action of muscle proteins. *Scientific American* 230:58-71.

Murray, M.P.; Duthie, E.H.; Gambert, S.T.; Sepic, S.B.; and Mollinger, L.A. 1985. Age-related differences in knee muscle strength in normal women. *Journal of Gerontology* 40:275-80.

Nakamura, Y., and Schwartz, A. 1972. The influence of hydrogen ion concentration calcium binding and release by skeletal muscle sarcoplasmic reticulum. *Journal of General Physiology* 59:22-32.

Narici, M.V.; Roi, G.S.; Landoni, L.; Minetti, A.E.; and Cerretelli, P. 1989. Changes in force, cross-sectional area and neural activation during strength training and detraining of the human quadriceps. *European Journal of Applied Physiology* 59:310-19.

National Strength and Conditioning Association. 1993. Position Statement and Literature Review. Anabolic-androgenic steroid use by athletes. *National Strength and Conditioning Association Journal* 15:9-28.

Nelson, G.A.; Arnall, D.A.; Loy, S.F.; Silvester, L.J.; and Conlee, R.K. 1990. Consequences of combining strength and endurance training regimens. *Physical Therapy* 70: 287-94.

Nelson, M.E.; Fiatarone, M.A.; Morganti, C.M.; Trice, I.; Greenberg, R.A.; and Evans, W.J. 1994. Effects of high-intensity strength training on multiple risk factors for osteoporotic fractures. *Journal of the American Medical Association* 272:1909-14.

Nelson, R.M.; Soderberg, G.L.; and Urbscheit, N.L. 1984. Alteration of motor-unit discharge characteristics in aged humans. *Physical Therapy* 64 (1): 29-34.

Nemoto, E.M.; Hoff, J.T.; and Sereringhaus, J.W. 1974. Lactate uptake and metabolism by brain during hyperlactacidemia and hypoglycemia. *Stroke* 5:48-53.

Newham, D.J. 1988. The consequences of eccentric contractions and their relationship to delayed onset muscle pain. *European Journal of Applied Physiology* 57:353-59.

Newham, D.J.; Jones, D.A.; and Clarkson, P.M. 1987. Repeated high-force eccentric exercise: Effects on muscle pain and damage. *Journal of Applied Physiology* 63:1381-86.

Newton, R.U.; Häkkinen, K.; Kraemer, W.J.; McCormick, M.; Volek, J.; Gordon, S.E.; Campbell, W.W.; and Evans, W.J. 1995. Resistance training and the development of muscle strength and power in young versus older men. In *XV Congress of the International Society of Biomechanics,* 672-73. Finland: University of Jyväskylä.

Newton, R.U.; Humphries, B.J.; Murphy, A.J.; Wilson, G.J.; and Kraemer, W.J. 1994. Biomechanics and neural activation during fast bench press movements: Implications for power training. National Strength and Conditioning Association Conference, New Orleans, 16-18 June.

Newton, R.U., and Kraemer, W.J. 1994. Developing explosive muscular power: Implications for a mixed methods training strategy. *Journal of Strength and Conditioning Research* 16:20

Newton, R.U.; Kraemer, W.J.; Häkkinen, K.; Humphries, B.J.; and Murphy, A.J. 1996. Kinematics, kinetics, and muscle activation during explosive upper body movements: Implications for power development. *Journal of Applied Biomechanics* 12:31-43.

Newton, R.U., and Wilson, G.J. 1993a. The kinetics and kinematics of powerful upper body movements: The effect of load. Abstracts of the International Society of Biomechanics XIVth Congress, Paris, 4-8 July, p. 1510.

Newton, R.U., and Wilson, G.J. 1993b. Reducing the risk of injury during plyometric training: The effect of dampeners. *Sports Medicine, Training and Rehabilitation* 4:1-7.

Nielsen, B.; Nielsen, K.; Behrendt-Hansen, M.; and Asmussen, E. 1980. Training of "functional muscular strength" in girls 7-19 years old. In *Children and exercise IX*, eds. K. Berg and B. Eriksson, 69-77. Baltimore, MD: University Park Press.

Norris, D.O. 1980. *Vertebrate endocrinology.* Philadelphia: Lea and Febiger.

Nosaka, K.; Clarkson, P.M.; McGuiggin, M.E.; and Byrne, J.M. 1991. Time course of muscle damage after high force eccentric exercise. *European Journal of Applied Physiology* 63:70-76.

Noth, J. 1992. Motor units. In *Strength and power in sport*, ed. P.V. Komi, 21-28. Oxford: Blackwell Scientific.

NSCA. *See* National Strength and Conditioning Association.

Nutik, G., and Cruess, R.L. 1974. Estrogen receptors in bone: An evaluation of the uptake of estrogen into bone cells. *Proceedings of the Society of Experimental Biology and Medicine* 146:265-68.

Nyburgh, K.H.; Bachrach, L.K.; Lewis, B.; Kent, K.; and Marcus, R. 1993. Low bone mineral density at axial and appendicular sites in amenorrheic athletes. *Medicine and Science in Sports and Exercise* 25:1197-1202.

O'Bryant, H.S.; Byrd, R.; and Stone, M.H. 1988. Cycle ergometry performance and maximum leg and hip strength adaptations to two different methods of weight-training. *Journal of Applied Sport Science Research* 2:27-30.

Ohtsuki, T. 1981. Decrease in grip strength induced by simultaneous bilateral exertion with reference to finger strength. *Ergonomics* 24:37-48.

O'Shea, P. 1966. Effects of selected weight training programs on the development of strength and muscle hypertrophy. *Research Quarterly* 37:95-102.

Osternig, L.R.; Robertson, R.N.; Troxel, R.K.; and Hansen, P. 1990. Differential responses to proprioceptive neuromuscular facilitation (PNF) stretch techniques. *Medicine and Science in Sports and Exercise* 22:106-11.

Oteghen, S.L. 1975. Two speeds of isokinetic exercise as related to the vertical jump performance of women. *Research Quarterly* 46:78-84.

Paffenbarger, R.S.; Hyde, R.T.; Wing, A.L.; and Steinmetz, C.H. 1984. A natural history of athleticism and cardiovascular health. *Journal of the American Medical Association* 252:491-95.

Page, B. 1966. Latest muscle building technique. *Muscle Builder* 14:20-21.

Pearson, A.C.; Schiff, M.; Mrosek, D.; Labovitz, A.J.; and Williams, G.A. 1986. Left ventricular diastolic function in weight lifters. *American Journal of Cardiology* 58:1254-59.

Pearson, D.R., and Costill, D.L. 1988. The effects of constant external resistance exercise and isokinetic exercise training on work-induced hypertrophy. *Journal of Applied Sport Science Research* 3:39-41.

Perrine, J.A., and Edgerton, V.R. 1975. Isokinetic anaerobic ergometry. *Medicine and Science in Sports* 7:78.

Petersen, S.; Wessel, J.; Bagnall, K.; Wilkens, H.; Quinney, A.; and Wenger, H. 1990. Influence of concentric resistance training on concentric and eccentric strength. *Archives of Physical Medicine and Rehabilitation* 71:101-5.

Petersen, S.R.; Miller, G.D.; Quinney, H.A.; and Wenger, H.A. 1987. The effectiveness of a mini-cycle on velocity-specific strength acquisition. *Journal of Orthopaedic and Sports Physical Therapy* 9:156-59.

Peterson, J.A. 1975. Total conditioning: A case study. *Athletic Journal* 56:40-55.

Pette, D., and Staron, R.S. 1990. Cellular and molecular diversities of mammalian skeletal muscle fibers. *Review of Physiology, Biochemistry and Pharmacology* 116:2-75.

Pfeiffer, R., and Francis, R. 1986. Effects of strength training on muscle development in prepubescent, pubescent and postpubescent males. *Physician and Sports Medicine* 14:134-43.

Phillips, S.K.; Bruce, S.A.; Newton, D.; and Woledge, R.C. 1992. The weakness of old age is not due to failure of muscle activation. *Journal of Gerontology: Medical Sciences* 47:45-49.

Pierce, K.; Rozenek, R.; and Stone, M.H. 1993. Effects of high volume weight training on lactate, heart rate, and perceived exertion. *Journal of Strength and Conditioning Research* 7:211-15.

Pipes, T.V. 1978. Variable resistance versus constant resistance strength training in adult males. *European Journal of Applied Physiology* 39:27-35.

Pipes, T.V. 1979. Physiological characteristics of elite body builders. *Physician and Sportsmedicine* 7:116-26.

Pizzimenti, M.A. 1992. Mechanical analysis of the Nautilus leg curl machine. *Canadian Journal of Sport Science* 17:41-48.

Ploutz, L.L.; Tesch, P.A.; Biro, R.L.; and Dudley, G.A. 1994. Effect of resistance training on muscle use during exercise. *Journal of Applied Physiology* 76:1675-81.

Polhemus, R.; Burkhart, E.; Osina, M.; and Patterson, M. 1981. The effects of plyometric training with ankle and vest weights on conventional weight training programs for men and women. *National Strength Coaches Association Journal* 2:13-15.

Poliquin, C. 1988. Five ways to increase the effectiveness of your strength training program. *National Strength and Conditioning Association Journal* 10 (3): 34-39.

Pollock, M.L.; Leggett, S.H.; Graves, J.E.; Jones, A.; Fulton, M.; and Cirulli, J. 1988. Effect of resistance training on lumbar extension strength. *American Journal of Sports Medicine* 17:624-29.

Pollock, M.L.; Wilmore, J.H.; and Fox, S.M. 1978. *Health and fitness through physical activity*. New York: Wiley.

Poole, H. 1964. Multi-poundage sets. *Muscle Builder* 14:20-21.

Powers, W.E.; Browning, F.M.; and Groves, B.R. 1978. The super overload: A new method for improving muscular strength. *Journal of Physical Education* (March/April): 10-12.

Prince, F.P.; Hikida, R.S.; and Hagerman, F.C. 1977. Muscle fiber types in women athletes and non-athletes. *Pflugers Archives* 371:161-65.

Prior, J.C.; Vigna, Y.M.; and McKay, D.W. 1992. Reproduction for the athletic female: New understandings of physiology and management. *Sports Medicine* 14:190-99.

Pullo, F.M. 1992. A profile of NCAA Division I strength and conditioning coaches. *Journal of Applied Sport Science Research* 6:55-62.

Rack, D.M.H., and Westbury, D.R. 1969. The effects of length and stimulus rate on isometric tension in the cat soleus muscle. *Journal of Physiology* 204:443-60.

Ramsay, J.A.; Blimkie, C.J.R.; Smith, K.; Garner, S.; MacDougall, J.D.; and Sale, D.G. 1990. Strength training effects in prepubescent boys. *Medicine and Science in Sports and Exercise* 22:605-14.

Rarick, G.L., and Larson, G.L. 1958. Observations on frequency and intensity of isometric muscular effort in developing static muscular strength in post-pubescent males. *Research Quarterly* 29:333-41.

Rasch, P. 1971. Isometric exercise and gains of muscular strength. In *Frontiers of fitness*, ed. R. Shepard, 98-111. Springfield, IL: Charles C Thomas.

Rasch, P., and Morehouse, L. 1957. Effect of static and dynamic exercises on muscular strength and hypertrophy. *Journal of Applied Physiology* 11:29-34.

Rasch, P.J., and Pierson, W.R. 1964. One position versus multiple positions in isometric exercise. *American Journal of Physical Medicine* 43:10-12.

Rasch, P.J.; Preston, W.R.; and Logan, G.A. 1961. The effect of isometric exercise upon the strength of antagonistic muscles. *Internationale Zeitschrift fur Angewandte Physiologie Einschliesslich Arbitsphysiologie* 19:18-22.

Richford, C. 1966. *Principles of successful body building*. Alliance, NE: Iron Man Industries.

Rieger, J. 1985. Upgrading your conditioning facility: Equipment evaluation and selection. *Cardinal Conditioning, University of Louisville Athletics and Sports Medicine* 4:1-4.

Rizzardo, M.; Bay, G.; and Wessel, J. 1988. Eccentric and concentric torque and power of the knee extensors of females. *Canadian Journal of Sport Science* 13:166-69.

Rogers, M.A., and Evans, W.J. 1993. Changes in skeletal muscle with aging: Effects of exercise training. In *Exercise and sport sciences reviews*, ed. J.O. Holloszy, vol. 21. Baltimore: Williams and Wilkins.

Rooney, K.J.; Herbert, R.D.; and Balnave, R.J. 1994. Fatigue contributes to the strength training stimulus. *Medicine and Science in Sports and Exercise* 26:1160-64.

Roth, D.A.; Stanley, W.C.; and Brooks, G.A. 1988. Induced lactacidemia does not affect postexercise O_2 consumption. *Journal of Applied Physiology* 65:1045-49.

Rowe, T.A. 1979. Cartilage fracture due to weight lifting. *British Journal of Sports Medicine* 13:130-31.

Rowell, L.B.; Kranning, K.K.; Evans, T.O.; Kennedy, J.W.; Blackman, J.R.; and Kusumi, F. 1966. Splanchnic removal of lactate and pyruvate during prolonged exercise in man. *Journal of Applied Physiology* 21:1773-83.

Roy, R.R., and Edgerton, V.R. 1992. Skeletal muscle architecture and performance. In *Strength and power in sport*, ed. P.V. Komi, 115-29. Oxford: Blackwell Scientific.

Rudman, D.; Feller, A.G.; Nagraj, H.S.; Gergans, G.A.; Lalitha, P.Y.; Goldberg, A.F.; Schlenker, R.A.; Cohn, L.; Rudman, I.W.; and Mattson, D.E. 1990. Effects of human growth hormone in men over 60 years old. *New England Journal of Medicine* 323:1-6.

Rupnow, A. 1985. Upper body strength—helping kids with the battle. *Journal of Physical Education, Recreation and Dance* 56:60-63.

Ryan, J.R., and Salciccioli, G.G. 1976. Fractures of the distal radial epiphysis in adolescent weight lifters. *Sports Medicine* 4:26-27.

Ryushi, T.; Häkkinen, K.; Kauhanen, H.; and Komi, P.V. 1988. Muscle fiber characteristics, muscle cross-sectional area and force production in strength athletes, physically active males and females. *Scandinavian Journal of Sports Science* 10:7-15.

Sailors, M., Berg, K. 1987. Comparison of responses to weight training in pubescent boys and men. *Journal of Sports Medicine* 27:30-37.

Sale, D.G. 1989. Strength training in children. In *Perspectives in exercise science and sports medicine*, eds. C.V. Gisolfi and D.R. Lamb, 165-216. Carmel, IN: Benchmark Press.

Sale, D.G. 1992. Neural adaptation to strength training. In *Strength and power in sport*, ed. P.V. Komi, 249-65. Oxford: Blackwell Scientific.

Sale, D.G.; MacDougall, J.D.; Alway, S.E.; Sutton, J.R. 1987. Voluntary strength and muscle characteristics in untrained men and female and male body builders. *Journal of Applied Physiology* 62:1786-93.

Sale, D.G.; MacDougall, J.D.; Jacobs I.; and Garner, S. 1990. Interaction between concurrent strength and endurance training. *Journal of Applied Physiology* 68:260-70.

Sale, D.G.; MacDougall, J.D.; Upton, A.R.M.; and McComas, A.J. 1983. Effect of strength training upon motorneuron excitability in man. *Medicine and Science in Sports and Exercise* 15:57-62.

Sale, D.G.; Moroz, D.E.; McKelvie, R.S.; MacDougall, J.D.; and McCartney, N. 1993. Comparison of blood pressure response to isokinetic and weight-lifting exercise. *European Journal of Applied Physiology* 67:115-20.

Sale, D.G.; Moroz, D.E.; McKelvie, R.S.; MacDougall, J.D.; and McCartney, N. 1994. Effect of training on the blood pressure response to weight lifting. *Canadian Journal of Applied Physiology* 19:60-74.

Saltin, B., and Åstrand, P.O. 1967. Maximal oxygen consumption uptake in athletes. *Journal of Applied Physiology* 23:353-58.

Schantz, P. 1982. Capillary supply in hypertrophied human skeletal muscle. *Acta Physiologica Scandinavica* 114:635-37.

Schantz, P.; Randall-Fox, E.; Hutchison, W.; Tyden, A.; and Åstrand, P.O. 1983. Muscle fibre type distribution, muscle cross-sectional area and maximal voluntary strength in humans. *Acta Physiologica Scandinavica* 117:219-26.

Schantz, P.; Randall-Fox, E.; Norgen, P.; and Tyden, A. 1981. The relationship between the mean muscle fibre area and the muscle cross-sectional area of the thigh in subjects with large differences in thigh girth. *Acta Physiologica Scandinavica* 113:537-39.

Scharf, H.-P.; Eckhardt, R.; Maurus, M.; and Puhl, W. 1994. Metabolic and hemodynamic changes during isokinetic muscle training. *International Journal of Sports Medicine* 15:S56-S59.

Schmidtbleicher, D., and Gollhofer, A. 1982. Neuromuskulare Untersuchungen zur Bestimmung individueller Belastungsgrossen fur ein Tiefsprungtraining. *Leistungssport* 12:298-307.

Schmidtbleicher, D.; Gollhofer, A.; and Frick, U. 1988. Effects of a stretch-shortening type training on the performance capability and innervation characteristics of leg extensor muscles. In *Biomechanics XI-A*, eds. G. de Groot, A. Hollander, P. Huijing, and G. van Ingen Schenau, vol. 7-A, 185-89. Amsterdam: Free University Press.

Schultz, R.W. 1967. Effect of direct practice and repetitive sprinting and weight training on selected motor performance tasks. *Research Quarterly* 38:108-18.

Scoles, G. 1978. Depth jumping! Does it really work? *Athletic Journal* 58:48-75.

Seaborne, D., and Taylor, A.W. 1984. The effect of speed of isokinetic exercise on training transfer to isometric strength in the quadriceps. *Journal of Sports Medicine* 24:183-88.

Secher, N.H. 1975. Isometric rowing strength of experienced and inexperienced oarsmen. *Medicine and Science in Sports* 7:280-83.

Secher, N.H.; Rorsgaard, S.; and Secher, O. 1978. Contralateral influence on recruitment of curarized muscle fibers during maximal voluntary extension of the legs. *Acta Physiologica Scandinavica* 130:455-62.

Serresse, O.; Lortie, G.; Bouchard, C.; and Boulay, M.R. 1988. Estimation of the contribution of the various energy systems during maximal work of short duration. *International Journal of Sports Medicine* 9 (6): 456-60.

Servedio, F.J.; Bartels, R.L.; Hamlin, R.L.; Teske, D.; Shaffer, T.; and Servedio, A. 1985. The effects of weight training using Olympic style lifts on various physiological variables in pre-pubescent boys. *Medicine and Science in Sports and Exercise* 17:158.

Sewall, L., Micheli, L. 1986. Strength training for children. *Journal of Pediatric Orthopedics* 6:143-46.

Sharkey, B. 1984. *Physiology of fitness.* Champaign, IL: Human Kinetics.

Sheehan, G. 1985. Health vs. fitness. *The Runner* (June):14-15.

Shellock, F.G., and Prentice, W.E. 1985. Warming-up and stretching for improved physical performance and prevention of sports related injuries. *Sports Medicine* 2:267-78.

Siegal, J.; Camaione, D.; and Manfredi, T. 1989. The effects of upper body resistance training in prepubescent children. *Pediatric Exercise Science* 1:145-54.

Silvester, L.J.; Stiggins, C.; McGown, C.; and Bryce, G. 1984. The effect of variable resistance and free-weight training programs on strength and vertical jump. *National Strength and Conditioning Association Journal* 5:30-33.

Sinning, W.E. 1974. Body composition assessment of college wrestlers. *Medicine and Science in Sports* 6:139-45.

Smith, M.J., and Melton, P. 1981. Isokinetic versus isotonic variable resistance training. *American Journal of Sports Medicine* 9 (4):275-79.

Spence, D.W.; Disch, J.G.; Fred, H.C.; and Coleman, A.E. 1980. Descriptive profiles of highly skilled women volleyball players. *Medicine and Science in Sports and Exercise* 12:299-302.

Speroff, L., and Redwine, D.B. 1980. Exercise and menstrual function. *Physician and Sportsmedicine* 8:42-48.

Spirits, P.; Pelliccia, A.; Proschan, M.A.; Granata, M.; Spataro, A.; Bellone, P.; Caselli, G.; Biffi, A.; Vecchio, C.; and Macron, B.J. 1994. Morphology of the "athletes heart" assessed by echocardiography in 947 elite athletes representing 27 sports. *American Journal of Cardiology* 74:802-6.

Spitzer, J.J. 1974. Effect of lactate infusion on canine myocardial free fatty acid metabolism in vivo. *American Journal of Physiology* 22:213-17.

Sprynarova, S., and Parizkova, J. 1971. Functional capacity and body composition in top weight lifters, swimmers, runners, and skiers. *International fur Angewandte Physiologie* 29:184-94.

Stalder, M.A.; Noble, B.J.; and Wilkerson, J.G. 1990. The effects of supplemental weight training for ballet dancers. *Journal of Applied Sport Science Research* 4:94-102.

Staff, P.H. 1982. The effect of physical activity on joints, cartilage, tendons and ligaments. *Scandinavian Journal of Social Medicine* 290(suppl.):59-63.

Stanforth, P.R.; Painter, T.L.; and Wilmore, J.H. 1992. Alteration in concentric strength consequent to powercise and universal gym circuit training. *Journal of Applied Sport Science Research* 6:152-57.

Stanley, W.C. 1991. Myocardial lactate metabolism during exercise. *Medicine and Science in Sports and Exercise* 23:920-24.

Staron, R.S.; Hagerman, F.C.; and Hikida, R.S. 1981. The effects of detraining on an elite power lifter. *Journal of Neurological Sciences* 51:247-57.

Staron, R.S.; Hikida, R.S.; and Hagerman, F.C. 1983. Reevaluation of human muscle fast-twitch subtypes: Evidence for a continuum. *Histochemistry* 78:33-39.

Staron, R.S., and Johnson, P. 1993. Myosin polymorphism and differential expression in adult human skeletal muscle. *Comparative Biochemical Physiology* 106B:463-75.

Staron, R.S.; Karapondo, D.L.; Kraemer, W.J.; Fry, A.C.; Gordon, S.E.; Falkel, J.E.; Hagerman, F.C.; and Hikida, R.S. 1994. Skeletal muscle adaptations during the early phase of heavy-resistance training in men and women. *Journal of Applied Physiology* 76:1247-55.

Staron, R.S.; Leonardi, M.J.; Karapondo, D.L.; Malicky, E.S.; Falkel, J.E.; Hagerman, F.C.; and Hikida, R.S. 1991. Strength and skeletal muscle adaptations in heavy-resistance-trained women after detraining and retraining. *Journal of Applied Physiology* 70:631-40.

Staron, R.S.; Malicky, E.S.; Leonardi, M.J.; Falkel, J.E.; Hagerman, F.C.; and Dudley, G.A. 1989. Muscle hypertrophy and fast fiber type conversions in heavy resistance-trained women. *European Journal of Applied Physiology and Occupational Physiology* 60:71-79.

Stauber, W.T.; Clarkson, P.M.; Fritz, V.K.; and Evans, W.J. 1990. Extracellular matrix disruption and pain after eccentric muscle action. *Journal of Applied Physiology* 69:868-74.

Steben, R.E., and Steben, A.H. 1981. The validity of the stretch-shortening cycle in selected jumping events. *Journal of Sports Medicine* 21:28-37.

Steinhaus, A.H. 1954. Some selected facts from physiology and the physiology of exercise applicable to physical rehabilitation. Paper presented to the Study Group on Body Mechanics, Washington, DC.

Stoessel, L.; Stone, M.H.; Keith, R.; Marple, D.; and Johnson, R. 1991. Selected physiological, psychological and performance characteristics of national-caliber United States women weightlifters. *Journal of Applied Sport Science Research* 5:87-95.

Stone, M.H. 1992. Connective tissue and bone response to strength training. In *Strength and power in sport,* ed. P.V. Komi, 279-90. Oxford: Blackwell Scientific.

Stone, M.H.; Fleck, S.J.; Triplett, N.R.; and Kraemer, W.J. 1991. Physiological adaptations to resistance training exercise. *Sports Medicine* 11:210-31.

Stone, M.H.; Johnson, R.C.; and Carter, D.R. 1979. A short term comparison of two different methods of resistance training on leg strength and power. *Athletic Training* 14:158-60.

Stone, M.H.; Nelson, J.K.; Nader, S.; and Carter, D. 1983. Short-term weight training effects on resting and recovery heart rates. *Athletic Training* (Spring): 69-71.

Stone, M.H.; O'Bryant, H.; and Garhammer, J.G. 1981. A hypothetical model for strength training. *Journal of Sports Medicine and Physical Fitness* 21:342-51.

Stone, M.H.; O'Bryant, H.; Garhammer, J.G.; McMillian, J.; and Rozenek, R. 1982. A theoretical model for strength training. *National Strength and Conditioning Association Journal* 4:36-39.

Stone, M.H.; Wilson, G.D.; Blessing, D.; and Rozenek, R. 1983. Cardiovascular responses to short-term Olympic style weight training in young men. *Canadian Journal of Applied Sport Science* 8:134-39.

Stowers, T.; McMillian, J.; Scala, D.; Davis, V.; Wilson, D.; and Stone, M. 1983. The short-term effects of three different strength-power training methods. *National Strength and Conditioning Association Journal* 5:24-27.

Straub, W.F. 1968. Effect of overload training procedures upon velocity and accuracy of the overarm throw. *Research Quarterly* 39:370-79.

Sugiura, T.; Matoba, H.; Miyata, H.; Kawai, Y.; and Murakami, N. 1992. Myosin heavy chain isoform transition in aging fast and slow muscles of the rat. *Acta Physiological Scandinavica* 144:419-23.

Swegan, D.B. 1957. The comparison of static contraction with standard weight training and effect on certain movement speeds and endurance. PhD dissertation, Pennsylvania State University.

Syrovy, I., and Gutmann, E. 1970. Changes in speed of contraction and ATPase activity in striated muscle during old age. *Experimental Gerontology* 5:31-35.

Talag, T.S. 1973. Residual muscular soreness as influenced by concentric, eccentric and static contractions. *Research Quarterly* 44:458-61.

Tanner, J.M. 1964. *The physique of the Olympic athlete.* London: Allen and Unwin.

Tarnopolsky, M.A.; MacDougall, J.D.; and Atkinson, S.A. 1988. Influence of protein intake and training status on nitrogen balance and lean body mass. *Journal of Applied Physiology* 64:187-93.

Tatro, D.L.; Dudley, G.A.; and Convertino, V.A. 1992. Carotid-cardiac baroreflex response and LBNP tolerance following resistance exercise. *Medicine and Science in Sports and Exercise* 24:789-96.

Tesch, P.A. 1987. Acute and long-term metabolic changes consequent to heavy-resistance exercise. *Medicine and Sport Science* 26:67-89.

Tesch, P.A. 1992a. Short- and long-term histochemical and biochemical adaptations in muscle. In *Strength and power in sport,* ed. P.V. Komi, 239-48. Oxford: Blackwell Scientific.

Tesch, P.A. 1992b. Training for bodybuilding. In *Strength and power in sport,* ed. P.V. Komi, 370-80. Oxford: Blackwell Scientific.

Tesch, P.A., and Dudley, G.A. 1993. *Muscle meets magnet.* Stockholm: P.A. Tesch.

Tesch, P.A.; Dudley, G.A.; Duvoisin, M.R.; Hather, B.M.; and Harris, R.T. 1990. Force and EMG signal patterns during repeated bouts of concentric or eccentric muscle actions. *Acta Physiologica Scandinavica* 138:263-71.

Tesch, P.A.; Hjort, H.; and Balldin, U.I. 1983. Effects of strength training on G tolerance. *Aviation, Space, and Environmental Medicine* 54:691-95.

Tesch, P.A., and Larsson, L. 1982. Muscle hypertrophy in body builders. *European Journal of Applied Physiology* 49:301-306.

Tesch, P.A.; Thorsson, A.; and Colliander, E.B. 1990. Effects of eccentric and concentric resistance training on skeletal muscle substrates, enzyme activities and capillary supply. *Acta Physiologica Scandinavica* 140:575-80.

Tesch, P.A.; Thorsson, A.; and Kaiser, P. 1984. Muscle capillary supply and fiber type characteristics in weight and power lifters. *Journal of Applied Physiology* 56:35-38.

Tharion, W.J.; Rausch, T.M.; Harman, E.A.; and Kraemer, W.J. 1991. Effects of different resistance exercise protocols on mood states. *Journal of Applied Sport Science Research* 5:60-65.

Thepaut-Mathieu, C.; Van Hoecke, J.; and Martin, B. 1988. Myoelectrical and mechanical changes linked to length specificity during isometric training. *Journal of Applied Physiology* 64:1500-5.

Thistle, H.G.; Hislop, H.J.; Moffroid, M.; and Lowman, E.W. 1967. Isokinetic contraction: A new concept in resistive exercise. *Archives of Physical Medicine and Rehabilitation* 48:279-82.

Thompson, C.W., and Martin, E.T. 1965. Weight training and baseball throwing speed. *Journal of the Association of Physical and Mental Rehabilitation* 19:194-96.

Thompson, D.B., and Chapman, A.E. 1988. The mechanical response of active human muscle during and after stretch. *European Journal of Applied Physiology* 57:691-97.

Thompson, P.D.; Sadanian, A.; Cullinane, E.M.; Bodziony, K.S.; Catlin, D.H.; Torek-Both, G.; and Douglas, P.S. 1992. Left ventricular function is not impaired in weight-lifters who use anabolic steroids. *Journal of the American College of Cardiology* 19:278-82.

Thorstensson, A. 1977. Observations on strength training and detraining. *Acta Physiologica Scandinavica* 100:491-93.

Thorstensson, A.; Karlsson, J.; Viitasalo, J.; Luhtanen, P.; and Komi, P. 1976. Effect of strength in training on EMG of human skeletal muscle. *Acta Physiologica Scandinavica* 98:232-36.

Thrash, K., and Kelly, B. 1987. Flexibility and strength training. *Journal of Applied Sport Science Research* 4:74-75.

Timonen, S., and Procope, B.J. 1971. Premenstrual syndrome and physical exercise. *Acta Obstetrica et Gynaecologica Scandinavica* 50:331-37.

Timson, B.F.; Bowlin, B.K.; Dudenhoeffer, G.A.; and George, J.B. 1985. Fiber number, area, and composition of mouse soleus muscle following enlargement. *Journal of Applied Physiology: Respiratory, Environmental and Exercise Physiology* 58:619-24.

Tipton, C.M.; Matthes, R.D.; Maynard, J.A.; and Carey, R.A. 1975. The influence of physical activity on ligaments and tendons. *Medicine and Science in Sports* 7:34-41.

Todd, T. 1978. *Inside powerlifting*. Chicago: Contemporary Books.

Todd, T. 1985. Historical perspective: The myth of the muscle-bound lifter. *National Strength and Conditioning Association Journal* 7:37-41.

Tomberline, J.P.; Basford, J.R.; Schwen, E.E.; Orte, P.A.; Scott, S.C.; Laughman, R.K.; and Ilstrud, D.M. 1991. Comparative study of isokinetic eccentric and concentric quadriceps training. *Journal of Orthopaedic and Sports Physical Therapy* 14:31-36.

Torg, J.S.; Pollack, H.; and Sweterlitsch, P. 1972. The effect of competitive pitching on the shoulders and elbows of preadolescent baseball pitchers. *Pediatrics* 49:267-72.

Totten, L., and Javorek, I. 1988. General physical training for the weightlifter. In *US Weight Lifting Federation coaching manual*, vol. 2. Colorado Springs, CO: U.S. Weightlifting Federation.

Trivedi, B., and Danforth, W.H. 1966. Effect of pH on the kinetics of frog muscle phosphofructokinase. *Journal of Biological Chemistry* 241:4110-12.

Tucci, J.T.; Carpenter, D.M.; Pollock, M.L.; Graves, J.E.; and Leggett S.H. 1992. Effect of reduced frequency of training and detraining on lumbar extension strength. *Spine* 17:1497-1501.

Turto, H.; Lindy, S.; and Halme, J. 1974. Protocollagen proline hydroxylase activity in work-induced hypertrophy of rat muscle. *American Journal of Physiology* 226:63-65.

Vandervoot, A.A.; Sale, D.G.; and Moroz, J. 1984. Comparison of motor unit activation during unilateral and bilateral leg extension. *Journal of Applied Physiology: Respiratory, Environmental and Exercise Physiology* 56:46-51.

Verhsoshanski, V. 1967. Are depth jumps useful? *Track and Field* 12:9.

Vermeulen, A.; Rubens, R.; and Verdonck, L. 1972. Testosterone secretion and metabolism in male senescence. *Journal of Clinical Endocrinology* 34:730-35.

Vitcenda, M.; Hanson, P.; Folts, J.; and Besozzi, M. 1990. Impairment of left ventricular function during maximal isometric dead lifting. *Journal of Applied Physiology* 69:2062-66.

Volpe, S.L.; Walberg-Rankin, J.; Rodman, K.W.; and Sebolt, D.R. 1993. The effect of endurance running on training adaptations in women participating in a weight lifting program. *Journal of Strength and Conditioning Research* 7:101-107.

Vorobyev, A.N. 1978. *A textbook on weightlifting*. Trans. J. Bryant. Budapest: International Weightlifting Federation.

Vrijens, J. 1978. Muscle strength development in the pre- and post-pubescent age. *Medicine and Sports* (Basel) 11:152-58.

Walberg, J.L., and Johnston, C.S. 1991. Menstrual function and eating behavior in female recreational weight lifters and competitive body builders. *Medicine and Science in Sports and Exercise* 23:30-36.

Walberg-Rankin, J.; Franke, W.D.; and Gwazdauskas, F.C. 1992. Response of beta-endorphin and estradiol to resistance exercise in females during energy balance and energy restriction. *International Journal of Sports Medicine* 13:542-47.

Waldman, R., and Stull, G. 1969. Effects of various periods of inactivity on retention of newly acquired levels of muscular endurance. *Research Quarterly* 40:393-401.

Ward, J., and Fisk, G.H. 1964. The difference in response of the quadriceps and biceps brachii muscles to isometric and isotonic exercise. *Archives of Physical Medicine and Rehabilitation* 45:612-20.

Warren, B.J.; Stone, M.H.; Kearney, J.T.; Fleck, S.J.; Johnson, R.L.; Wilson, G.D.; and Kraemer, W.J. 1992. Performance measures, blood lactate and plasma ammonia as indicators of over work in elite junior weightlifters. *International Journal of Sports Medicine* 13:372-76.

Wasserman, D.H.; Connolly, C.C.; and Pagliassotti, M.J. 1991. Regulation of hepatic lactate balance during exercise. *Medicine and Science in Sports and Exercise* 23:912-19.

Weider, J. 1954. Cheating exercises build the biggest muscles. *Muscle Builder* 3:60-61.

Wells, C.L. 1978. The female athlete: Myths and superstitions put to rest. In *Toward an understanding of human performance*, ed. E.J. Burke, 37-40. Ithaca, NY: Movement Press.

Wells, J.B.; Jokl, E.; and Bohanen, J. 1973. The effect of intense physical training upon body composition of adolescent girls. *Journal of the Association for Physical and Mental Rehabilitation* 17:63-72.

Weltman, A.; Janney, C.; Rians, C.; Strand, K.; Berg, B.; Tippit, S.; Wise, J.; Cahill, B.; and Katch, F. 1986. The effects of hydraulic resistance strength training in prepubertal males. *Medicine and Science in Sports and Medicine* 18:629-38.

Westcott, W. 1992. A new look at youth fitness. *American Fitness Quarterly* 11:16-19.

Wickiewicz, T.L.; Roy, R.R.; Powell, P.L.; Perrine, J.J.; and Edgerton, B.R. 1984. Muscle architecture and force-velocity relationships in humans. *Journal of Applied Physiology: Respiratory, Environmental and Exercise Physiology* 57:435-43.

Widholm, O. 1979. Dysmenorrhea during adolescence. *Acta Obstetrica et Gynaecologica Scandinavica* 87:61-66.

Williams, D. 1991. The effect of weight training on performance in selected motor activities for preadolescent males (Abstract). *Journal of Applied Sport Science Research* 5:170.

Williams, M., and Stutzman, L. 1959. Strength variation throughout the range of joint motion. *Physical Therapy Review* 39:145-52.

Willoughby, D.S. 1993. The effects of mesocycle-length weight training programs involving periodization and partially equated volumes on upper and lower body strength. *Journal of Strength and Conditioning Research* 7: 2-8.

Wilmore, J.H. 1974. Alterations in strength, body composition, and anthropometric measurements consequent to a 10-week weight training program. *Medicine and Science in Sports* 6:133-38.

Wilmore, J.H., and Costill, D.L. 1994. *Physiology of sport and exercise*. Champaign, IL: Human Kinetics.

Wilmore, J.H.; Parr, R.B.; Girandola, R.N.; Ward, P.; Vodak, P.A.; Barstow, T.J.; Pipes, T.V.; Romero, G.T.; and Leslie, P. 1978. Physiological alterations consequent to circuit weight training. *Medicine and Science in Sports* 10:79-84.

Wilson, G.J.; Newton, R.U.; Murphy, A.J.; and Humphries, B.J. 1993. The optimal training load for the development of dynamic athletic performance. *Medicine and Science in Sports and Exercise* 25:1279-86.

Wilt, F. 1968. Training for competitive running. In *Exercise physiology*, ed. H.B. Falls, 395-414. New York: Academic Press.

Withers, R.T. 1970. Effect of varied weight-training loads on the strength of university freshmen. *Research Quarterly* 41:110-14.

Wolinsky, F.D., and Fitzgerald, J.F. 1994. Subsequent hip fracture among older adults. *American Journal of Public Health* 84:1316-18.

Wright, J.E. 1980. Anabolic steroids and athletics. In *Exercise and sport science reviews*, eds. R.S. Hutton and D.I. Miller, 149-202. The Franklin Institute.

Yarasheski, K.E.; Campbell, J.A.; Smith, K.; Rennie, M.J.; Holloszy, J.O.; and Bier, D.M. 1992. Effect of growth hormone and resistance exercise on muscle growth in young men. *American Journal of Applied Physiology* 262:E261-67.

Yarasheski, K.E.; Zachwieja, J.J.; and Bier, D.M. 1993. Acute effects of resistance exercise on muscle protein synthesis rate in young and elderly men and women. *American Journal of Applied Physiology* 265:210-14.

Yates, J.W., and Kamon, E. 1983. A comparison of peak and constant angle torque-velocity curves in fast and slow twitch populations. *European Journal of Applied Physiology* 51:67-74.

Yesalis, C.E. 1993. *Anabolic steroids in sport and exercise*. Champaign, IL: Human Kinetics.

Young, A., and Skelton, D.A. 1994. Applied physiology of strength and power in old age. *International Journal of Sports Medicine* 15:149-51.

Young, A.; Stokes, M.; and Crowe, M. 1984. Size and strength of the quadriceps muscles of old and young women. *European Journal of Clinical Investigation* 14:282-87.

Young, W.B. 1993. Training for speed/strength: Heavy versus light loads. *National Strength and Conditioning Association Journal* 15:34-42.

Young, W.B., and Bilby, G.E. 1993. The effect of voluntary effort to influence speed of contraction on strength, muscular power and hypertrophy development. *Journal of Strength and Conditioning Research* 7:172-78.

Yudkin, J., and Cohen, R.D. 1974. The contribution of the kidney to the removal of a lactic acid load under normal and acidotic conditions in conscious rat. *Clinical Science and Molecular Medicine* 46:9.

Zemper, E.D. 1990. Four year study of weight room injuries in a national sample of college football teams. *National Strength and Conditioning Association Journal* 12:32-34.

Zernicke, R.F., and Loitz, B.J. 1992. Exercise-related adaptations in connective tissue. In *Strength and power in sport*, ed. P.V. Komi, 77-95. Oxford: Blackwell Scientific.

Zinovieff, A. 1951. Heavy resistance exercise: The Oxford technique. *British Journal of Physical Medicine* 14:129-32.

Zrubak, A. 1972. Body composition and muscle strength of body builders. *Acta Facultatis Rerum Naturalium Universitatis Comenianae Anthropologia* 11:135-44.

Index

About the Authors

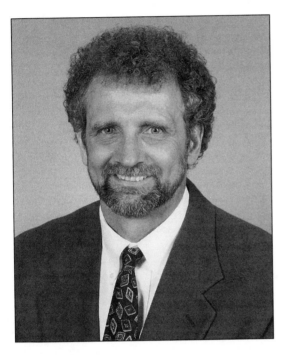

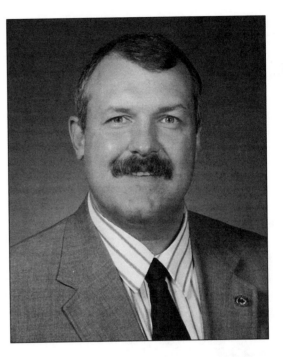

Steven J. Fleck earned a PhD in exercise physiology from the Ohio State University in 1978. He has headed the physical conditioning program of the U.S. Olympic Committee, served as strength coach for the German Volleyball Association, and coached high school track, basketball, and football. Dr. Fleck is a past vice president of basic and applied research for the National Strength and Conditioning Association (NSCA) and is a fellow of the American College of Sports Medicine. He was honored in 1991 as the NSCA Sport Scientist of the Year.

Dr. Fleck is the president of Fleck's Rx, a consulting firm that advises elite athletes, coaches, and fitness enthusiasts on training programs. At home in Colorado Springs, Colorado, he enjoys weight training, rock climbing, hiking, and Alpine skiing.

William J. Kraemer earned a PhD in physiology from the University of Wyoming in 1984. He holds multiple appointments at the Pennsylvania State University, where he is professor of applied physiology, director of research in the Center for Sports Medicine, associate director of the Center for Cell Research, and faculty member in the Kinesiology Department and the Noll Physiological Research Center. He is also editor-in-chief of the *Journal of Strength and Conditioning Research*.

The former head of the Exercise Biochemistry Laboratory at the U.S. Army Research Institute of Environmental Medicine, Dr. Kraemer is also a past president, vice president, and committee chair of the NSCA. This association honored him in 1992 as its Sport Scientist of the Year and in 1994 gave him its highest award, the Lifetime Achievement Award, making him at that time the second person ever to earn the honor. He is a fellow of the American College of Sports Medicine and a member of both the American Physiological Society and the Endocrine Society. For recreation he enjoys painting, fishing, weight training, and running.

MORE STRENGTH TRAINING BOOKS FROM HK

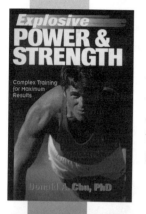

1996 • Paperback • 200 pp
Item PCHU0643 • ISBN 0-87322-643-7
$15.95 ($23.95 Canadian)

The best in sports conditioning now combines plyometric, resistance, and sprint training. *Explosive Power and Strength* not only offers these three training methods in one, but also shows how to create individualized, sports-specific programs. The book features 33 resistance and 45 plyometric exercises with 115 detailed illustrations, plus three ready-to-use workouts for each of 11 sports.

1994 • Hardback •560 pp
Item BNSC0694 • ISBN 0-87322-694-1
$50.00 ($74.95 Canadian)

In *Essentials of Strength Training and Conditioning*, the leaders in exercise sciences explore the scientific principles, concepts, and theories as well as the practical how-tos of strength training and conditioning. For the first time, students and professionals can turn to a single source for up-to-date, comprehensive information on a full range of strength and conditioning topics.

1994 • Paperback • 208 pp
Item PBAE0618 • ISBN 0-87322-618-6
$19.95 ($29.95 Canadian)

This instructor guide is the only resource available with step-by-step approaches on how to plan, prepare, implement, and evaluate a technically sound and safe total-body weight training program. The book also provides the flexibility to set up and plan lessons according to each teaching situation.

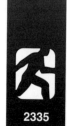

HUMAN KINETICS
The Information Leader in Physical Activity
www.humankinetics.com

2335

Prices are subject to change.